OBSTETRICS AND GYNECOLOGY

Just the Facts

OBSTETRICS AND GYNECOLOGY
Just the Facts

Patrick Duff, MD

Professor and Residency Program Director
Department of Obstetrics and Gynecology
Associate Dean for Student Affairs
University of Florida College of Medicine
Gainesville, Florida

Rodney K. Edwards, MD, MS

Assistant Professor
Division of Maternal-Fetal Medicine
Department of Obstetrics and Gynecology
University of Florida College of Medicine
Gainesville, Florida

John D. Davis, MD

Associate Professor and Director
Division of Gynecologic Surgery
Department of Obstetrics and Gynecology
University of Florida College of Medicine
Gainesville, Florida

Alice Rhoton-Vlasak, MD

Clinical Assistant Professor
Division of Reproductive Endocrinology and Infertility
Department of Obstetrics and Gynecology
University of Florida College of Medicine
Gainesville, Florida

McGraw-Hill

Medical Publishing Division

New York   Chicago   San Francisco   Lisbon   London   Madrid   Mexico City
Milan   New Delhi   San Juan   Seoul   Singapore   Sydney   Toronto

Obstetrics and Gynecology: *Just the Facts*

1 2 3 4 5 6 7 8 9 0   QDP/QDP   0 9 8 7 6 5 4

ISBN 0-07-136978-3

Notice

Medicine is an ever-changing science. As new research and clinical experience broaden our knowledge, changes in treatment and drug therapy are required. The authors and the publisher of this work have checked with sources believed to be reliable in their efforts to provide information that is complete and generally in accord with the standards accepted at the time of publication. However, in view of the possibility of human error or changes in medical sciences, neither the authors nor the publisher nor any other party who has been involved in the preparation or publication of this work warrants that the information contained herein is in every respect accurate or complete, and they disclaim all responsibility for any errors or omissions or for the results obtained from use of the information contained in this work. Readers are encouraged to confirm the information contained herein with other sources. For example and in particular, readers are advised to check the product information sheet included in the package of each drug they plan to administer to be certain that the information contained in this work is accurate and that changes have not been made in the recommended dose or in the contraindications for administration. This recommendation is of particular importance in connection with new or infrequently used drugs.

This book was set in Times New Roman by Macmillan India.
The editors were Andrea Seils and Mary E. Bele.
The production supervisor was Richard Ruzycka.
The cover designer was Aimee Nordin.
The index was prepared by Andover Publishing Services.
Quebecor/Dubuque was printer and binder.

This book is printed on acid-free paper.

Library of Congress Cataloging-in-Publication Data

Obstetrics & gynecology : just the facts / edited by Patrick Duff... [et al.].—1st ed.
    p. ; cm.
  Includes bibliographical references.
  ISBN 0-07-136978-3
    1. Gynecology—Handbooks, manuals, etc. 2. Obstetrics—Handbooks, manuals, etc. I.
  Title: Obstetrics and gynecology. II. Duff, W. Patrick.
    [DNLM: 1. Genital Diseases, Female—Handbooks. 2. Pregnancy
Complications—Handbooks. 3. Gynecology—Handbooks. 4. Obstetric Surgical
Procedures—Handbooks.   WQ 39 O137 2004]
RG110.O267 2004
618—dc22
                                                        2004049966

CONTENTS

PREFACE

This book presents a concise but comprehensive review of the key clinical facts in obstetrics and gynecology. It is intended as a primary reference for nurse-practitioners, nurse-midwives, medical students, family practitioners, and internists who provide obstetric and gynecologic care. It also is intended as a convenient review text for residents and practitioners in obstetrics and gynecology who are preparing for certification and licensure examinations. We sincerely hope that you will find this text to be of value as you work to promote women's health.

Patrick Duff, MD
Rodney K. Edwards, MD, MS
John D. Davis, MD
Alice Rhoton-Vlasak, MD

We dedicate this book to the individuals who keep us excited about our specialty and who sustain our commitment to the educational mission of academic medicine—our students.

OBSTETRICS

1 PRECONCEPTION COUNSELING

Rodney K. Edwards

BACKGROUND

- Many women are not aware that certain medical conditions, drugs, and environmental exposures may have adverse effects on them and their fetuses.
- Organogenesis begins approximately 17 days after fertilization, about the time of the first missed menstrual cycle. Therefore any measures aimed at optimizing the environment for the developing embryo/fetus are more likely to be effective if begun prior to the time when the pregnant woman seeks prenatal care.
- The best time to provide information to women about pregnancy is prior to conception. Such a **preconception counseling visit** should include an assessment of prior obstetric history, risk of genetic disease, current medical conditions, status of immunity to certain infections and need for immunizations, nutritional status, and risk of exposure to teratogenic agents. After such an assessment, a candid conversation with the patient will provide her with objective information regarding the implications of a potential pregnancy for her and her fetus.
- Since 50 percent of all pregnancies are unplanned, every visit that a woman of reproductive age makes to a medical care provider should, at least in part, be a preconception counseling visit.

OBSTETRIC HISTORY

- One common reason women seek preconception counseling is that they have had a previous pregnancy with an adverse outcome.

- A detailed obstetric history can help to identify the condition(s) that contributed to the prior bad result. As an example, a history of painless cervical dilation in the second trimester is consistent with the diagnosis of incompetent cervix. A history of recurrent pregnancy loss due to fetal death in the late first or early second trimester should prompt an evaluation for antiphospholipid antibody syndrome or a genetic thrombophilia.

GENETIC EVALUATION

- Personal and family histories (of both the prospective mother and father) may alert the clinician to an increased risk of certain genetic diseases. Construction of a **pedigree** is invaluable during this assessment.
- Certain ethnic groups have an increased risk of specific genetic diseases. Table 1-1 lists some of these diseases for which carrier screening is available.
- Increased maternal age (>35 years) is associated with an increased risk of aneuploidy. Increased paternal age (>55 years) is associated with an increased risk of new mutations for autosomal dominant conditions (eg, achondroplasia, neurofibromatosis).
- For couples with significant genetic risk, counseling should include a discussion not only of preconception screening but also of prenatal diagnosis. Referral to a geneticist or genetic counselor may be warranted.

MEDICAL CONDITIONS

- **Diabetes mellitus** is one of the most common medical conditions that can complicate pregnancy.
  ○ Achieving strict glycemic control prior to pregnancy decreases the risk of congenital anomalies,

TABLE 1-1   Common Genetic Diseases for which Carrier Screening Is Available

DISEASE	TRANSMISSION	OFFER TESTING FOR
Tay-Sachs disease	Autosomal recessive	Eastern European Jewish or French Canadian descent
Cystic fibrosis	Autosomal recessive	Eastern European Jewish descent, Caucasian, Other
Sickle cell anemia	Autosomal recessive	African, Mediterranean, or Middle Eastern descent
β-Thalassemia	Heterozygotes minimally to moderately affected. Homozygotes severely affected	Mediterranean descent
α-Thalassemia	Heterozygotes mildly affected. Homozygotes die in utero	Indian, Pakistani, Southeast Asian, or Filipino descent

preeclampsia, macrosomia, intrauterine growth restriction, and fetal death in utero.

- Target levels for glucose monitoring are fasting values below 95 mg/dL and 1-h postprandial values below 135 mg/dL.
- The preconception period is the ideal time to teach the patient about the importance of adhering to an appropriate meal plan, properly obtaining and recording capillary blood glucose values, using carbohydrate oral intake or glucagon for hypoglycemia, and administering insulin injections corrrectly.
- Women with **congenital heart disease** have an increased risk (3 to 10 percent) of having an infant with congenital heart disease. In addition, pregnancy may pose a significant threat to the health of such women (see Chap. 7B).
- Women with **epilepsy** face an increased risk of having an infant with a congenital anomaly. In addition, common anticonvulsant medications increase the risk of congenital anomalies.
  - **Diphenylhydantoin,** in as many as 10 percent of infants exposed as fetuses, produces a syndrome (the "hydantoin syndrome") characterized by microcephaly, mental retardation, abnormal facies, growth restriction, and hypoplastic nails. This drug also increases the risk for cardiac defects and cleft lip and palate.
  - **Valproic acid** and **carbamazepine** are associated with approximately a 1 percent risk of neural tube defects. Both drugs are also associated with an increased risk of craniofacial abnormalities.
  - **Trimethadione** has been associated with abnormalities similar to those of the hydantoin syndrome. In addition, V-shaped eyebrows, a high arched palate, and abnormal dentition may be seen.
- A history of **chronic hypertension** should prompt an assessment of baseline renal function.

- If the patient has significant proteinuria (>500 mg/ 24 h), pregnancy will cause her to be at risk not only for an adverse perinatal outcome (see Chap. 11) but also for worsening renal function.
  - **Angiotensin converting enzyme (ACE) inhibitors** and angiotensin receptor antagonists are considered teratogenic during all trimesters of pregnancy. Exposed fetuses may develop renal dysplasia.
- If a woman has **chronic renal disease,** her prognosis with pregnancy largely depends on the degree of renal insufficiency and the presence of hypertension.
  - Pregnancy is reasonably safe in women who are normotensive and have mild degrees of renal insufficieny.
  - For women with coexisting hypertension and/or a serum creatinine over 2.5 mg/dL, preeclampsia and preterm delivery occur in the majority of cases.
- Women with less common medical conditions may present for preconception counseling visits. The clinician may have to consult the medical literature prior to addressing the risks of a given medical condition and/or its treatment to pregnant women and fetuses.

INFECTIONS/IMMUNIZATIONS

- Screening for immunity to common infections and offering vaccinations against these infections is an important part of preconception care.
  - Pregnancy should be avoided, typically for 1 month, following the administration of live attenuated vaccines.
  - In a patient deemed to be at sufficiently high risk of infection, toxoid or inactivated vaccine preparations are considered safe for administration during pregnancy.
  - Passive immunization with immune globulin preparations, when appropriate, also is safe during pregnancy.
  - Immunizations are discussed in more detail in Chap. 34.
- Women at high risk of viral **hepatitis** should be offered vaccination. Vaccines are available for hepatitis A and B. Both of these vaccines are killed virus vaccines.
- Approximately 90 percent of adults are immune to **varicella**.
  - However, infections in adults are more severe than those in children, and pregnant women who develop varicella infections seem to be particularly vulnerable to pneumonia.
  - Furthermore, fetal varicella infections result in congenital anomalies in 1 to 2 percent of cases.

- Varicella immunoglobulin G (IgG) titers can be obtained to identify nonimmune patients. Essentially all adults with and most without a history of clinical infection in childhood are immune to varicella.
- A live attenuated vaccine against varicella is available.
- Women should be tested for immunity to **rubella,** and those without immunity to this infection should be vaccinated.
  - Fetal infection with rubella can be devastating, causing systemic effects most notably in the central nervous system (deafness, microcephaly, mental retardation).
  - Infection may occur in as many as 50 percent of fetuses whose nonimmune mothers develop the infection early in the first trimester. By the end of the first trimester, the risk to the fetus decreases to about 10 percent; in cases of maternal infection after the first trimester, the risk that the fetus will develop congenital rubella syndrome is approximately 1 percent.
  - Although no cases of congenital rubella syndrome have been associated with the rubella vaccine, it is a live attenuated virus. Therefore, women should be advised to use effective contraception for 1 month following vaccination.
- All patients should be counseled regarding ways to minimize the likelihood of developing **toxoplasmosis.**
  - *Toxoplasma gondii* is a unicellular parasite that can cause fetal infections characterized by cerebral calcifications, chorioretinitis, hydrocephalus, and potentially other sequelae.
  - Fetal infection occurs in 60 to 65 percent of cases of maternal infection in the third trimester and approximately 20 to 25 percent of cases of maternal infection during the first and second trimesters. However, fetal infections that occur earlier in pregnancy tend to be more severe.
  - The two most common ways to acquire toxoplasmosis are by handling raw or undercooked meats and coming into contact with cat feces containing infectious oocysts. Therefore pregnant women should adhere to frequent hand washing during food preparation and should avoid cat litter.
- Unfortunately, there is no evidence that screening for **cytomegalovirus** or **parvovirus** prevents fetal infections with these two viruses. Furthermore, cytomegalovirus can cause recurrent infections that may adversely affect the fetus. Universal precautions should be emphasized for those women at high risk of developing infections with these viruses (elementary school teachers, day care workers, and health care workers).

- Screening for infection with the **human immunodeficiency virus** (HIV) should be offered to all women at preconception visits. Screening for other sexually transmitted diseases should be offered based on an assessment of the given woman's risk.

NUTRITIONAL CONSIDERATIONS

- Appropriate **weight gain** during pregnancy reduces perinatal morbidity. Such outcomes as preterm delivery, fetal growth abnormalities, and increased cesarean delivery rates are associated with insufficient or excessive weight gain during pregnancy. Table 1-2 displays recommended ranges of weight gain.
- All women who are capable of becoming pregnant should consume 0.4 mg of **folic acid** daily in order to reduce the risk of neural tube defects in infants. One prenatal vitamin taken daily provides the recommended amount of folic acid and is also a good multivitamin choice for women of reproductive age. Women who have delivered a previous infant with a neural tube defect should consume 4 mg of folic acid daily for 1 month prior to conception and throughout the first trimester of pregnancy.
- Very high doses of **vitamin A** may cause renal and craniofacial defects in fetuses. The daily dose of vitamin A should be no greater than 5000 IU. Some readily available vitamin supplements contain amounts of this vitamin far in excess of this recommended maximum.
- Women with **phenylketonuria,** an autosomal recessive genetic disease, should adhere to dietary restriction of phenylalanine. Excessive blood levels of this amino acid are associated with significant risks of mental retardation, congenital heart disease, and growth restriction in the fetus.
- Counseling regarding the harmful effects of tobacco, alcohol, and illicit drugs is appropriate during preconception visits. **Alcohol** is the most common nongenetic cause of mental retardation.

TABLE 1-2 Weight Gain Recommended during Pregnancy

PREPREGNANCY WEIGHT	RECOMMENDED WEIGHT GAIN
Underweight BMI[a] <20	30–40 lb
Appropriate weight BMI 20–26	25–35 lb
Overweight BMI >26	15–25 lb

[a]BMI=body mass index (weight in kilograms divided by the square of height in meters).

TERATOGENS

- Approximately 3 percent of infants are born with major congenital anomalies.
  - For an exposure to cause a gross structural defect, it must occur during the period of organogenesis. Later exposures may still cause problems but are associated with finer defects or functional impairments.
  - It is reassuring that approximately 95 percent of the 200 most frequently prescribed drugs appear to be safe in pregnancy.
  - However, some drugs and environmental agents are thought to be responsible for about 5 percent of congenital anomalies. Some of these agents are listed earlier in this chapter. This section describes some of the other known teratogens.
- Although **danazol** can cause virilization of a female fetus when it is taken during the first trimester, there are no data that reliably implicate oral contraceptives or medroxyprogesterone acetate as being teratogenic.
- Although ingestion of the synthetic estrogen **diethylstilbestrol** by pregnant women should be rare today, this drug may cause genitourinary abnormalities in infants exposed to it in utero.
- **Warfarin** may cause fetal midface abnormalities such as hypoplasia of the nasal bridge, stippling of the epiphyses, and central nervous system abnormalities. This drug is considered teratogenic when administered at any time during gestation. However, exposure during the first trimester is more likely to cause adverse fetal effects than exposure later in gestation.
- **Heparin,** including low-molecular-weight formulations, is not associated with an increased risk of congenital anomalies.
- Approximately 1 percent of fetuses exposed to **lithium** in utero have congenital anomalies. Cardiac defects, particularly Ebstein's anomaly, are most closely associated with fetal exposure to this medication.
- **Antineoplastic or other cytotoxic agents** are obviously potentially teratogenic to the developing fetus. Whenever possible, these agents should be avoided during pregnancy, particularly during the first trimester. However, in selected circumstances (eg, a pregnant patient with an aggressive malignancy), the benefit of treatment may outweigh the risk to the fetus.
- Like high doses of vitamin A, the derivatives of this vitamin (eg, isotretinoin and etretinate) cause birth defects. Approximately one-third of fetuses exposed

TABLE 1-3   Estimated Fetal Radiation Exposure from Commonly Performed Radiologic Procedures

PROCEDURE	FETAL EXPOSURE
Ultrasound	0 rads
Magnetic resonance imaging	0 rads
Plain film of the chest (two views)	0.02–0.07 millirads
Abdominal film (one-view "KUB"[a])	0.1 rad
Mammography	0.01–0.02 rad
Barium enema	2–4 rads
Computed tomography	
Head or chest	<1 rad
Abdomen and pelvis	3.5 rads
Pelvimetry	0.25 rad

[a]KUB=kidneys, ureter, bladder.

to **isotretinoin** in utero develop serious abnormalities, including blindness, deafness, hydrocephalus, microtia, microphthalmia, thymic agenesis, and cardiac defects. **Etretinate,** an oral agent used to treat psoriasis, causes fetal abnormalities similar to those observed with isotretinoin, even when intake precedes the pregnancy by up to 18 months. Conversely, topical use of tretinoin is not associated with a risk of teratogenicity because it is not absorbed systemically.

- Multiple **chemical agents** are associated with spontaneous abortion, restriction of fetal growth, and neurologic abnormalities. Some of these chemicals include methyl mercury, lead, organic solvents, and polychlorinated biphenyls.
- **Maternal hyperthermia** increases the risk of neural tube defects. Therefore pregnant women should not use hot tubs or saunas, particularly early in gestation.
- Finally, **ionizing radiation** can cause adverse fetal effects, such as growth restriction and mental retardation. However, teratogenic effects do not occur at doses below 5 rads. Although avoidance of radiation during pregnancy is desirable, appropriate medical care of the pregnant woman may make it unavoidable. Table 1-3 lists estimates of fetal radiation exposure from commonly performed radiologic procedures.

BIBLIOGRAPHY

American College of Obstetricians and Gynecologists. Preconceptional care. *ACOG Tech Bull* No. 205, May 1995.

Kuller JA, Strauss RA, Cefalo RC. Preconceptional and prenatal care. In: Ling FW, Duff P, eds. *Obstetrics & Gynecology: Principles for Practice.* New York: McGraw-Hill, 2001.

2 GAMETOGENESIS AND FERTILIZATION

Rodney K. Edwards

MALE GAMETOGENESIS

- Spermatogenesis is the process whereby sperm are formed within the **seminiferous tubules** in the testes.
- **Leydig cells**, which lie between the seminiferous tubules, produce testosterone in response to stimulation by **luteinizing hormone** (LH). Testosterone production is essential for spermatogenesis. However, its exact effect on developing sperm is unknown.
- Sperm are made continuously in the testes from puberty until death. The process is divided into three phases: mitosis, meiosis, and transformation. The entire cycle takes approximately 64 days, and waves of cells along the seminiferous tubules are at varying stages of the cycle.
  - The stem cells in the seminiferous tubules are called **spermatogonia**. These **diploid** (46 chromosomes) cells undergo mitotic division to produce **primary spermatocytes**. These cells are destined to become mature sperm, while the remaining population of spermatogonia continue to serve as stem cells.
  - Primary spermatocytes undergo the first meiotic division, producing **haploid** (23 chromosomes) **secondary spermatocytes**.
  - These secondary spermatocytes undergo the second meiotic division to form **spermatids**.
  - Spermatids become **mature sperm** by undergoing transformation, or spermiogenesis, whereby most of the cytoplasm is lost and flagella are developed.
- **Sertoli cells** have differentiating sperm cells embedded in their cytoplasm. Adjacent Sertoli cells form the blood-testis barrier through a series of tight junctions, isolating maturing sperm from the bloodstream. In addition, Sertoli cells secrete the fluid that transports spermatozoa through the seminiferous tubules and into the epididymis.
- Spermatogenesis is presented pictorially in Fig. 2-1.

FEMALE GAMETOGENESIS

- The number of oocytes a given woman has is maximal at about 20 weeks of fetal life. This number is approximately 6 to 7 million. Atresia of the oocytes also begins in the first half of fetal life. By birth, there are only 1 to 2 million oocytes remaining in the ovary. By puberty, only 300,000 of the original oocytes remain,

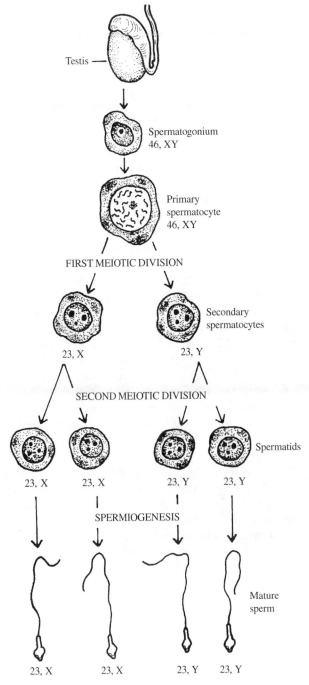

FIG. 2-1 Normal spermatogenesis. This process usually begins at puberty and continues throughout the rest of a man's life. Note that four mature sperm form from one primary spermatocyte.

and only 400 to 500 of them will eventually ovulate during the course of a woman's reproductive life.
- Oogenesis differs from spermatogenesis in that only one final daughter oocyte forms from each precursor cell. The remainder of the genetic material is discarded in **polar bodies**.

- At approximately 8 weeks of gestation, **primary oocytes** in the female fetus begin the first meiotic division. These primary oocytes arrest division in the diplotene stage of prophase of the first meiotic division until the time of ovulation. They are therefore diploid cells. Differentiating to this point protects them from undergoing atresia, the fate of the majority of the **oogonia** that do not proceed to the primary oocyte stage.
- After puberty, once ovulatory cycles are established, a cohort of follicles begins growing over several months in a gonadotropin-independent fashion. Later, the growth of these **primordial follicles** becomes dependent on follicle-stimulating hormone (FSH). As the oocyte grows, the surrounding **granulosa cells** also grow, changing from single- to multi-layered.
- During the **preantral follicle** stage, the granulosa cells continue to proliferate. In addition, **theca cells** in the stroma adjacent to the granulosa cells begin to proliferate. LH stimulates theca cells to produce androgens. These androgens are converted to estrogens by aromatase in the granulosa cells under stimulation by FSH. This local production of estrogen causes the microenvironment in the follicle to favor continued growth and differentiation. One of the cohort of preantral follicles is destined to become a preovulatory follicle. The remainder of the follicles undergo atresia.
- **Preovulatory follicles** contain an antrum that is filled with granulosa cell secretions. The oocyte remains connected to the follicle by a stalk of specialized granulosa cells called the **cumulus oophorus**.
- Estrogen is inhibitory to LH secretion at lower concentrations. However, when the estrogen concentration is high for more than 48 h, it produces a surge in the secretion of LH. This **LH surge** results in luteinization of the granulosa cells and triggering of ovulation 10 to 12 h after the LH peak.
- Shortly before ovulation, the primary oocyte completes the first meiotic division. Unlike the corresponding stage of spermatogenesis, here the division of cytoplasm is unequal. Almost all of the cytoplasm goes with the haploid **secondary oocyte**. The other daughter cell is the first polar body. This small, non-functioning cell soon degenerates.
- After ovulation, the granulosa cells remaining in the follicle secrete progesterone. This follicle is invaded by blood vessels and becomes the **corpus luteum**. The progesterone secreted from the corpus luteum into the bloodstream supports the endometrium during the luteal phase. If pregnancy occurs, human chorionic gonadotropin (hCG) stimulates the corpus luteum to continue producing progesterone until the developing placenta can synthesize enough progesterone to maintain the pregnancy (at about 5 weeks of gestation).
- Oogenesis is presented pictorially in Fig. 2-2.

FERTILIZATION

- Fertilization occurs in the ampulla of the fallopian tube.
- Only one out of every million sperm deposited in the vagina reaches that portion of the tube.
  - The effects of estrogen, which is secreted in abundance in the late follicular phase, enhance sperm

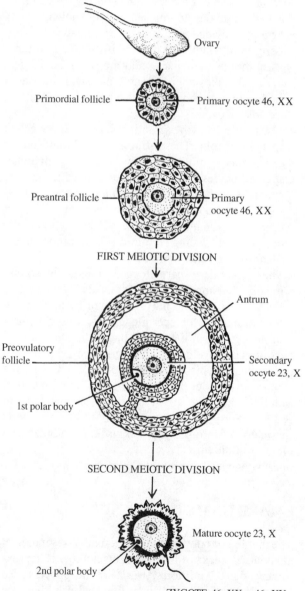

FIG. 2-2 Normal oogenesis. This process usually begins at puberty and continues until menopause. Note that only a single mature ovum forms from one primary oocyte.

transport. This hormone causes the cervical mucus to be thin, watery, and copious in amount. In addition, estrogen primes the reproductive tract for the effects of other mediators, such as prostaglandins and oxytocin.
- ◦ Both prostaglandins in semen and oxytocin released from the pituitary during intercourse stimulate uterine contractions that help propel sperm toward and into the tubes.
- ◦ Sperm appear in the fallopian tubes 5 to 60 min after ejaculation.
- ◦ These sperm are usually fertile for 1 to 2 days, but they may remain so for up to 4 days.
- At the time of ovulation, the fimbria is in close contact with the ovary. The ovum and its surrounding granulosa cells are swept into the fallopian tube by beating cilia on the surface of the fimbria.
- ◦ The ovum can be fertilized only during the first 6 to 24 h after ovulation.
- ◦ As soon as a sperm penetrates the ovum, the ovum completes the second meiotic division. The second polar body is extruded, and the fertilized ovum begins to divide.
- Progesterone, secreted by the corpus luteum, inhibits the muscular contractions of the proximal fallopian tube, thus allowing the conceptus to pass into the uterine cavity.
- ◦ It takes approximately 4 days for the conceptus to travel from the site of fertilization in the ampulla to the uterine cavity.
- ◦ By the time the conceptus reaches the uterine cavity, it is at the blastocyst stage, consisting of about 100 cells.

IMPLANTATION

- At the time of maximal progesterone secretion by the corpus luteum, about 5 to 7 days after fertilization, implantation of the conceptus in the endometrial lining occurs.
- By the time of implantation, the conceptus consists of an inner mass of cells destined to become the embryo and an outer rim of **trophoblast** that will give rise to the placenta and fetal membranes.
- ◦ The trophoblast invades the endometrium, anchoring the conceptus to the uterine wall and burying it within the endometrium.
- ◦ As the trophoblast continues to grow and differentiate into placenta, endometrial blood vessels are invaded, projections of the trophoblast that will become placental villi develop, and the histologic structures necessary to conduct maternal-to-fetal diffusion are formed.

BIBLIOGRAPHY

Palter SF, Olive DL. Reproductive physiology. In: Berek JS, Adashi EY, Hillard PA, eds. *Novak's Gynecology*, 12th ed. Baltimore: Williams & Wilkins, 1996.

Speroff L, Glass RH, Kase NG. *Clinical Gynecologic Endocrinology and Infertility*, 6th ed. Baltimore: Lippincott Williams & Wilkins, 1999.

3   FETAL PHYSIOLOGY

Rodney K. Edwards

AMNIOTIC FLUID DYNAMICS

- In the first trimester, the origin of amniotic fluid is uncertain. It may represent an ultrafiltrate of maternal plasma through the fetal membranes or of fetal plasma through the nonkeratinized fetal skin. By the second trimester, the fetus is thought to be the source.
- Amniotic fluid becomes progressively more hypotonic throughout pregnancy. Hypotonic fetal urine production begins by 12 weeks of gestation and increasingly contributes to amniotic fluid. By 20 weeks of gestation, increasing keratinization of the fetal skin removes the contribution of transudation across the skin.
- The purpose of amniotic fluid is to cushion the fetus and umbilical cord, protect the fetus from trauma, and allow musculoskeletal development. Inspiration and swallowing of amniotic fluid are necessary for normal pulmonary and gastrointestinal development.
- **Polyhydramnios**, an excessive amount of amniotic fluid, may be due to congenital anomalies (particularly those involving upper gastrointestinal obstruction or impaired swallowing), diabetes, hydrops fetalis, and multiple gestations. It may also be idiopathic.
- **Oligohydramnios**, an abnormally low volume of amniotic fluid, may be due to renal agenesis, obstruction of the fetal urinary tract, or uteroplacental insufficiency (with coexisting restriction of fetal growth).

FETAL CIRCULATION

- The fetal circulation differs significantly from that of the child or adult. In part, these differences are necessary because the placenta, not the lungs, is the respiratory organ for the fetus. Also, these differences allow selective delivery of more highly oxygenated blood to the heart and brain. Figure 3-1 shows the major features of the fetal circulation.

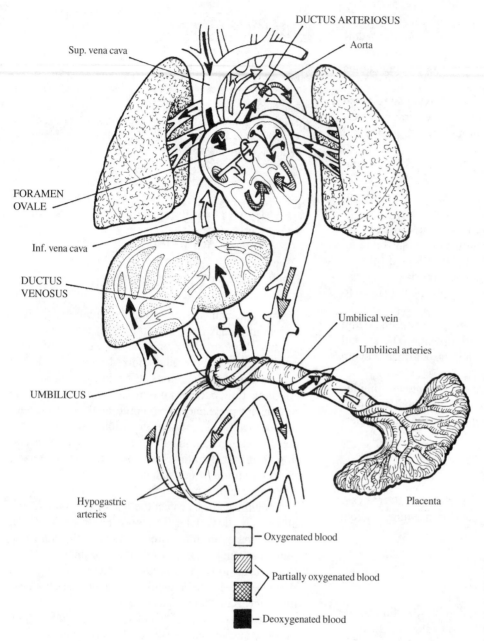

DUCTUS ARTERIOSUS

Sup. vena cava

Aorta

FORAMEN
OVALE

Inf. vena cava

DUCTUS
VENOSUS

Umbilical vein

Umbilical arteries

UMBILICUS

Hypogastric
arteries

Placenta

☐ — Oxygenated blood

▨ ⟩ Partially oxygenated blood
▩

■ — Deoxygenated blood

FIG. 3-1 The fetal circulation. Note that oxygenated blood is delivered to the fetus via the umbilical vein. In addition, there are three major shunts that do not exist in the adult: the ductus venosus, foramen ovale, and ductus arteriosus.

- Oxygenated blood is delivered to the fetus from the umbilical vein. The **ductus venosus** allows this oxygenated blood to bypass the liver and enter the inferior vena cava directly. Selective streaming minimizes mixing of this blood with the deoxygenated blood flowing from the hepatic veins into the inferior vena cava.
- During fetal life, the ventricles work in parallel rather than in series. Well-oxygenated blood is directed to the left ventricle, which supplies the brain and heart, and less oxygenated blood is directed to the right ventricle, which supplies the rest of the body. This separation is facilitated by the structure of the right atrium and interatrial septum. The crista dividens, part of the interatrial

septum, directs the well-oxygenated blood coming from the medial part of the inferior vena cava across the **foramen ovale** and into the left atrium and ventricle. Blood from the superior vena cava and lateral part of the inferior vena cava is directed toward the right ventricle.
- Because pulmonary vascular resistance is very high, less than 15 percent of the blood exiting the right ventricle goes to the lungs. The remainder of the output from the right ventricle is shunted through the **ductus arteriosus** into the descending aorta.
- After birth, the umbilical vessels, ductus venosus, foramen ovale, and ductus arteriosus constrict or close. In addition, the pulmonary vascular resistance decreases.

The lungs then function as the respiratory organ, and the ventricles work in series rather than in parallel.

ACID-BASE EQUILIBRIUM

- Two groups of acids are formed by fetal metabolism—carbonic and noncarbonic acids.
  - Carbonic acid is formed by the hydration of carbon dioxide (CO_2) during oxidative metabolism. Since CO_2 diffuses rapidly across the placenta, respiratory acidosis corrects rather quickly.
  - Noncarbonic acids, such as lactate and hydroxybutyrate, are formed during anaerobic glycolysis. These acids diffuse across the placenta more slowly than does CO_2. Therefore it takes longer to correct metabolic acidosis.
- The fetal pH is directly related to the concentration of bicarbonate and inversely related to the concentration of CO_2. Bicarbonate and hemoglobin are the two most important buffers in fetal blood, allowing a relatively constant pH. A **base deficit** exists when the amount of buffer is below the normal level.
- **Respiratory acidosis** results from the rise in CO_2 that occurs when blood flow from the placenta to the fetus is impeded (eg, umbilical cord compression). If reduced perfusion persists, hypoxia develops and leads to anaerobic metabolism and the production of noncarbonic acids.
- Examination of umbilical cord blood gas values provides information regarding the acid-base balance of the newborn at the time of delivery. Table 3-1 presents blood-gas criteria with which to classify fetal/newborn acidemia. Of note, major neurologic morbidity due to birth asphyxia rarely occurs unless the umbilical artery pH is less than 7.00. However, as many as two-thirds of term infants with pH values below this threshold will be admitted to the regular newborn nursery and have no apparent sequelae.

HEMATOPOIETIC SYSTEM

- Hematopoiesis occurs predominately in the yolk sac until 8 weeks of gestation. During the late first trimester and the second trimester, the liver is the principal site of red blood cell synthesis. By 26 weeks, the bone marrow becomes the major site of hematopoiesis. The spleen and lymph nodes are minor sites. Fetal erythropoiesis is under fetal control exclusively; maternal erythropoietin does not cross the placenta.
- Hemoglobin is a tetramer of two copies each of two different peptide chains. Normal adult hemoglobin, **hemoglobin A**, is made up of α and β chains. **Fetal hemoglobin**, made up of α and γ chains, binds oxygen with more affinity than does hemoglobin A. As shown in Fig. 3-2, this difference shifts the oxygen dissociation curve of the fetus to the left, aiding transfer of oxygen from mother to fetus. The major reason for this difference is the lower affinity of fetal hemoglobin for 2,3-diphosphoglycerate (2,3-DPG).
- The majority of antibodies in the fetal circulation are immunoglobulin G (IgG) acquired transplacentally from the mother. The bulk of IgG transport does not occur until the last 4 weeks of gestation, thus contributing to the increased susceptibility of preterm fetuses to infection. Since IgM cannot cross the placenta, appreciable levels of this class of antibody in the fetal or umbilical cord blood suggest the presence of congenital infection.

PULMONARY SYSTEM

- There are three stages of fetal lung development.
  - During the **pseudoglandular stage**, the bronchial tree is formed. This stage ends by about 16 weeks of gestation, and the most distal structure is the terminal bronchiole.

TABLE 3-1   Blood-Gas Criteria for the Classification of Fetal/Neonatal Acidemia

TYPE OF ACIDEMIA	PCO$_2$[a]	BASE DEFICIT
Respiratory	High	Normal
Metabolic	Normal	High
Mixed	High	High

[a]PCO$_2$ = partial pressure of carbon dioxide.

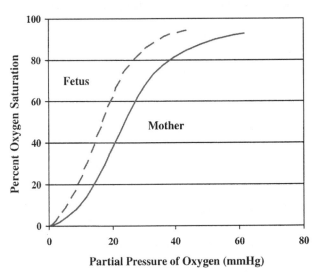

FIG. 3-2 The fetal oxygen dissociation curve is shifted to the left, owing to the increased affinity of fetal hemoglobin for oxygen.

○ From 16 to 25 weeks, during the **canalicular stage**, the terminal bronchioles give rise to the respiratory bronchioles and saccular ducts.

○ Alveoli are formed during the **terminal sac stage**. At birth, only about 15 percent of the adult complement of alveoli are present, and this stage of lung development continues until about 8 years of age.

• In addition to the presence of alveoli, ex utero oxygenation and respiration require the presence of **surfactant**.

○ This material is a soap-like substance composed mostly of phospholipids. Surfactant is synthesized in type II pneumocytes, which line the alveoli. It decreases surface tension at the air-tissue interface and prevents alveolar collapse during expiration.

○ Preterm infants may produce insufficient amounts of surfactant and develop respiratory distress syndrome. The advent of neonatal surfactant therapy has reduced the sequelae of neonatal respiratory disease. In addition, glucocorticoids administered to the pregnant woman at risk of preterm delivery reduce the incidence of respiratory distress syndrome and other complications of prematurity.

GASTROINTESTINAL SYSTEM

• Fetal swallowing begins by the end of the first trimester. Although not a significant factor early in pregnancy, swallowing substantially regulates the volume of amniotic fluid later in gestation. Much of the water in swallowed amniotic fluid is absorbed across the fetal small bowel; the unabsorbed material (meconium) is transported as far as the distal colon.

• **Meconium** consists of water, desquamated fetal cells, lanugo, hair, vernix, and bile pigments. Defecation of meconium in utero may represent simply maturation of the gastrointestinal tract, as this event occurs in more than 10 percent of births beyond 39 weeks of gestation. However, the passage of meconium may occur as a result of colonic muscular contraction caused by either vagal stimulation due to umbilical cord compression or arginine vasopressin release resulting from hypoxia.

• The ability of the liver to conjugate bilirubin is limited but improves near term. Glycogen storage in the fetal liver is minimal during the second trimester; but by term, levels are two to three times those in the adult.

ENDOCRINE SYSTEM

• Fetal thyroid physiology is independent of maternal thyroid hormones. Neither thyroid-stimulating hormone nor thyroxine crosses the placenta in appreciable amounts. The placenta concentrates iodide on the fetal side; during the second and third trimesters, the fetal thyroid concentrates iodide to a greater degree than the maternal thyroid. This fact causes the administration of radioactive iodine during pregnancy to be particularly hazardous.

• Fetal pancreatic function is discussed in Chap. 7C.

• At term, the fetal adrenal glands weigh as much as those of an adult. More than 85 percent of the organ is composed of a fetal zone that is not found in adult glands. The daily production of steroids by the fetal adrenal glands at term is three to four times that in a resting adult.

BIBLIOGRAPHY

Fetal growth and development. In: Cunningham FG, Gant NF, Leveno KJ, et al, eds. *Williams Obstetrics*, 21st ed. New York: McGraw-Hill, 2001.

Ross MG, Ervin MG, Novak D. Placental and fetal physiology. In: Gabbe SG, Niebyl JR, Simpson JL, eds. *Obstetrics: Normal and Problem Pregnancies*, 4th ed. New York: Churchill Livingstone, 2002.

4   MATERNAL PHYSIOLOGY

Patrick Duff

INTRODUCTION

• This chapter reviews the major maternal physiologic changes that occur during pregnancy.

• In each section, the key clinical implications of these physiologic changes are highlighted.

PLACENTAL FUNCTION

• The placenta is composed of two principal cell lines.

○ **Synctiotrophoblasts**

○ **Cytotrophoblasts**

• The synctiotrophoblast synthesizes two hormones of great importance in pregnancy.

○ **Human chorionic gonadotropin** (HCG) stimulates the corpus luteum to synthesize estradiol and progesterone during the first trimester.

○ **Human placental lactogen (HPL)**

▪ Stimulates lipolysis, which provides the mother with an alternate fuel source, thus sparing glucose for use by the fetus.

- ▪ Antagonizes the effect of insulin, thus creating a diabetogenic effect.
- Substances in the maternal blood cross the placental membrane by several different mechanisms (Table 4-1).

TABLE 4-1   Mechanisms of Placental Transfer

SUBSTANCE	MECHANISM OF PLACENTAL TRANSFER
Oxygen, carbon dioxide, water, most electrolytes	Simple diffusion
Glucose	Facilitated diffusion
Iron, amino acids	Active transport
Most drugs, immunoglobulins	Pinocytosis

CHANGES IN THE SKIN

- **Striae gravidarum** ("stretch marks") tend to appear as uterine size increases.
- **Vascular spiders** and **palmar erythema** result from increased serum estrogen concentrations.
- **Hirsutism** and **acne** may become apparent to the patient. These changes result primarily from the increased serum concentration of progesterone.
- **Hyperpigmentation** in certain areas of the skin is due to increased production of melanocyte-stimulating hormone (MSH), which, in turn, results from the increased serum concentration of estrogens.
  - ○ Nipple
  - ○ Areola
  - ○ Axilla
  - ○ Umbilicus
  - ○ Linea nigra
  - ○ Face (**melasma**, the "mask of pregnancy")

CHANGES IN THE BREAST

- Overall, the breasts enlarge in size.
- The cystic consistency of the breast increases.
- The superficial venous pattern becomes more prominent.
- The areola darkens.
- The sebaceous glands of the breast (**follicles of Montgomery**) hypertrophy.
- Colostrum may be secreted late in pregnancy.

CHANGES IN THE ABDOMINAL WALL

- The uterus enlarges progressively throughout a normal pregnancy.

- The rectus muscles become progressively separated as the uterus enlarges (**diastasis recti**).
- Because of the separation of the rectus muscles, an infraumbilical midline incision is the fastest and easiest way to perform a laparotomy in a pregnant woman.

CHANGES IN THE GENITAL TRACT

VAGINA

- The vascularity of the vagina increases.
- The vagina becomes increasingly distensible.
- The upper vaginal vault becomes almost cyanotic in appearance in early pregnancy (**Chadwick's sign**).
- The capillary bed of the vagina becomes increasingly permeable, resulting in a characteristic white discharge (**leukorrhea of pregnancy**).

CERVIX

- The cervix becomes increasingly vascularized and edematous.
- Columnar epithelium from the endocervical canal is typically everted onto the exocervix (**ectopy**).

UTERUS

- Uterine blood flow increases dramatically during pregnancy. At term, 15 to 20 percent of cardiac output perfuses the uterus.
  - ○ Approximately 5 percent of the blood flow perfuses the myometrium.
  - ○ Ten to 15 percent perfuses the endometrium.
  - ○ Eighty percent perfuses the placenta.
- The amount of structural protein and connective tissue in the uterus increases progressively throughout gestation.

CARDIOVASCULAR SYSTEM

- Because of elevation of the diaphragm, the heart is raised and rotated slightly to the left on its longitudinal axis. As a result, the electrocardiogram (ECG) will demonstrate a slight left-axis deviation.
- Heart rate increases by about 5 to 15 percent during a normal singleton pregnancy.
- Stroke volume increases approximately 25 to 30 percent.
- Cardiac output increases by approximately 35 to 50 percent.

- Cardiac output increases even more during labor.
  - Early first stage—15 to 20 percent
  - Late first stage—30 to 35 percent
  - Second stage—35 to 40 percent
- Because of increased blood flow through the pulmonary artery and aorta, grade 1 or 2 systolic ejection murmurs are common in pregnancy.
- The demand for increased cardiac output may pose particular difficulty for patients with certain cardiac diseases. Patients with any of the following disorders have a significantly increased risk of mortality during pregnancy.
  - Mitral stenosis
  - Aortic stenosis
  - Ischemic heart disease
  - Marfan's syndrome
  - Eisenmenger's syndrome
  - Primary pulmonary hypertension

PULMONARY PHYSIOLOGY

- During pregnancy, the maternal respiratory rate increases slightly.
- **Tidal volume** (the amount of air exchanged with normal inspiration and expiration) increases from about 450 to 600 mL.
- Therefore the **minute ventilation** (respiratory rate × total volume) increases.
- **Inspiratory reserve volume** (the amount of air that can be inspired at the end of a normal inspiration) remains constant in pregnancy—about 2050 mL.
- **Inspiratory capacity** (sum of inspiratory reserve volume plus tidal volume) increases from about 2500 to 2650 mL.
- **Expiratory reserve volume** (the amount of air that can be expired at the end of a normal expiration) decreases in pregnancy from approximately 700 to 550 mL.
- **Residual volume** (the amount of air remaining in the lung at the end of maximal expiration) decreases from 1000 to about 800 mL.
- **Functional residual capacity** (the sum of expiratory reserve volume plus residual volume) decreases in pregnancy from about 1700 to 1350 mL.
- **Vital capacity** (the sum of expiratory reserve volume plus tidal volume plus inspiratory reserve volume) remains constant in pregnancy—about 3200 mL.
  - Measurement of vital capacity with a spirometer is a valuable test in assessing pregnant patients with cardiopulmonary disease.
- Arterial blood gases are altered in pregnancy.
  - Increased minute ventilation leads to an increased pH and decreased P_{CO_2}.
  - The kidney compensates for these changes by increasing bicarbonate excretion. Therefore the serum HCO_3 decreases.
  - The resulting blood gas alteration in pregnancy is a **partially compensated respiratory alkalosis**.

HEMATOPOIETIC SYSTEM

RED CELLS

- Blood volume increases 30 to 50 percent.
- Red cell number increases by about 30 percent.
- Plasma volume increases by almost 50 percent.
- Because the plasma volume increases more than the red cell mass, the maternal hematocrit tends to decrease in pregnancy (**physiologic or dilutional anemia of pregnancy**).
- Iron deficiency still is the most common cause of anemia in pregnancy, but dilutional anemia is the second most common cause.
- Other important causes of anemia include:
  - Folate deficiency
  - Hemoglobinopathy
  - Blood loss
  - B_{12} deficiency

WHITE CELLS

- The total white blood cell count increases up to the range of 10,000 to 14,000/mm^3.
- The white cell count may rise above 20,000/mm^3 during labor.
- Because of these changes, an elevated white blood cell count is not necessarily an indicator of infection.

PLATELET COUNT

- The platelet count usually remains normal during pregnancy.
- In isolated instances the platelet count may decline in late pregnancy in the absence of any hematopoietic disorder. This condition is termed **benign gestational thrombocytopenia**.

COAGULATION SYSTEM

- During pregnancy the liver increases its synthesis of coagulation factors I, II, VII, VIII, IX, and X.
- The placenta actively synthesizes tissue thromboplastin (coagulation factor III).

- Enlargement of the uterus causes marked increases in venous pressures in the veins of the lower extremities and pelvis.
- Because of these changes, there is an increased risk of venous thromboembolism in pregnancy.

GASTROINTESTINAL SYSTEM

- Progesterone inhibits smooth muscle peristalsis in the gastrointestinal tract.
- The possible clinical consequences of delayed gastrointestinal motility include:
  - Delayed gastric emptying, resulting in early satiety.
  - Relaxation of the cardioesophageal sphincter, leading to gastroesophageal reflux.
  - Delayed colonic emptying, leading to constipation.
  - Biliary tract stasis, resulting in an increased frequency of cholelithiasis, cholecystitis, and pancreatitis.
- As pregnancy progresses, the appendix may change its location from a right-lower-quadrant organ to a mid- or even upper-quadrant organ. This alteration in anatomic location may lead to delay in the diagnosis of appendicitis in pregnant women.

RENAL SYSTEM

- Renal blood flow increases approximately 30 to 40 percent during pregnancy.
- The glomerular filtration rate (GRF) increases to approximately 100 to 150 mL/min.
- Because of increased renal blood flow and increased GFR, the blood urea nitrogen concentration (BUN), serum creatinine, and serum uric acid decrease in pregnancy.
- Drugs that are processed by renal excretion (eg, aminoglycosides, antiseizure medications) may require dosage increases to maintain therapeutic serum concentrations in pregnancy.
- Progesterone inhibits ureteral peristalsis. As a result, lower urinary tract infections in pregnancy are more likely to progress to upper tract infections (see Chap. 25).

ENDOCRINE SYSTEM

- The endocrine changes of major clinical importance in pregnancy relate primarily to thyroid gland physiology.
- The liver increases synthesis of thyroid binding globulin (TBG).

- To compensate for the increased serum concentration of TBG, the thyroid gland increases synthesis of T_3 and T_4.
- However, the serum concentrations of free T_3 and T_4 remain constant during pregnancy.
- Similarly, the serum concentration of thyroid-stimulating hormone (TSH) remains unchanged in pregnancy.
- T_3, T_4, and TSH do not cross the placenta. The fetus is entirely autonomous with respect to thyroid hormone production.

BIBLIOGRAPHY

Capeless E, Fry AG. Maternal physiology. In: Ling FW, Duff P, eds. *Obstetrics & Gynecology. Principles for Practice.* New York: McGraw-Hill, 2001.

5   PRENATAL CARE
Patrick Duff

PURPOSE

- A major purpose of prenatal care is to identify patients at high risk for adverse pregnancy outcomes and to target them for intensive management.
- A second major objective is to screen seemingly low-risk patients for unusual complications such as karyotype abnormalities, congenital malformations, gestational diabetes, or genitourinary tract infection. Once identified, these women can then receive specialized care.

FIRST PRENATAL APPOINTMENT— HISTORY

- The first prenatal appointment should be scheduled as soon as practical after the patient has a positive pregnancy test.
- The patient's menstrual history should be carefully documented.
  - First day of last menstrual period (LMP)
  - Interval between cycles and regularity of cycles
- The estimated date of confinement (EDC) or estimated due date (EDD) can be determined by use of **Naegele's rule**.

- Subtract 3 from the month of the LMP
- Add 7 to the day of the LMP
- For example, if LMP is 5/20, EDC is 2/27
- During this appointment, a detailed history should be taken to identify conditions that place the patient at increased risk for adverse pregnancy outcome. Examples of key historic and demographic features are summarized below:

AGE

- Women who are 35 years of age or older are at increased risk of having an infant with a genetic abnormality. They should be scheduled for genetic counseling.
- Patients who are less than 17 years of age are at increased risk for problems such as:
  - Sexually transmitted diseases
  - Unstable social situation
  - Poor nutrition
  - Anemia

RACE

- Caucasian patients are at increased risk of carrying the gene for cystic fibrosis and should be offered testing for the most common mutations.
- African-American patients are at increased risk of carrying the gene for sickle cell disease and of having gestational diabetes. They should be screened for both disorders.
- Hispanic patients are at increased risk of having gestational diabetes and should be screened for this condition.

RELIGION

- Jewish women of Eastern European ancestry are at increased risk of carrying the gene for Tay-Sachs disease and should be offered testing for this disorder.
- Women who are Jehovah's Witnesses typically are averse to blood transfusion. In view of the fact that hemorrhage is a recognized major obstetric complication (eg, abruptio placentae, placenta previa, postpartum uterine atony), knowledge of the patient's attitude toward transfusion is essential.
- Patients who are Roman Catholic usually strongly oppose abortion. Knowledge of this conviction is of great importance if the clinician needs to counsel the patient about a life-threatening fetal abnormality.
- Muslim women may have a decided preference for a female physician.

PAST MEDICAL HISTORY

- The clinician should inquire about childhood illnesses that may lead to subsequent morbidity in adulthood (eg, rheumatic fever resulting in rheumatic heart disease).
- The patient should be queried about viral illnesses and vaccinations.
  - Measles
  - Mumps
  - Rubella
  - Polio
  - Varicella (chickenpox)
- Adult medical illnesses should be recorded, particularly those with a potentially negative impact on pregnancy, such as:
  - Diabetes
  - Hypertension
  - Collagen vascular disease
  - Hemoglobinopathy
  - Cardiopulmonary disease
  - Renal disease
- A history of sexually transmitted diseases should be documented. Some diseases (eg, gonorrhea and chlamydial infection) may predispose to tubal injury and possible ectopic pregnancy. Others (eg, syphilis, HIV, hepatitis B) pose a major risk to the fetus or neonate.
- The patient should be asked about major surgical procedures, particularly procedures affecting the genital tract such as:
  - Prior cesarean delivery
  - Prior tubal surgery
- A list of the patient's medications should be recorded. Prescription drugs, over-the-counter medications, and herbal preparations should be included. An assessment should be made of the risk that any of these medications pose to the fetus.
- A history of drug allergies should be recorded. The nature and severity of the allergy should be clearly defined, and a careful distinction should be made between an expected side effect (eg, nausea related to narcotics) and a true allergy (eg, an anaphylactic reaction to penicillin).

PAST OBSTETRIC HISTORY

- The patient should be asked about her prior pregnancies.
  - Complications—eg, placenta previa, abruptio placentae, or preterm delivery
  - Method of delivery—cesarean vs. vaginal
- The patient should be queried about prior abortions.
  - Spontaneous vs. elective vs. indicated
  - Technique of abortion
  - Complications

FAMILY HISTORY

- A history of well-recognized recessive, dominant, and sex-linked disorders should be documented.
- The patient should be queried about a history of multifactorial defects, such as:
  - Neural tube defect
  - Cleft lip and/or palate
  - Congenital heart defects

SOCIAL HISTORY

- The patient's type of employment should be identified, and a determination should be made as to whether her work poses any hazard to her or her fetus.
- The patient should be asked about the use of tobacco products. If she smokes, she should receive strong support for cessation of smoking.
  - Counseling
  - Nicotine replacement
  - Pharmacologic therapy (eg, bupropion)
- The patient's use of alcohol should be documented. She should be strongly advised against alcohol ingestation at **any** time during pregnancy.
- The patient should be questioned about the use of illicit drugs such as marijuana, cocaine, and heroin. Women who abuse drugs should be referred to a drug treatment center.

FIRST PRENATAL APPOINTMENT— PHYSICAL EXAMINATION

- Once the patient's complete history has been recorded, a comprehensive physical examination should be performed. Particular attention should be directed to confirming that uterine size is consistent with the patient's menstrual dates.
- The laboratory tests to be performed at the first prenatal appointment are summarized in Table 5-1.
- All patients should receive a prescription for a balanced multivitamin preparation that includes folic acid (400 to 1000 µg) and elemental iron (60 mg).

SUBSEQUENT PRENATAL APPOINTMENTS

- As a general rule, appointments for low-risk patients should be scheduled every 4 to 6 weeks until 36 weeks of gestation and weekly thereafter.

TABLE 5-1 Laboratory Tests Performed at First Prenatal Appointment

TEST	PURPOSE OF TEST
Complete blood count	Evaluate for anemia, white cell abnormality, and thrombocytopenia
Rubella serology; IgG antibody	Confirm immunity to rubella. If patient is not immune, she should be vaccinated postpartum.
Serologic test for syphilis	Identify infected patient and treat her to prevent congenital infection.
HIV serology	Identify infected patient and begin antiretroviral therapy to improve maternal well-being and prevent perinatal transmission of infection.
Hepatitis B surface antigen	Identify chronic carrier of hepatitis B and target her infant for immunoprophylaxis with hepatitis B immune globulin and hepatitis B vaccine
One-hour glucose challenge test	Identify **high-risk** patient who has gestational diabetes and begin early treatment to prevent fetal macrosomia.
Urine culture	Identify the 5 to 10% of patients who have asymptomatic bacteriuria and treat them to prevent symptomatic UTI.
Blood type and antibody screen	Identify women who are Rh-negative and who will benefit from immunoprophylaxis with Rh-immune globulin. Identify women who are isoimmunized to antigens such as D, Kell, Kidd, Duffy.
Cytomegalovirus serology and toxoplasmosis serology	These tests should be performed only in immunocompromised women or women who have symptoms suggestive of infection. Both of these microorganisims can cause congenital infection, which can be detected by a combination of ultrasound and amniocentesis.
Tuberculin skin test	This test should be performed only in high risk patients. Those who have a positive test should have a chest x-ray to determine if they have active disease.
Nucleic acid probe for gonorrhea and chlamydial infection	Identify patient with gonorrhea or chlamydia and treat her to prevent perinatal transmission of infection.
Abdominal or endovaginal ultrasound	This test should be performed if the FHT cannot be heard, if the patient has an unsure LMP, or if she has any history of first-trimester bleeding.

Key: FHT, fetal heart tones; LMP, last menstrual period.

- High-risk patients may require appointments every other week until 28 weeks of gestation and weekly thereafter.
- Patients at extremely high risk may require weekly evaluation throughout pregnancy.
- The following should be routine features of the prenatal appointment:
  - **Assessment of weight.** As a general rule, patients should gain about 0.5 lb per week for the first 20 weeks of gestation and 1.0 lb per week thereafter.

○ **Assessment of blood pressure.** Blood pressure >140/90 mmHg **after** 20 weeks may be an indication of gestational hypertension or preeclampsia.

○ **Assessment of fundal height**
  ▪ The expected fundal height at gestational ages up to 20 weeks is summarized in Fig. 5-1.
  ▪ Beyond 20 weeks. the expected fundal height in centimeters above the pubic symphysis is approximately equal to the gestational age ± 2 cm. For example, at 28 weeks, the uterus should measure 26 to 30 cm.

CORRELATION OF UTERINE SIZE WITH GESTATIONAL AGE (<20 WEEKS)

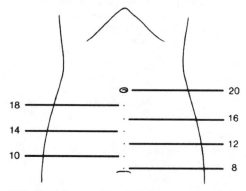

FIG. 5-1 Schematic drawing showing approximate fundal height at gestational ages up to 20 weeks.

▪ Principal causes for fundal height that is greater than expected include:
  ▫ Incorrect dates
  ▫ Uterine anomaly
  ▫ Multiple gestation
  ▫ Large fetus
  ▫ Molar pregnancy
▪ Principal causes for fundal height that is less than expected include:
  ▫ Incorrect dates
  ▫ Fetal death
  ▫ Oligohydramnios
  ▫ Fetal growth restriction

○ **Documentation of fetal heart tones (FHT) and fetal movement**
  ▪ FHT usually can be heard with the doptone at 12 to 14 weeks.
  ▪ Fetal movement is typically perceived by the patient at 16 to 20 weeks.

○ **Assessment for peripheral and facial edema**
  ▪ Mild pretibial edema is common in pregnancy, especially in the third trimester.
  ▪ Severe pretibial edema and swelling of the face and hands may be one of the first manifestations of preeclampsia.

○ **Urinalysis**
  ▪ **Proteinuria**—a possible manifestation of urinary tract infection, renal disease, or preeclampsia.
  ▪ **Glucosuria**—a possible manifestation of diabetes.

TABLE 5-2   Selected Laboratory Tests That Should Be Performed during Prenatal Appointments

GESTATIONAL AGE	TEST	PURPOSE
15 to 18 weeks	Serum analyte screening	Screen for neural tube defect, trisomy 18, and trisomy 21
18 to 20 weeks	Ultrasound examination	Confirm gestational age
		Determine placental location
		Assess amniotic fluid volume
		Identify multiple gestation
		Identify major anatomic malformations
24 to 28 weeks	One-hour glucose challenge test	Screen patient for gestational diabetes.
24 to 28 weeks	Saline microscopy and pH assessment of vaginal secretions	Screen for bacterial vaginosis in women at high risk for preterm delivery
28 weeks	Hematocrit	Evaluate for anemia
	Antibody screen if patient is Rh-negative	Document absence of isoimmunization before administering Rh immune globulin
35 to 37 weeks	Genital tract culture for group B streptococci	Identify colonized women who will benefit from intrapartum antibiotic prophylaxis
35 to 37 weeks	Nucleic acid probes for gonorrhea and chlamydial infection and serology for syphilis	These tests should be performed in women who tested positive earlier in pregnancy to be certain that there is no reinfection or persistence of infection.

- **Leukocyte esterase and nitrites**—positive test may be indicative of UTI.

FURTHER ESSENTIALS

- Selected laboratory tests should be performed during follow-up prenatal appointments. These tests are summarized in Table 5-2.
- At each appointment patients should be reminded of the importance of good general health habits and balanced nutrition.
- During the third trimester, a portion of each appointment should be devoted to a discussion of the delivery plan:
  - Use of electronic monitors and intravenous infusions
  - Type of anesthesia.
  - Use of an episiotomy
  - Family members in attendance at delivery
  - Methods of infant feeding
  - Circumcision of a male infant
  - Subsequent method of birth control

BIBLIOGRAPHY

Kuller JA, Strauss RA, Cefalo RC. Preconceptional and prenatal care. In: Ling FW, Duff P, eds. *Obstetrics & Gynecology. Principles for Practice*. New York: McGraw-Hill, 2001.

6 SPONTANEOUS ABORTION

Rodney K. Edwards

BACKGROUND

- The term **abortion** is defined as the termination of pregnancy, by any means, prior to the point when the fetus is capable of living outside the uterus.
- **Spontaneous abortion** occurs in the absence of medical or surgical measures. The colloquial term for spontaneous abortion is **miscarriage**.
- Strictly defined, spontaneous abortions occur prior to 20 weeks of gestation. After 20 weeks, such a termination of pregnancy is technically a preterm delivery.

EPIDEMIOLOGY

- Ten to 15 percent of clinically recognized pregnancies result in spontaneous abortion. However, when "chemical pregnancies" are also considered, where the serum value of the beta subunit of human chorionic gonadotropin (β-hCG) is positive but there is no recognized intrauterine gestation on ultrasound, the rate of spontaneous abortion exceeds 30 percent of all pregnancies.
- The likelihood of spontaneous abortion increases with advancing maternal age (Fig. 6-1).

ETIOLOGY

- Fetal factors
  - Morphologic abnormalities or absence of the embryo or fetus are present in approximately 70 percent of spontaneous abortions prior to 10 weeks of gestation. When the embryo is absent, this situation sometimes is referred to as a "blighted ovum," or anembryonic gestation.
  - Chromosomal abnormalities are present in 50 to 60 percent of embryos and fetuses that are spontaneously aborted at less than 10 weeks of gestation.
    - The most common group of chromosomal abnormalities is the autosomal trisomies (eg, trisomy 21, or Down's syndrome).
    - The most common single abnormality is monosomy X (Turner's syndrome).
    - This relationship between fetal aneuploidy and spontaneous abortion explains the association

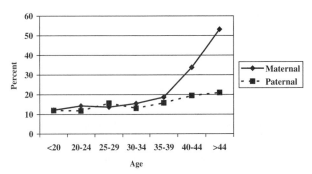

FIG. 6-1 The frequency of spontaneous abortion increases with maternal but not paternal age. (Data from Warburton D, Fraser FC. Spontaneous abortion risks in man: data from reproductive histories collected in a medical genetics unit. *Am J Hum Genet* 1964;16:1–25.)

between maternal age and increased risk of spontaneous abortion (Fig. 6-1).

- Genetic abnormalities other than aneuploidy also contribute to some cases of spontaneous abortion (eg, single gene mutations or polygenic factors).

- Maternal factors
  - Both spontaneous abortions and congenital anomalies are more common in women with pregestational diabetes mellitus; the incidence of each is related to the degree of glycemic control (see also Chap. 7C).
  - Thyroid abnormalities are more closely associated with infertility than with spontaneous abortion.
  - Insufficient secretion of progesterone by the corpus luteum, or "luteal phase defect," has been implicated as a possible cause of spontaneous abortion. However, it is often difficult to determine whether a low serum progesterone value is a cause or consequence of an abnormal pregnancy. Therefore this condition, and the frequency with which it occurs, is controversial.
  - In cattle, microorganisms such as *Brucella abortus* and *Campylobacter fetus* cause spontaneous abortions. However, evidence that these or other microorganisms cause spontaneous abortions in humans is inconclusive.
  - Certain environmental exposures increase the likelihood of spontaneous abortion.
    - Smoking and alcohol use both increase the risk.
    - Toxins such as lead, mercury, formaldehyde, ethylene oxide, benzene, and large doses of ionizing radiation also increase the risk.
    - Caffeine consumption increases the risk of spontaneous abortion. However, the risk is significantly increased only with heavy intake. There is no evidence that moderate consumption of caffeine causes spontaneous abortions.
  - Autoantibodies, such as lupus anticoagulant and anticardiolipin, can cause spontaneous abortion by inducing placental thrombosis and infarction. Patients with one of these antibodies and a significant clinical event (thromboembolic event or recurrent pregnancy loss) are said to have the antiphospholipid syndrome.
  - Spontaneous abortion and other complications of pregnancy, such as intrauterine fetal demise and preeclampsia, are more common in women with certain genetic thrombophilias (eg, factor V Leiden mutation).
  - Some müllerian abnormalities, such as a uterine septum, may cause spontaneous abortions. Some acquired uterine abnormalities, such as uterine synechiae, are also associated with spontaneous abortions.
  - Incompetent cervix is a cause of both spontaneous abortion in the second trimester and preterm delivery. This entity is discussed in Chap. 9.

CATEGORIES OF SPONTANEOUS ABORTION

- **Threatened abortion** is a diagnosis that is made clinically whenever bleeding and/or cramping occurs in the first half of pregnancy.
  - Approximately half of these women will eventually abort.
  - Rh-immune globulin should be administered to Rh-negative women with threatened abortion or any of the other categories of spontaneous abortion discussed in this section.
  - There is no proven benefit to any treatment for this condition.
- When cervical dilation occurs in the first trimester or rupture of the membranes occurs in the first half of pregnancy, an **inevitable abortion** is said to be present.
  - Women with this condition will usually abort spontaneously and/or develop chorioamnionitis.
  - Rarely, women with premature rupture of the membranes early in the second trimester do not abort or become infected. Infants born to these women still are at very high risk of mortality due to pulmonary hypoplasia.
- Prior to 10 weeks of gestation, the embryo or fetus and the placenta are usually expelled together. An **incomplete abortion** occurs whenever part but not all of the products of conception are passed.
  - Vaginal bleeding may occur in this situation and can be profuse.
  - Uterine curettage is indicated to evacuate the remaining products of conception from the endometrial cavity.
- Women who spontaneously have cramping and bleeding and pass all products of conception have a **complete abortion**.
  - A transvaginal ultrasound examination confirms the absence of remaining products of conception in the endometrial cavity.
  - On occasion, clotted blood and other debris will be present in the endometrial cavity. If the area of such debris in the sagittal plane of the uterus is less than 6 cm^2, it will usually pass spontaneously. If the area is greater than 6 cm^2, uterine curettage is usually indicated.
- A **missed abortion** occurs when fetal death does not quickly lead to spontaneous abortion. Since there are no symptoms, the fetal death is not recognized until several weeks after it has occurred.

TABLE 6-1 Diagnostic Evaluation for Couples with Recurrent Pregnancy Loss

CAUSE	DIAGNOSTIC TEST(S)	APPROXIMATE PROBABILITY OF ABNORMAL TEST	POSSIBLE TREATMENT
Endocrine (diabetes; hypothyroidism)	Fasting glucose or glucose tolerance testing; thyroid-stimulating hormone	<5%	Glycemic control; levothyroxine
Genetic (eg, unbalanced translocation)	Maternal and paternal karyotype	3–5%	Donor gametes
Environmental toxins	Medical history	5%	Avoid exposure (eg, stop smoking)
Uterine abnormality	Hysterosalpingogram; sonohysterogram	15–20%	Excision of septum or synechiae
Antiphospholipid syndrome (APS)	Anticardiolipin antibody; test for lupus anticoagulant[a]	15–25%	Aspirin; heparin and aspirin
Thrombophilia	Laboratory evaluation[b]	5%	Aspirin; heparin and aspirin

[a]Tests commonly used to screen for lupus anticoagulant include the activated partial thromboplastin time, dilute Russell viper venom time, and the kaolin clotting time.
[b]The extent of the laboratory evaluation that should be conducted to screen for a thrombophilia in women with RPL is controversial. An appropriate battery of tests might include some or all of the following: DNA tests for factor V Leiden mutation, the prothrombin gene mutation, and plasminogen activator inhibitor-1; activity assays for antithrombin III, protein C, and protein S; and a fasting homocysteine level.

RECURRENT ABORTION

- **Recurrent pregnancy loss** (RPL), formerly known as habitual abortion, has classically been defined as the occurrence of three or more consecutive spontaneous abortions.
  - Some physicians advocate initiating an evaluation after two such losses.
  - There is controversy about what constitutes a pregnancy loss—whether the loss(es) must be clinically recognized pregnancies or if "chemical pregnancies" also count.
- The risk of RPL varies according to maternal age (see Fig. 6-1) and obstetric history. Couples with RPL and a prior successful pregnancy have a 70 percent chance of eventually producing another live-born child. Even couples with RPL who have never delivered a live-born child have a 50 percent chance of eventually delivering one.
- Although a possible cause can be found in most cases, at least 35 percent of cases of RPL are idiopathic. Possible causes are listed under "Etiology" earlier in this chapter. In addition, possible causes, diagnostic tests, and potential therapies are presented in Table 6-1.

BIBLIOGRAPHY

Abortion. In: Cunningham FG, Gant NF, Leveno KJ, et al, eds. *Williams Obstetrics*, 21st ed. New York: McGraw-Hill, 2001.
Kutteh WH. Recurrent pregnancy loss. In: Ling FW, Duff P, eds. *Obstetrics & Gynecology: Principles for Practice.* New York: McGraw-Hill, 2001.

7 MAJOR MEDICAL COMPLICATIONS OF PREGNANCY

A Asthma

Patrick Duff

DEFINITION

- Asthma is a chronic disorder characterized by bronchial hyperresponsiveness and airway inflammation.
- Inflammation in the airways causes recurrent episodes of wheezing, chest tightness, dyspnea, and coughing.
- These episodes are associated with widespread and variable airflow obstruction, which is reversible with treatment.

EPIDEMIOLOGY

- Asthma is usually classified on the basis of its severity (Table 7A-1).
- A variety of environmental allergens, microbes, and even medications (eg, aspirin) may trigger asthmatic episodes.
- In addition, asthma may be precipitated by stress, exercise, and exposure to cold temperatures.

CLINICAL MANIFESTATIONS

- The principal clinical manifestations of asthma are as follows:

TABLE 7A-1   Classification of Asthma

DEGREE OF SEVERITY	CLINICAL MANIFESTATIONS	OBJECTIVE MEASURES OF PULMONARY FUNCTION
Severe persistent	Continual symptoms Frequent exacerbations Frequent nighttime symptoms Physical activity limited	$FEV_1 \leq 60\%$ of predicted value Variability in PEF >30%
Moderate persistent	Daily symptoms Exacerbations >2 times/week Activity limited by exacerbations Nighttime symptoms >2 times/week	FEV_1 61–79% of predicted value Variability in PEF >30%
Mild persistent	Symptoms >2 times/week but <1 time/daily Nighttime symptoms <2 times/week Activity may be limited by exacerbations	$FEV_1 \geq 80\%$ of predicted value Variability in PEF 20–30%
Mild intermittent	Symptoms ≤2 times/week Exacerbations are brief Asymptomatic and normal level of activity between exacerbations	FEV_1 >80% of predicted value Variability in PEF <20%

Key: FEV_1=forced expiratory volume in 1 s; PEF=peak expiratory flow.
Table 7A-1 is adapted from data presented in Naureckas ET, Solway J. Mild asthma. *N Engl J Med* 2001;345:1257–1262.

- ○ Dyspnea
- ○ Chest tightness
- ○ Inspiratory and expiratory wheezing
- ○ Prolongation of the expiratory phase of respiration
- ○ Cough—particularly pronounced in the early morning and at night
- The clinical manifestations vary with the severity of the underlying disease and with the patient's ability to avoid environmental allergens and comply with medication regimens.

DIAGNOSIS

- The diagnosis of asthma is established primarily by history and physical examination.
- Pulmonary function testing is of value in classifying the severity of asthma (see Table 7A-1).

EFFECT OF ASTHMA ON PREGNANCY

- Patients with mild intermittent and mild persistent asthma usually have few maternal or fetal complications during pregnancy.
- Patients with moderate and severe asthma, particularly those who require oral steroids, are more likely to experience complications such as the following:
  - ○ Preterm delivery
  - ○ Intrauterine growth restriction
  - ○ Gestational diabetes

- Poorly controlled severe asthma, progressing to status asthmaticus, may be a life-threatening condition for both the mother and fetus.

MANAGEMENT

MILD INTERMITTENT ASTHMA

- Daily medication is not required.
- The patient should use a short-acting inhaled beta$_2$ agonist such as metaproterenol (2 to 3 puffs, up to a maximum of 12 puffs per day), as needed for symptoms.
- The beta$_2$ agonist should also be used prophylactically in anticipation of activities (eg, exercise) or exposure (eg, cold) that precipitate symptoms.

MILD PERSISTENT ASTHMA

- Daily medication is required.
- One drug of choice is an inhaled corticosteroid such as triamcinolone (100 μg per spray, 4 puffs twice daily, up to a maximum of 16 puffs per day).
- Patients should also use a short-acting inhaled beta$_2$ agonist as needed for symptoms or in anticipation of activities or exposures that precipitate symptoms.
- An alternative treatment regimen is the combination of fluticasone, an inhaled corticosteroid, plus salmeterol, a long-acting beta$_2$ agonist. This combination is marketed as the Advair Diskus®. It should be

administered as one inhalation twice daily and is of particular value in patients with prominent nocturnal symptoms. It is available in three different dosing regimens:
  ○ Fluticasone (100 µg) plus salmeterol (50 µg)
  ○ Fluticasone (250 µg) plus salmeterol (50 µg)
  ○ Fluticasone (500 µg) plus salmeterol (50 µg)
- Patients using salmeterol plus fluticasone may still need to use a short-acting inhaled beta₂ agonist as needed for symptoms.

MODERATE AND SEVERE ASTHMA

- Patients with moderate or severe asthma require daily treatment with multiple medications.
- These individuals should use an inhaled corticosteroid and regular doses of an inhaled beta₂ agonist. They also may find the combination of salmeterol and fluticasone (see above) to be of value.
- In addition, patients with moderate to severe asthma may require regularly scheduled doses of other agents, such as the following:
  ○ Oral theophylline (bronchodilator)
  ○ Oral corticosteroids (anti-inflammatory agent)
  ○ Cromolyn sodium (mast cell stabilizer)
  ○ Anticytokine medications
    ▪ Zileuton
    ▪ Montelukast
    ▪ Zafirlukast

ACUTE ASTHMATIC ATTACK

- An acute asthmatic attack is a life-threatening medical emergency that requires immediate attention in the emergency department or on an inpatient ward.
- Emergency treatment includes the following:
  ○ Monitoring of maternal oxygenation with either pulse oximetry or arterial blood gas determinations
  ○ Administration of oxygen by face mask
  ○ Rehydration with intravenous fluids
  ○ Intravenous or oral corticosteroids
  ○ Administration of a beta₂ agonist by nebulizer
  ○ Administration of a bronchodilator such as terbutaline subcutaneously
  ○ Administration of broad spectrum antibiotics to treat for possible underlying infection
  ○ Continuous fetal heart rate monitoring to assess for evidence of fetal hypoxia.
- Patients with asthma should maintain a good state of hydration.
- They should remain well rested and eat a well-balanced diet.

- They should avoid known allergens and exposures. If such encounters cannot be avoided, these patients should administer prophylactic doses of short-acting inhaled beta₂ agonists.
- Affected patients should receive the influenza vaccine annually, during the period from late October through January.
- Patients should also receive the pneumococcal vaccine.

BIBLIOGRAPHY

Busse WW, Lemanske RF. Asthma. *N Engl J Med* 2001;344:350–362.
Drazer JM, Israel E, O'Byrne PM. Treatment of asthma with drugs modifying the leukotriene pathway. *N Engl J Med* 1999;340:197–205.
Naureckas ET, Solway J. Mild asthma. *N Engl J Med* 2001;345:1257–1262.
Tan KS, Thomson NC. Asthma in pregnancy. *Am J Med* 2000;109:727–733.

B Cardiac Disease

Rodney K. Edwards

CARDIOVASCULAR CHANGES IN PREGNANCY

- Blood volume increases to 40 to 50 percent above nonpregnant levels by 32 weeks of gestation. Women with multiple gestations show even greater increases. Plasma volume expands to a greater degree than red cell volume. Table 7B-1 displays the circulatory changes during pregnancy.
- Hematocrit declines because of the proportionately greater rise in plasma volume than in red cell volume (see Table 7B-1). In the latter part of pregnancy, hematocrit values increase as erythropoiesis continues while plasma volume stabilizes.

TABLE 7B-1 Circulatory Changes during Normal Pregnancy

PARAMETER	CHANGE
Plasma volume	Starting by 6 weeks, increases an average of 50% over baseline values by 32 weeks
Red cell volume	Starting after the first trimester, increases 20% over baseline values by term
Blood volume	Starting by 6 weeks, increases an average of 40% by 32 weeks

- Cardiac output rises to 30 to 50 percent over baseline values by 20 to 24 weeks. The early increase in cardiac output is due to a larger stroke volume; stroke volume later exhibits a modest decline, as heart rate rises 10 to 20 percent later in pregnancy. During the second half of pregnancy, the supine position causes the cardiac output to be significantly decreased, owing to diminished venous return.
- Blood pressure declines in midpregnancy due to decreased total peripheral resistance and the rise in cardiac output. Women who fail to demonstrate a decline in blood pressure are more likely to develop preeclampsia.
- During labor, with each contraction, up to 500 mL of blood is "autotransfused" into the maternal circulation, resulting in increased blood pressure and cardiac output.

DIAGNOSIS OF CARDIAC DISEASE IN PREGNANCY

- Many signs and symptoms seen in normal pregnancy may be confused with those of underlying cardiac disease. Fatigue, mild dyspnea, orthopnea, peripheral edema, systolic outflow murmurs, palpitations, and cardiomegaly on chest radiography are normal in pregnancy.
- Dyspnea that limits activity, exertional angina, syncope, diastolic murmurs, and dysrhythmias do not normally occur in pregnancy and warrant further investigation.

GENERAL MANAGEMENT PRINCIPLES

- Regional anesthesia causes a fall in cardiac output and blood pressure due to vasodilation. It can be used safely in most patients with cardiac disease.
- Identification of women with significant cardiac disease prior to conception allows appropriate counseling. Some cardiac conditions are associated with a significant risk of mortality, and pregnancy may be ill advised in affected patients (Table 7B-2).
- Antibiotic prophylaxis against bacterial endocarditis should be administered to women with significant structural cardiac disease and an appropriate indication (Table 7B-3). Vaginal delivery as an indication is controversial. Manual extraction of the placenta and cesarean delivery **are** indications.
- Infants born to women with congenital cardiac defects have a 3 to 10 percent risk of having structural heart defects. Fetal echocardiography is indicated in these patients.

TABLE 7B-2 Cardiac Disease and Maternal Mortality Risk

GROUP	EXAMPLES
Low risk: <1% mortality	Atrial or ventricular septal defect
	Pulmonic or tricuspid valvular disease
	Corrected tetralogy of Fallot
	Porcine valve
	Mild mitral stenosis
	Patent ductus arteriosus
Moderate risk: 5–15% mortality	Aortic stenosis
	Coarctation of the aorta
	Moderate to severe mitral stenosis or mitral stenosis with atrial fibrillation
	Mechanical heart valve
	Uncorrected tetralogy of Fallot
	Prior myocardial infarction
High risk: 25–50% mortality	Primary pulmonary hypertension
	Eisenmenger's syndrome
	Marfan's syndrome with aortic root involvement

TABLE 7B-3 Antibiotic Prophylactic Regimens for Bacterial Endocarditis

INDICATION	REGIMEN
Labor and delivery	Ampicillin 2 g IV and gentamicin 1.5 mg/kg IV in the active phase of labor; repeat 8 h later
Patients with beta-lactam allergies	Replace ampicillin in above regimen with vancomycin 1 g IV
Alternative oral regimen for use with "low-risk" procedure or indication	Amoxicillin 3 g orally before procedure and 1.5 g 6 h later

SPECIFIC VALVULAR DISEASES

- **Mitral stenosis** is the most common form of rheumatic heart disease in pregnant women.
  - The primary symptom is easy fatigability.
  - Due to the risk of mortality with pregnancy, symptomatic patients should undergo surgical correction prior to pregnancy.
  - This condition results in fixed cardiac output, shortened diastolic filling time, and elevated left atrial and pulmonary capillary pressure.
  - Limiting activity and cautious diuresis are the mainstays of treatment. If left atrial enlargement is present or if atrial fibrillation develops, anticoagulation is indicated. Surgical treatment (valvuloplasty or valve replacement) may be necessary if medical therapy does not alleviate symptoms.
  - During labor and delivery, invasive hemodynamic monitoring may be helpful. However, it is important to remember that pulmonary capillary wedge pressure may not accurately reflect left ventricular filling pressure in these patients and should not be relied upon.

- Epidural anesthesia, avoidance of tachycardia, supplemental oxygen, semi-Fowler's positioning, avoidance of the Valsalva maneuver, and operative vaginal delivery are all advised for these patients.
- The puerperium is the most hazardous time for these women. They may need diuretics in order to prevent pulmonary edema.
- **Aortic stenosis** is uncommon during pregnancy.
  - Due to a fixed stroke volume, exertion may result in decreased oxygen delivery to the cerebral and coronary vessels. Compensatory left ventricular hypertrophy occurs and increases the oxygen requirements of the myocardium.
  - Pregnancy is contraindicated if the valve area is less than 1 cm^2. Patients with angina, dyspnea, and syncope have a 5-year mortality rate approaching 50 percent.
  - Management goals include avoiding tachycardia and maintaining filling pressures in a narrow therapeutic window, avoiding both decreased cardiac output and pulmonary edema. Regional anesthesia should be used with extreme caution.
  - Valve replacement, valvulotomy, or balloon valvuloplasty may be needed in cases refractory to medical therapy.
- **Mitral regurgitation** may be due to mitral valve prolapse, rheumatic fever, or aortic outflow obstruction.
  - Symptoms are due to reduced ventricular output and may include fatigue and dyspnea. Atrial enlargement may lead to atrial fibrillation in long-standing cases.
  - The goal of management is reduction of left ventricular afterload. Epidural analgesia is recommended.
- **Aortic regurgitation** rarely causes left ventricular failure until the fourth or fifth decades of life. Therefore failure complicates pregnancy in less than 10 percent of cases.
  - Management goals include reduction in afterload and activity restriction. If heart failure develops, digoxin and diuretics may be required.
  - Epidural anesthesia is recommended.
  - Bradycardia increases regurgitation across the valve and is poorly tolerated.

CONGENITAL LESIONS

- Small **ventricular septal defects** (VSDs) are generally well tolerated.
  - If left-to-right shunting increases to a critical level, pulmonary vascular resistance rises and reverse shunting with cyanosis may occur (see Eisenmenger's syndrome below).

- Epidural anesthesia may not be tolerated if it is associated with a significant drop in systemic pressure.
  - Cyanosis developing during labor signals right-to-left shunting and should be treated with supplemental oxygen and measures to increase vascular resistance. Invasive hemodynamic monitoring should be considered in such cases.
- **Atrial septal defects** (ASDs) are common congenital heart lesions found in adults.
  - The most common form is the ostium secundum defect.
  - It may be associated with mitral prolapse or regurgitation.
  - Right-sided failure and arrhythmias are generally not observed until the fourth or fifth decade of life.
  - This lesion is generally well tolerated, and no specific therapy is required in most gravidas.
  - Invasive monitoring is rarely needed. Epidural anesthesia is preferred, as it minimizes increases in peripheral resistance that would enhance left-to-right shunting.
- **Patent ductus arteriosus** (PDA) shunts blood from the high-pressure aorta to the lower-pressure pulmonary artery.
  - Most patients have these lesions corrected during childhood.
  - However, as with ASDs, patients with small lesions tolerate pregnancy well and have a benign course until middle age.
- **Tetraology of Fallot** is defined as the presence of right ventricular outflow obstruction, VSD, right ventricular hypertrophy, and an aorta overriding the VSD. Right-to-left shunting with cyanosis is usually present.
  - With **uncorrected** lesions, there is a reduced life expectancy and pregnancy is uncommon. If pregnancy occurs, spontaneous abortion, intrauterine growth restriction, and cardiac failure frequently occur.
  - With **corrected** lesions, pregnancy is usually well tolerated. However, there is an increased incidence of intrauterine growth restriction.
  - Management during labor and delivery should include supplemental oxygen and efforts to maintain venous return. Narcotics or pudendal block are preferred for analgesia for vaginal delivery; general anesthesia is preferred for cesarean delivery.
- Severe **coarctation of the aorta** is usually corrected during infancy.
  - This diagnosis should be suspected when there is a blood pressure gradient between the upper and lower extremities or when there is isolated hypertension in the right upper extremity.
  - As with aortic stenosis, stroke volume is relatively fixed.

○ Coexistent cerebral berry aneurysms are relatively common.

○ Patients with prior repair should be evaluated for aortic narrowing.

DEVELOPMENTAL CARDIAC LESIONS

- **Eisenmenger's syndrome** is defined as a right-to-left shunt (via ASD, VSD, or PDA) **and** elevated pulmonary vascular resistance.
  ○ Maternal and fetal mortality rates are high (12 to 70 percent and 50 percent, respectively).
  ○ Cyanosis, chest pain, syncope, and hemoptysis are poor prognostic signs.
  ○ Termination of pregnancy should be discussed.
  ○ For those women who continue pregnancy, management includes limitation of activity, consideration of anticoagulation, maintenance of preload, supplemental oxygen, and avoidance of hypovolemia.
- **Marfan's syndrome** is an autosomal dominant genetic disorder that results in weakened connective tissue.
  ○ Cardiac manifestations include weakness of the aortic root and mitral valve prolapse.
  ○ The maternal mortality rate in pregnancy is as high as 50 percent in those women with a dilated aortic root prior to pregnancy.
  ○ An aortic root diameter >40 mm is a threshold above which there is a significant risk of aortic dissection. However, this threshold may fail to predict dissection.
  ○ Management centers on avoiding hypertension and the force of ventricular systole transmitted to the aortic wall via use of beta blockade. Regional anesthesia is generally well tolerated.
  ○ Signs and symptoms of aortic dissection include chest pain, hypertension (or hypotension if the dissection is large or ruptures), tachycardia, and a loud murmur of aortic insufficiency.
- **Mitral valve prolapse** is the most common heart lesion found in women of childbearing age. The incidence is approximately 12 percent.
  ○ Most patients are asymptomatic and have uneventful pregnancies.
  ○ Endocarditis prophylaxis is not indicated unless there is coexistent mitral insufficiency.
- **Idiopathic hypertrophic subaortic stenosis** causes obstruction to left ventricular outflow due to a hypertrophied interventricular septum.
  ○ Ventricular systole narrows the outflow tract. This narrowing is improved with increased left ventricular end-diastolic volume.

○ Symptoms are similar to those of aortic stenosis.

○ This genetic condition is autosomal dominant with variable penetrance.

○ The increased blood volume associated with pregnancy may actually improve outflow obstruction. However, ventricular failure and supraventricular tachyarrhythmias may develop.

○ Management should include beta blockade, avoidance of hypovolemia, and minimization of expulsive efforts in the second stage of labor with operative vaginal delivery.

OTHER CARDIAC DISEASES

- **Peripartum cardiomyopathy** is an idiopathic condition that results in congestive heart failure and a dilated cardiomyopathy.
  ○ It occurs in the last month of pregnancy or first 5 months postpartum.
  ○ Treatment includes bed rest, sodium restriction, digoxin, and diuretics.
  ○ Half of these women have persistent cardiomegaly and symptoms for more than 6 months.
  ○ This condition frequently recurs and future pregnancies are contraindicated.
- **Ischemic cardiac disease** is uncommon in women of childbearing age.
  ○ It may be seen in pregnant women of increased maternal age, those who smoke, and those who have diabetes.
  ○ Treatment during gestation includes decreased activity, nitrates, and beta blockade.
  ○ The mortality rate with myocardial infarction is highest if it occurs during the third trimester and/or if delivery occurs within 2 weeks.
  ○ During labor and delivery, supplemental oxygen and regional anesthesia should be used. Cesarean delivery should be performed for obstetric indications.

BIBLIOGRAPHY

Clark SL. Structural cardiac disease in pregnancy. In: Clark SL, Phelan JP, Cotton DB, eds. *Critical Care Obstetrics,* 2nd ed. Boston: Blackwell Scientific Publications, 1991.

Landon M. Medical complications of pregnancy: cardiac disease. In: Ling FW, Duff P, eds. *Obstetrics & Gynecology: Principles for Practice.* New York: McGraw-Hill, 2001.

Shulman ST, Amren DP, Bisno AL, et al. Prevention of bacterial endocarditis. *Circulation* 1984;70:1125A.

C   Diabetes

Patrick Duff

CLASSIFICATION

- In nonpregnant patients, diabetes usually is classified as **juvenile-onset (type I)** vs. **adult-onset (type II) diabetes.**
- In pregnant patients, diabetes is classified as **pregestational** vs. **gestational.**
  - Patients with pregestational diabetes essentially always require insulin.
  - Some patients with gestational diabetes may be treated with diet alone. Others require oral hypoglycemic agents or insulin.

GESTATIONAL DIABETES

EPIDEMIOLOGY

- Gestational diabetes occurs in 1 to 4 percent of pregnancies.
- Recognized risk factors include the following:
  - Age >25 years
  - Family history of diabetes
  - African-American race
  - Hispanic race
  - Prior history of a macrosomic infant
  - Prior history of an unexplained stillbirth
  - History of an infant with multiple congenital anomalies
  - Prior or present history of polyhydramnios
- The principal diabetogenic hormone of pregnancy is human placental lactogen (HPL), which is produced by the synctiotrophoblast of the placenta. Serum concentrations of HPL reach their zenith in the third trimester. Hence patients are at greatest risk for gestational diabetes in the last trimester of pregnancy.
- Patients should be divided into three risk categories for purposes of screening.
  - Patients at *low risk* (ie, Caucasian women of ideal body weight who are under 25 years of age) do not require screening.
  - Patients at *intermediate risk* (ie, one relatively minor risk factor) should be screened at 24 to 28 weeks.
  - Patients at *high risk* (one or more major risk factors) should be screened on the initial prenatal visit and, if negative, again at 28 to 32 weeks.
- The best-validated screening test is the 1-h glucose challenge test.
  - The glucose load is 50 g of glucola (200 calories).

- The test may be performed in the fasting or non-fasting state.
- The cutoff for the 1-h glucose determination is 135 mg%.
- If the 1-h glucose challenge test is abnormal, the patient should have a 3-h glucose tolerance test after a 100-g glucose meal (400 calories).
  - The 3-h test should be administered in the fasting state.
  - The cutoff values for the test are as follows:
    - Fasting blood sugar—95 mg%
    - 1-h postprandial—180 mg%
    - 2-h postprandial—155 mg%
    - 3-h postprandial—140 mg%
  - The diagnosis of gestational diabetes is confirmed if the fasting blood sugar is abnormal or if two of the other three values are elevated.

COMPLICATIONS

- The principal maternal complications include the following:
  - Increased risk of UTI
  - Increased risk of preeclampsia
  - Poor glycemic control
- The principal fetal/neonatal complications are as follows:
  - Macrosomia—which, in turn, is associated with a higher risk of cesarean delivery and shoulder dystocia.
  - Neonatal hypoglycemia

MANAGEMENT

- The mainstay of management is a diabetic diet.
  - The diet initially should consist of 30 calories per kilogram of ideal body weight.
  - The calories should be distributed as approximately 50 percent carbohydrate, 30 to 35 percent fat, and 15 to 20 percent protein.
  - The goal of glycemic control is to maintain the fasting blood sugar ≤90 mg% and the 1-h postprandial glucose ≤135 mg% without causing overt symptoms of hypoglycemia.
- If diet therapy fails to achieve glycemic control, the patient should be treated with glyburide.
  - Glyburide is a newer sulfonylurea that does not cross the placenta.
  - The starting dose is 2.5 mg orally in the morning.
  - The dose may be increased in stepwise fashion to a maximum of 20 mg/day.
  - Although the drug is usually administered as a single dose in the morning, some patients may benefit from divided doses in the morning and evening.

- If diet and glyburide do not achieve appropriate glycemic control, insulin is indicated (see below).
- Patients with gestational diabetes should have serum amalyte screening at approximately 15 to 16 weeks of gestation to test for trisomy 18, trisomy 21, and neural tube defects.
- They should also have at least one ultrasound examination at 18 to 20 weeks to confirm gestational age, assess amniotic fluid volume, and evaluate for anomalies. A second ultrasound examination should be performed near term if macrosomia is suspected.
- Antepartum fetal heart rate testing is not routinely indicated. However, patients who have a hypertensive disorder, who have a history of a poor obstetric outcome, or who reach 40 weeks of gestation should have testing.
- As a matter of routine, delivery should take place at approximately 38 to 39 weeks of gestation when the cervix becomes favorable for induction of labor.
- Primary cesarean delivery should be considered if the estimated fetal weight exceeds 4250 to 4500 g or if there is a prior history of a traumatic vaginal delivery.

PREGESTATIONAL DIABETES

EPIDEMIOLOGY

- Less than 1 percent of pregnant women have pregestational diabetes.
- Essentially, all patients with pregestational diabetes require insulin to maintain euglycemia.
- The longer the duration of diabetes and the more brittle the glucose control, the higher the rate of maternal and fetal complications in pregnancy.

COMPLICATIONS OF PREGESTATIONAL DIABETES

- The principal maternal complications of pregestational diabetes are as follows:
  - Increased risk of diabetic ketoacidosis
  - Increased risk of preeclampsia
  - Increased risk of urinary tract infection, respiratory tract infection, and skin infection
  - Increased risk of spontaneous abortion
- The major fetal and neonatal complications associated with pregestational diabetes include
  - Increased risk of congenital anomalies
    - The overall frequency of major anomalies is 3 to 5 percent.
    - Cardiac and neural tube defects are the most common anomalies.

- The pathognomonic anomaly is sacral agenesis (caudal regression syndrome or sirenomelia).
  - Fetal growth disorders
    - Long-standing insulin dependency is typically associated with fetal intrauterine **growth restriction** (IUGR).
    - Insulin dependency of shorter duration is more likely to be associated with fetal macrosomia.
  - Neonatal metabolic derangements
    - Hypoglycemia
    - Hypocalcemia
    - Hypokalemia
    - Hyperbilirubinemia
  - Neonatal cardiomyopathy
  - Increased risk of respiratory distress syndrome

MANAGEMENT

INSULIN THERAPY
- Patients with pregestational diabetes should receive the same diet outlined previously for patients with gestational diabetes. Typically, the calories are distributed as follows:
  - Breakfast—2/7
  - Lunch—2/7
  - Dinner—2/7
  - Bedtime snack—1/7
- Patients should maintain a relatively precise schedule for meals and administration of insulin.
- Most patients can maintain acceptable glucose control by administering a combination of an insulin with an intermediate duration of action (NPH) and another with a short duration of action (regular).
  - A reasonable estimate for determining a patient's total insulin requirement is 0.6 to 1.0 U/kg of ideal body weight per day. The lower dosing range is for patients in the first two trimesters of pregnancy. The higher dosing range is more appropriate in the final trimester.
  - Two-thirds of the daily dose should be NPH. Two-thirds of this dose should be administered before breakfast and one-third before dinner.
  - One-third of the total daily insulin dose should be regular insulin. One-half to two-thirds of this dose should be administered with the morning NPH and one-third to one-half with the evening NPH.
  - For patients who have nocturnal hypoglycemia or who have a persistently elevated fasting blood sugar, the evening dose of NPH may be moved to bedtime. The dose of regular insulin should still be given prior to dinner.
  - Some patients may benefit from the use of use of very short acting insulin (lispro insulin) to correct wide fluctuations in postprandial glucose concentrations.

○ Other patients may be so brittle that they require an insulin pump to maintain acceptable glycemic control. The pump provides a basal infusion of longer-acting insulin and permits the programming of infusions of very short acting insulin coincident with meals.

○ The goals of glucose control are the same as those outlined previously.

ANTEPARTUM SURVEILLANCE

• An endovaginal ultrasound examination should be performed at approximately 6 weeks of gestation to confirm fetal viability.

• Serum analyte screening should be performed at 15 to 16 weeks of gestation to test for an open neural tube defect, trisomy 18, and trisomy 21.

• A targeted ultrasound and fetal echocardiogram should be performed at approximately 20 weeks to assess for anatomic malformations.

• Additional ultrasound examinations should be performed as indicated if fetal growth restriction or macrosomia is suspected.

• Weekly antepartum testing of the fetal heart rate or biophysical profile testing is indicated beginning at about 32 weeks of gestation.

• On a routine basis, delivery should be performed at 37 to 39 weeks, depending on the results of fetal testing and the precision of maternal glucose control.

• When delivery is planned before 38 weeks, studies of the maturity of the fetal lung should be performed.

• Mode of delivery should be based upon the following considerations:
  ○ History of prior deliveries
  ○ Estimated size of the fetus
  ○ Cervical examination
  ○ Assessment of ability of the fetus to tolerate labor

• A pediatrician should attend the delivery because of the increased risk of neonatal hypoglycemia.

BIBLIOGRAPHY

Freinkel N, Dooley SL, Metzger BE. Care of the pregnant woman with insulin-dependent diabetes mellitus. *N Engl J Med* 1985;313:96–101.

Kjos SL, Buchanan TA. Gestational diabetes mellitus. *N Engl J Med* 1999;341:1749–1756.

Langer O, Conway DL, Berkus MD, et al. A comparison of glyburide and insulin in women with gestational diabetes. *N Engl J Med* 2000;343:1134–1138.

D Gastrointestinal Disease

Rodney K. Edwards

GASTROINTESTINAL MOTILITY DISORDERS

• Mild to moderate **nausea and vomiting** are the most frequent complaints in the first half of pregnancy.
  ○ 70 to 90 percent of women are affected.
  ○ Symptoms usually begin by 4 to 6 weeks of gestation, peak at 10 to 12 weeks, and resolve by 14 to 16 weeks.
  ○ The term morning sickness is used colloquially, since symptoms typically are worse early in the day. However, symptoms can occur at any time of the day.
  ○ Mild to moderate nausea and vomiting cause no increase in pregnancy complications.
  ○ Treatment consists of ingesting small, frequent meals rich in carbohydrates. If pharmacologic therapy is needed, pyridoxine (vitamin B_6) 50 mg once or twice daily should be first-line therapy. The combination of pyridoxine and doxylamine was previously marketed in the United States for treating pregnancy-related nausea. Despite convincing evidence that the drug Bendectin did not cause birth defects, it was removed from the market in the 1980s due to the cost to the company of defending lawsuits claiming birth defects. Doxylamine is still available over the counter as Unisom Sleep Tabs. One-half to one tablet can be taken once or twice daily. In refractory cases, metoclopramide (5 to 10 mg orally every 6 to 8 h) and/or phenothiazines (eg, prochlorperazine 5 to 10 mg orally or rectally every 6 to 8 h) may be used.

• **Hyperemesis gravidarum** is characterized by vomiting that is severe enough to result in dehydration, hypokalemia, acidosis, and significant weight loss.
  ○ This condition affects 1 to 2 percent of pregnant women and has a peak incidence in the late first trimester.
  ○ It is a diagnosis of exclusion; other causes of vomiting should be ruled out.
  ○ Hospitalization, intravenous hydration, and parenteral antiemetic medications are needed. In refractory cases, oral intake may not be possible for a prolonged period of time, making total parenteral nutrition necessary.

• **Gastroesophageal reflux disease** (GERD) is common during pregnancy, affecting over half of gravid women.
  ○ It is most common during the third trimester.

○ Symptoms are exacerbated by the recumbent position, ingestion of acidic foods, caffeine, and large or late-night meals.
○ Treatment initially should involve avoiding exacerbating factors, elevation of the head of the bed, and antacids. If these measures are insufficient, treatment with an H_2-receptor antagonist or proton pump inhibitor is indicated.
• **Constipation** is a complaint of up to one-third of pregnant women.
○ Symptoms tend to be worse in the first and third trimesters.
○ The treatments of choice are increased fluid intake, increased dietary fiber, bulk-forming fiber preparations, and stool softeners such as docusate.

PEPTIC ULCER DISEASE

• Women with this condition usually improve during pregnancy. Only about 1 in 8 women with preexisting peptic ulcer disease will report either the same or worsening symptoms during pregnancy.
• Symptoms are often similar to those of GERD; antacids and elevation of the head of the bed may improve symptoms caused by peptic ulcer disease. Women who do not improve should be referred to a gastroenterologist for endoscopy.
• In cases refractory to dietary modification, antacids, and H_2 antagonists, proton pump inhibitors and antibiotic therapy against *Helicobacter pylori* may be considered.

INFLAMMATORY BOWEL DISEASE

• The etiology of both Crohn's disease and ulcerative colitis is unknown. The peak incidence for both of these conditions is during the third and fourth decade. Both conditions are associated with intestinal inflammation of a nonspecific, chronic, relapsing nature.
• **Crohn's disease** can affect any part of the gastrointestinal tract, with the small bowel and colon most often involved.
○ It has an incidence of 1 in 20,000 to 1 in 50,000.
○ Epidemiologic studies suggest that women with Crohn's disease are less likely to conceive.
○ When conception does occur, women with active disease or first presentation during pregnancy have an increased risk of spontaneous abortion.
○ Most patients have no change in disease activity during pregnancy.
• **Ulcerative colitis** affects only the colon and rectum.

○ This condition is much more common than Crohn's disease, affecting 1 in 1000 to 1 in 2500 women in the reproductive years.
○ Compared with Crohn's disease, ulcerative colitis is associated with more acute symptoms, including cramping, bloody stools, diarrhea, and weight loss.
○ This condition does not seem to affect fertility or pregnancy outcome, particularly if it is quiescent at the time of conception.
• Aspirin derivatives, such as sulfasalazine, are the mainstay of pharmacologic treatment for the inflammatory bowel diseases.
○ When needed, courses of systemic corticosteroids also can be given safely during pregnancy.
○ Newer medications, aimed at specific proinflammatory substances, are now available. However, there is little information regarding the safety of these drugs during pregnancy.

APPENDICITIS

• Appendicitis is the most common surgical emergency during pregnancy that does not involve the uterus. Its incidence is approximately 1 per 1500 deliveries.
• The diagnosis of appendicitis during pregnancy is challenging. Because the enlarging uterus displaces the appendix from its usual location at McBurney's point, the classic presentation may not occur (Fig. 7D-1). In addition, anorexia and a mild leukocytosis are common in pregnancy.
• Most large series report a rate of false-positive clinical diagnosis of at least 20 percent. This high rate is acceptable in pregnancy because the fetal loss rate approaches 50 percent if perforation occurs, compared to less than 2 percent in the absence of perforation. Furthermore, maternal mortality is increased when the diagnosis is delayed.

HEPATITIS

• Hepatitis is one of the most common and contagious viral infections. There are six known, distinct types of hepatitis virus: A, B, C, D, E, and G. Key features of these viruses are summarized in Table 7D-1.
• Hepatitis A and E are transmitted by the fecal-oral route.
○ Both of these viruses are RNA viruses.
○ Neither is associated with a chronic carrier state.
○ Hepatitis A occurs in epidemics in the United States. Hepatitis E is rare in this country but is endemic in developing countries.

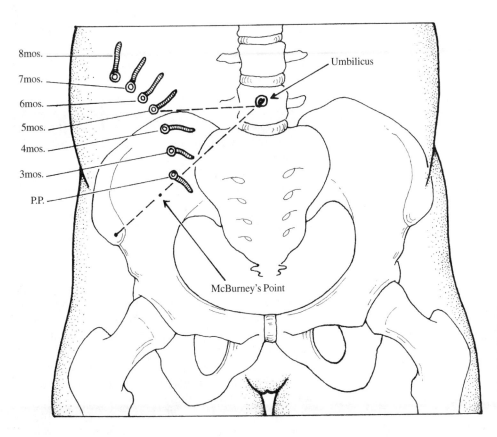

8mos.

7mos.

6mos.

5mos.

4mos.

3mos.

P.P.

Umbilicus

McBurney's Point

FIG. 7D-1 Change in the position of the appendix during pregnancy. (Modified from Baer JL, Reis RA, Arens RA. Appendicitis in pregnancy with changes in position and axis of the normal appendix in pregnancy. *JAMA* 1932;98:1359.)

TABLE 7D-1   Summary of Key Facts Relating to Hepatitis in Pregnancy

HEPATITIS	VIRAL TYPE	TRANSMISSION	DIAGNOSTIC TEST	CHRONIC CARRIER STATE	VACCINE	VERTICAL TRANSMISSION
A	RNA	Fecal-oral	Virus-specific IgM	No	Yes; inactivated	Very rare
B	DNA	Parenteral, sexual, or perinatal	Surface antigen	Yes; 10–15%	Yes; passive and active recombinant	Common, but most cases prevented by immunoprophylaxis
C	RNA	Parenteral, sexual, or perinatal	Hepatitis C antibody	Yes; common	No	More likely if hepatitis C RNA-positive
D	RNA	Parenteral, sexual, or perinatal	Antigen and IgM antibody	Possible if coinfected with hepatitis B	No	Uncommon
E	RNA	Fecal-oral	Antibody	No	No	Very rare

Key: RNA = ribonucleic acid; DNA = deoxyribonucleic acid; IgM = immunoglobulin M.

- ○ A vaccine against hepatitis A is available. The vaccine is formalin-inactivated and is safe for use in pregnancy.
- Hepatitis B is transmitted parenterally, by sexual contact, or perinatally.
  - ○ It is a DNA virus that is the most common cause of viral hepatitis in the United States.
  - ○ Ten to 15 percent of infected patients become chronically infected. A minority of these chronically infected patients eventually develop chronic active hepatitis, cirrhosis, or hepatocellular carcinoma.
  - ○ In the absence of immunoprophylaxis, vertical transmission to the neonate occurs in 10 to 20 percent of women who are positive for surface antigen and approximately 90 percent who are positive for both surface antigen and e antigen.
  - ○ Infants born to women who are positive for hepatitis B surface antigen should receive a combination of passive immunization with hepatitis B immune globulin and the recombinant hepatitis B vaccine. This combination prevents approximately 90 percent of neonatal hepatitis B infections.
  - ○ The hepatitis B vaccine is safe for use during pregnancy.
- Hepatitis C is transmitted parenterally, by sexual contact, or perinatally.

○ It is due to an RNA virus that is the most common cause of posttransfusion hepatitis or hepatitis in intravenous drug abusers.

○ Most patients infected with this virus are asymptomatic.

○ Chronic infection is more common with hepatitis C than with any other hepatitis virus.

○ No vaccine is available.

○ The vertical transmission rate depends on whether or not the pregnant woman has demonstrable serum levels of hepatitis C RNA. In women who have low or undetectable levels of RNA, the transmission rate is less than 10 percent. However, if the RNA level is high, the vertical transmission rate may be as high as 40 percent. Cesarean delivery prior to labor may offer some protection against vertical transmission in high-risk cases.

• Hepatitis D is due to an RNA virus that is dependent on coinfection with hepatitis B. Therefore the epidemiology of this virus is similar to that of the virus causing hepatitis B.

• Hepatitis G is due to a recently described RNA virus; although similar to hepatitis C, it is a much milder disease.

ACUTE FATTY LIVER

• This rare idiopathic condition usually presents with nausea and vomiting, followed by abdominal pain and headache. As the disease progresses, jaundice, mental status changes, coagulopathy, oliguria, and metabolic acidosis develop. The most common proximate causes of death are hemorrhage, renal failure, and hypoglycemia.

• The differential diagnosis includes hepatitis and severe preeclampsia with associated HELLP syndrome (hemolysis, elevated liver enzymes, low platelets).

• If the diagnosis of acute fatty liver is made, delivery and supportive care are indicated.

INTRAHEPATIC CHOLESTASIS OF PREGNANCY

• Intrahepatic cholestasis usually presents in the third trimester of pregnancy with intense pruritus and possibly mild jaundice.

• This condition is uncommon in the United States but complicates up to 10 percent of pregnancies in Chile. It is also somewhat common in Sweden. The condition tends to recur in subsequent pregnancies and when patients receive oral contraceptives.

• The diagnosis is made by demonstration of increased levels of serum bile acids, at least three times the upper limit of normal. Deposition of these bile acids in the skin may be the cause of pruritus.

• Although controversial, the rates of preterm birth and fetal death appear to be higher in pregnant women with cholestasis. It is prudent to do antenatal testing and deliver such patients at or near term, after documentation of fetal pulmonary maturity.

• Diphenhydramine or hydroxizine may offer some relief from the pruritus. Cholestyramine reduces the resorption of bile acids and can improve symptoms. Symptoms regress within days after delivery.

LIVER TRANSPLANTATION

• Pregnancy in women who have undergone liver transplantation is rare but is becoming more common. Immunosuppressive medications should be continued throughout pregnancy.

• As with renal transplant patients, rates of pregnancy-related hypertensive disorders and preterm delivery are high in women with liver transplants.

• Pregnancy should be undertaken in the liver transplant recipient only when there are no signs of rejection for a prolonged period of time. A prudent recommendation would be that women should be stable for at least 2 years after transplant.

CHOLECYSTITIS

• Pregnancy increases the likelihood of gallstone formation but not the occurrence of acute cholecystitis.

• Treatment of acute cholecystitis in pregnancy should include bowel rest, intravenous hydration, and parenteral analgesia.

• If possible, cholecystectomy should be postponed until after delivery. However, surgery during pregnancy should be undertaken in cases complicated by ascending cholangitis, common bile duct obstruction, or pancreatitis.

PANCREATITIS

• Acute pancreatitis occurs in 1 in 1000 to 1 in 4000 pregnancies. The most common causes are gallstones and hyperlipidemia. Medications, alcohol abuse, and trauma are other possible causes.

• Pregnancy predisposes to gallstone formation. Furthermore, serum lipids are increased during pregnancy. Therefore, pregnancy indirectly predisposes women to pancreatitis due to the two most common causes.

- In a patient with epigastric pain, elevated serum levels of amylase and lipase support the diagnosis. However, the severity of illness does not correlate with the degree of elevation of these enzymes.
- If acute pancreatitis occurs in the third trimester, more than half of such cases will be complicated by preterm labor.
- Treatment is primarily supportive, with bowel rest, intravenous hydration, and parenteral analgesia. If gallstones are the cause, surgery or ERCP can be performed.

BIBLIOGRAPHY

Duff P. Maternal and perinatal infection. In: Gabbe SG, Niebyl Jr, Simpson JL, eds. Obstetrics: *Normal and Problem Pregnancies,* 4th ed. New York: Churchill Livingstone, 2002.

Samuels P. Noninfectious hepatobiliary diseases. In: Ling FW, Duff P, eds. *Obstetrics & Gynecology: Principles for Practice.* New York: McGraw-Hill, 2001.

Steinlauf AF, Traube M. Gastrointestinal complications. In: Burrow GN, Duffy TP, eds. *Medical Complications during Pregnancy,* 5th ed. Philadelphia: Saunders, 1999.

E   Hematologic Disease

Rodney K. Edwards

ANEMIA

- During pregnancy, plasma volume expands 50 percent and the red blood cell (RBC) mass expands 30 percent. This hemodilution results in the **physiologic anemia** of pregnancy.
  - The hematocrit decreases from an average of 42 percent to 30 to 35 percent.
  - However, a hemoglobin concentration below 10.5 g/dL or a hematocrit below 30 percent should prompt a laboratory evaluation to assess the cause of the anemia.
  - The fetus usually does not become anemic from maternal nutritional deficiencies, since nutrients such as iron and folate are efficiently transferred to the fetus even against a concentration gradient.
- The initial laboratory evaluation of the anemic pregnant patient should include an assessment of the mean corpuscular volume (MCV). The MCV accompanies the hemoglobin and hematocrit values in an automated complete blood count (CBC). In addition, a reticulocyte count may be helpful in narrowing the possible causes of anemia.
  - A normal MCV is 80 to 95 fl. Until proven otherwise, a low MCV should be considered consistent with iron deficiency, and an elevated MCV should be considered consistent with folate deficiency.
  - A reticulocyte count that is elevated above the normal range of 1 to 2.5 percent indicates that RBC survival is shorter than the normal 100 to 120 days (eg, as a result of bleeding or hemolysis). A low or normal reticulocyte count in the setting of anemia indicates a relative deficiency of erythropoietin (eg, renal failure) or marrow dysfunction (eg, iron or folate deficiency).
- Second only to the physiologic anemia of pregnancy, **iron deficiency** is the most common cause of anemia in pregnancy.
  - Florid iron deficiency is characterized by a hypochromic (low mean corpuscular hemoglobin concentration) and microcytic (low MCV) anemia (Fig. 7E-1). However, in earlier stages of iron deficiency, the anemia may be normochromic and/or normocytic.
  - Demonstration of low levels of serum iron and ferritin confirm the diagnosis.
  - Pica, the craving for nonnutritional substances, sometimes occurs in patients with iron-deficiency anemia during pregnancy. This craving may lead to the consumption of such substances as ice, starch, or clay. In addition to substituting for iron-containing foods in the diet, these substances reduce iron intake by complexing with iron in the gut and

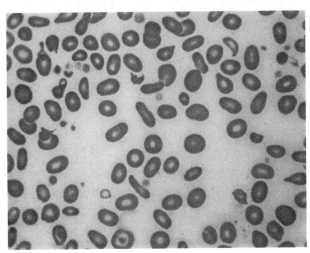

FIG. 7E-1 A peripheral blood smear from a patient with iron-deficiency anemia. Note the pale, hypochromic red blood cells. (Courtesy of Neil Harris, MD.; Department of Pathology; University of Florida; Gainesville.)

antagonizing absorption. Correction of the iron deficiency decreases the cravings.

○ The treatment of choice for iron-deficiency anemia or for iron supplementation is ferrous sulfate, 325 mg orally one to three times daily. Other iron preparations are less well absorbed. Constipation is a common side effect of this medication; it can be treated or prevented by taking docusate, 100 mg orally one to three times daily.

○ Although the contribution of anemia in general to pregnancy complications is controversial, there is a definite association between iron-deficiency anemia and preterm delivery and low birth weight.

• Table 7E-1 lists some of the other causes of anemia during pregnancy.

THROMBOEMBOLISM

• Pregnant women are five times more likely than nonpregnant women to experience venous thromboembolism (VTE). The absolute risk is 0.5 to 3 per 1000.

• Multiple changes in the coagulation system that increase the likelihood of thrombosis occur during pregnancy. These changes include increased concentrations of clotting factors, decreased concentration of protein S, decreased fibrinolytic activity, increased venous stasis, vascular injury associated with delivery, and increased activation of platelets.

• Risk factors for VTE in pregnancy include genetic thrombophilias (eg, factor V Leiden mutation, prothrombin gene mutation, hyperhomocystinemia, antithrombin-III deficiency, and protein C or S deficiency), antiphospholipid syndrome, prior history of VTE, trauma, prolonged immobilization, major surgery, atrial fibrillation, and mechanical heart valves.

• The treatment of choice for VTE in pregnancy is heparin. Neither unfractionated heparin nor low-molecular-weight heparins (LMWHs) cross the placenta.

○ The principal side effects of heparin include bleeding, osteoporosis, and heparin-induced thrombocytopenia. If laboratory monitoring is required, the activated partial thromboplastin time (aPTT) should be used. Depending on the indication, heparin may be given in prophylactic doses where the aPTT is *not* prolonged or in therapeutic doses where the aPTT is prolonged to 1.5 to 2 times baseline 8 h after a dose.

○ LMWHs have the same side effects as unfractionated heparin. However, data from nonpregnant individuals suggest that these side effects occur less commonly with LMWHs. In nonpregnant patients, these medications offer a dosing advantage over unfractionated heparin. However, during pregnancy, twice-daily dosing often is needed, and LMWHs are approximately 10 times as expensive as unfractionated heparin. If laboratory monitoring is required, the anti–factor Xa level should be used. The decision between prophylactic and therapeutic dosing, as with unfractionated heparin, depends on the indication. What constitutes a therapeutic anti–factor Xa level is controversial. However, levels of 0.3 to 0.6 are generally considered therapeutic.

○ Warfarin derivatives cross the placenta and have been associated with teratogenic effects (see Chap. 1). Their use in pregnancy is primarily in pregnant women with artificial heart valves. These women

TABLE 7E-1   Other Causes of Anemia during Pregnancy

CAUSE	CBC FINDINGS	RISK FACTORS	DIAGNOSTIC TEST(S)	TREATMENT
Folate deficiency	High MCV; hypersegmented neutrophils; pancytopenia	Multiple gestation; hemoglobinopathy; antifolate medications; alcohol abuse	Low RBC (not serum) folate level	Oral supplementation (1 mg is included in most prenatal vitamins)
B_{12} deficiency	High MCV; hypersegmented neutrophils	Inflammatory bowel disease; gastrectomy or gastric bypass; tropical sprue	Serum B_{12}	Intramuscular vitamin B_{12}
Sickle cell disease and variants	Low MCV; sickle forms	African descent	Hemoglobin electrophoresis	Folate supplements (2-5 mg/day); recognize and treat pain crisis; may need transfusion or exchange transfusion
Thalassemias	Low MCV; low MCHC; target cells	β: Mediterranean or African descent; α: Asian descent	Hemoglobin electrophoresis	Folate supplements (1-2 mg/day); avoid iron supplementation

CBC=complete blood count; MCV=mean corpuscular volume; MCHC=mean corpuscular hemoglobin concentration.

have unacceptably high rates of thrombosis on heparin or LMWH.
- The test of choice for diagnosis of pulmonary embolism in pregnant patients is either spiral computed tomography (CT) or a ventilation/perfusion scan. Both of these tests expose the mother and fetus to ionizing radiation. However, the dose to the fetus is small, and consideration of the diagnosis of pulmonary embolism outweighs the risk to the fetus. Doppler ultrasonography is the test of choice for diagnosis of deep venous thrombosis in the lower extremities.
- The use of regional anesthesia, either epidural or spinal, is controversial in patients receiving anticoagulation. Epidural and spinal anesthesia are generally considered safe in women on unfractionated heparin who have a normal aPTT and platelet count. However, patients receiving LMWH should not receive regional anesthesia until 24 h after the last dose.

THROMBOCYTOPENIA

- Since a CBC, rather than a hematocrit, is now obtained during routine prenatal screening, thrombocytopenia is diagnosed more commonly in pregnant women.
- In nonpregnant individuals, the normal platelet count is 150,000 to 400,000/μL. The lower limit of normal is arbitrary, and clinically significant bleeding rarely occurs unless the platelet count is less than 10,000/μL or less than 50,000/μL in association with trauma or surgery. The mean platelet count in pregnant women is lower than the mean value for nonpregnant individuals.
- **Gestational thrombocytopenia** accounts for about two-thirds of cases of thrombocytopenia during pregnancy. Approximately 6 to 8 percent of pregnant women are diagnosed with this condition.
  - The cause of gestational thrombocytopenia is unknown, and there are no diagnostic tests that definitively differentiate it from mild immune thrombocytopenic purpura (ITP).
  - Platelet counts almost always remain above 70,000/μL.
  - As there are no symptoms of bleeding, the thrombocytopenia is detected as part of routine screening.
  - These women have no history of thrombocytopenia outside of pregnancy.
  - Pregnant women with gestational thrombocytopenia and their fetuses/neonates are not at risk for bleeding complications.
  - Because the distinction between gestational thrombocytopenia and ITP cannot be made with certainty, the platelet count should be repeated every 1 to 2 months.

- **Alloimmune thrombocytopenia** is discussed in Chap. 15.
- **Immune thrombocytopenic purpura** (ITP) affects between 1 in 1000 and 1 in 10,000 pregnant women.
  - Autoantibodies of the IgG class cause increased platelet destruction in the reticuloendothelial system.
  - The diagnosis is one of exclusion. There are no pathognomonic symptoms, signs, or tests for ITP.
  - Thrombocytopenia can be severe and cause maternal hemorrhage, particularly in the peripartum period.
  - The treatment of choice is prednisone, usually started at a dose of 40 to 100 mg/day. Once a response is noted, the dose can be tapered. Refractory cases can be treated with intravenous immune globulin or splenectomy. Patients who relapse after splenectomy generally are considered incurable but may derive some benefit from certain chemotherapeutic agents, such as cyclophosphamide.
  - Since the antibodies involved in ITP are of the IgG class, they can cross the placenta and potentially can result in neonatal thrombocytopenia. Twelve to 15 percent of neonates born to women with ITP will have platelet counts below 50,000/μL. Fortunately, the risk of intracranial hemorrhage is much less than that reported for alloimmune thrombocytopenia.
  - The mode of delivery should be determined by traditional obstetric indications. Prophylactic cesarean delivery does not appear to reduce the risk of fetal or neonatal hemorrhage. In addition, most specialists in maternal-fetal medicine do not think that assessment of the fetal platelet count with percutaneous umbilical blood sampling is indicated for this condition.
- Preeclampsia is a common cause of thrombocytopenia in pregnant women. This condition is discussed in Chap. 11.
- Epidural anesthesia appears to be safe in women with platelet counts of at least 100,000/μL.

BIBLIOGRAPHY

American College of Obstetricians and Gynecologists. Thrombocytopenia in pregnancy. *ACOG Pract Bull* No. 6, September 1999.

American College of Obstetricians and Gynecologists. Thromboembolism in pregnancy. *ACOG Pract Bull* No. 19, August 2000.

Duffy TP. Hematologic Aspects of Pregnancy. In: Burrow GN, Duffy TP, eds. *Medical Complications During Pregnancy*, 5th ed. Philadelphia: Saunders, 1999.

F Neurologic Disease

Rodney K. Edwards

BACKACHE

- Postural backache is a complaint of almost every pregnant woman. The problem is caused by exaggeration of the lumbar lordosis that occurs in response to the expanding uterus.
- Pain is usually localized to the lumbar and sacroiliac areas but may also extend into the legs. The problem is exacerbated by anything that increases the lumbar lordosis (eg, high-heeled shoes).
- Oral acetaminophen, taken in four divided doses not to exceed 4 g per day, and warm compresses offer some relief. Swimming is an ideal exercise to strengthen the back, particularly prior to pregnancy in women with preexisting back pain or severe backache in a prior pregnancy.

LEG CRAMPS

- More than one-fourth of women experience leg cramps during the latter part of pregnancy. These cramps usually occur at night or immediately upon initiation of movement after awakening.
- The gastrocnemius is the muscle most often affected. However, the quadriceps, hamstrings, and gluteal muscles also can be involved.
- Evidence for an effective treatment for these leg cramps is lacking.

HEADACHE

- **Tension headaches** are the most common type of headaches experienced by pregnant women.
  - ○ Symptoms usually are worse late in the day and typically are maximal at the vertex or occiput.
  - ○ These headaches may be treated effectively with a combination of neck massage, acetaminophen, and heat or ice packs applied to the neck.
- Approximately 15 to 20 percent of women of childbearing age have **migraine headaches**.
  - ○ Classic migraine headaches are preceded by an *aura* that usually includes scintillations or scotomata. More than 80 percent of these women improve during pregnancy. Those patients most likely to improve are women who have catamenial (ie, menstrually associated) migraine headaches.
  - ○ Narcotics, acetaminophen, and phenothiazines (eg, prochlorperazine) can be used to treat acute pain.
  - ○ Nonsteroidal anti-inflammatory drugs should be avoided, particularly in the third trimester, due to their association with constriction of the ductus arteriosus and oligohydramnios. Likewise ergots, due to their oxytocic effects, should be avoided throughout pregnancy. Sumatriptan and related agents have not been studied in pregnancy. Because these agents are vasoconstrictors, it is probably prudent to avoid their use in pregnancy except in patients who fail to respond to other measures.
  - ○ Both beta blockers and calcium channel blockers may be used safely for prophylaxis in patients with frequent migraines. Selective serotonin reuptake inhibitors also are considered safe for use during pregnancy, but these agents must be taken for weeks prior to becoming effective.

CARPAL TUNNEL SYNDROME

- Weight gain and dependent edema are ubiquitous in pregnancy. Both of these factors predispose to compression of the median nerve as it passes through the carpal tunnel.
- Symptoms usually start in the third trimester and include pain, numbness, and tingling over the palmar aspect of the hand, thumb, index finger, middle finger, and lateral half of the ring finger. Patients often complain of being awakened by these symptoms. In severe cases, muscle weakness may occur.
- Most patients respond to the wearing of wrist splints at night, and symptoms usually resolve early in the postpartum period. Surgical decompression rarely is needed.

EPILEPSY

- Approximately 1 percent of people have a seizure disorder, and the vast majority of cases of epilepsy are idiopathic.
- Epilepsy itself and most anticonvulsant medications increase the likelihood of congenital abnormalities. Therefore, women with epilepsy ideally should undergo preconceptional counseling. (Preconception counseling for patients with epilepsy and the teratogenic potential of commonly prescribed anticonvulsant medications are discussed in Chap. 1.)
- Due to fear of teratogenic effects, women with epilepsy and/or their physicians may discontinue anticonvulsant medications when pregnancy is diagnosed.
  - ○ However, control of seizures is of primary importance for maximizing the likelihood of good outcome for both mother and fetus.

- When possible, pregnant women with epilepsy should be treated with only one medication.
  - Because of the physiologic changes that occur during pregnancy, doses of anticonvulsant medications often will need to be *increased* in pregnant women to maintain therapeutic levels.
  - Table 7F-1 lists the therapeutic levels of commonly prescribed anticonvulsant medications.
- There is an increased incidence of hemorrhagic disease of the newborn in the offspring of epileptic women. This problem is due to a deficiency of the vitamin K–dependent clotting factors. However, since virtually all infants receive 1 mg of vitamin K intramuscularly at birth, this problem rarely is seen today.
- Because of the increased incidence of malformations in infants born to women with epilepsy, maternal serum screening, targeted obstetric ultrasound examinations, and fetal echocardiography are indicated in these patients.

MYASTHENIA GRAVIS

- Autoantibodies of the IgG class, directed against the acetylcholine receptors in skeletal muscle, cause myasthenia gravis. The disease is manifest by fatiguability of ocular, facial, and oropharyngeal muscles.
- Thymectomy improves symptoms in the majority of patients, but many of them will still need medical therapy with an acetylcholinesterase inhibitor such as neostigmine or pyridostigmine. Occasionally, exacerbations will require treatment with plasmapheresis.
- As with most autoimmune diseases, some patients with myasthenia gravis improve during pregnancy. However, approximately equal numbers of women remain unchanged or worsen during pregnancy. Deterioration in the first 6 weeks postpartum is common.
- Because the uterus is composed of smooth muscle, the course of the first stage of labor is unaffected by myasthenia gravis. However, the second stage of labor, which requires voluntary expulsive efforts, may be prolonged, and operative vaginal delivery may be required.
- Several medications that are commonly used in pregnancy are contraindicated or should be used with caution in women with myasthenia gravis. These medications are listed in Table 7F-2.
- Neonatal myasthenia occurs in 10 to 25 percent of infants born to women with myasthenia gravis. A weak cry and poor sucking effort develop within the first 2 days of life and persist for several weeks.

TABLE 7F-1   Anticonvulsant Medications Commonly Used during Pregnancy[a]

MEDICATION	USUAL DOSE FOR NONPREGNANT INDIVIDUALS	THERAPEUTIC RANGE (μg/mL)
Phenytoin	300–400 mg/day in 1–3 doses	Total 10–20 Free 1–2
Carbamazepine	800–1200 mg/day in 2–4 doses	4–12
Valproate	600–1200 mg/day in 1–3 doses	50–100
Phenobarbital	120–180 mg/day in 2–3 doses	15–40
Primidone	750–1500 mg/day in 3 doses	5–15

[a]Note that the doses listed in this table may need to be exceeded in pregnant women in order to maintain therapeutic levels.

TABLE 7F-2   Medications to Avoid in Pregnant Women with Myasthenia Gravis

DRUG OR MEDICATION CLASS	USE IN OBSTETRICS	PROBLEM IN PATIENTS WITH MYASTHENIA
Magnesium sulfate	Tocolysis or seizure prophylaxis in preeclamptic patients	Contraindicated; accentuates neuromuscular blockade; may precipitate respiratory arrest
Glucocorticoids	Acceleration of fetal pulmonary maturity	Use with caution; may initially increase muscle weakness
Narcotics	Analgesia	Use with caution; myasthenia patients are extremely sensitive
Nondepolarizing muscle relaxants (eg, vecuronium)	General anesthesia	Contraindicated; prolonged paralysis can occur
Inhalational anesthetics	General anesthesia	Use with caution; may exacerbate myasthenia
Aminoglycosides (eg, gentamicin)	Treatment of puerperal infections	Use with extreme caution; can block motor endplate and cause myasthenic crisis

Respiratory assistance may be required. The condition is thought to be due to transplacental passage of IgG directed at the acetylcholine receptor.

MULTIPLE SCLEROSIS

- Multiple sclerosis is an idiopathic, multifocal demyelinating disease of the central nervous system. The course of the disease is chronic and characterized by exacerbations and remissions of varying duration.
- Relapses are less common during pregnancy but more common in the postpartum period. The disease does not seem to affect pregnancy outcomes adversely.
- When indicated, the mainstay of treatment during pregnancy is high-dose corticosteroids.

CORTICAL VEIN THROMBOSIS

- Cortical vein thrombosis occurs in approximately 1 in 10,000 pregnancies, most commonly in the postpartum period. Manifestations include headache, lethargy, nausea, vomiting, and seizures.
- The diagnosis is made with computed tomography (CT) or magnetic resonance imaging (MRI) scans of the head.
- Unless the woman has an underlying hypercoagulable condition, the issue of whether anticoagulation should be prescribed in future pregnancies is controversial.

SUBARACHNOID HEMORRHAGE

- Subarachnoid hemorrhages occur in fewer than 1 in 5000 pregnancies. However, this condition accounts for 10 percent of maternal deaths. Bleeding from a congenital arteriovenous (AV) malformation or rupture of a berry aneurysm in or near the circle of Willis causes most of these hemorrhages.
- This disorder should be suspected in any patient with localized signs of cerebral or meningeal irritation. The diagnosis is made by demonstration of subarachnoid blood on a CT scan of the head or examination of the cerebrospinal fluid (CSF). Magnetic resonance angiography or fluoroscopic angiography may be used to localize the site of bleeding.
- Those lesions amenable to such therapy should be treated surgically. Induced hypotension and hypothermia commonly are used during these procedures. Fetal monitoring should be employed intraoperatively, and blood pressure should be increased if fetal bradycardia occurs.
- Pregnant women who have undergone surgical repair of berry aneurysms or AV malformations can be delivered vaginally. It probably is best to avoid the Valsalva maneuver with the use of epidural anesthesia and operative vaginal delivery. Patients with uncorrected lesions probably are best served by delivery via cesarean prior to labor.
- Pregnancy is contraindicated in women with inoperable AV malformations. Such women should undergo preconception counseling.

PSEUDOTUMOR CEREBRI

- Patients with pseudotumor cerebri usually present with a headache and may have diplopia. Papilledema is present in essentially all patients, and obese women seem to be more predisposed to developing this condition.
- Diagnosis requires documentation of a normal CT or MRI scan of the head, an increased CSF pressure, and normal CSF composition.
- Analgesics are used to treat headache. The carbonic anhydrase inhibitor acetazolamide decreases CSF production in many patients. Serial lumbar puncture also has been advocated. In refractory cases where vision is threatened, lumboperitoneal shunting of CSF or fenestration of the optic nerve sheath may be necessary.
- Pregnancy outcome is unaffected by the presence of pseudotumor cerebri.
- Regional anesthesia has been used successfully in such patients. This condition is not an indication for cesarean delivery. However, the Valsalva maneuver should be avoided, and the second stage of labor should be shortened with a low or outlet operative vaginal delivery.

BIBLIOGRAPHY

Donaldson JO. Neurologic complications. In: Burrow GN, Duffy TP, eds. *Medical Complications during Pregnancy*, 5th ed. Philadelphia: Saunders, 1999.

Samuels P. Neurologic disorders. In: Ling FW, Duff P, eds. *Obstetrics & Gynecology: Principles for Practice*. New York: McGraw-Hill, 2001.

 Renal Disease

Rodney K. Edwards

RENAL CHANGES IN PREGNANCY

- The renal collecting system, including the renal pelves and ureters, dilates markedly during pregnancy. The dilation is greater on the right than on the

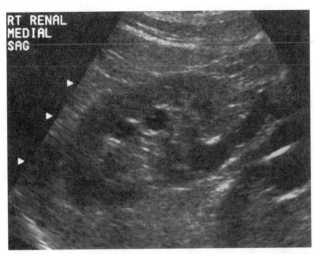

FIG. 7G-1 An ultrasound image of the right kidney obtained from a woman in the second trimester of pregnancy. Note the dilation of the calyces and proximal ureter. (Courtesy of Christopher Sistrom, MD, Department of Radiology, University of Florida College of Medicine, Gainesville.)

left and is due to hormonal influences (primarily the effect of progesterone) and mechanical compression by the expanding uterus. Figure 7G-1 shows an image of this dilation of the renal collecting system obtained by renal ultrasound.

- Both renal plasma flow (RPF) and the glomerular filtration rate (GFR) increase during pregnancy. The GFR increases to a greater degree than RPF, leading to lower blood urea nitrogen levels and serum creatinine levels during pregnancy. A serum creatinine value above 0.8 mg/dL is abnormal during pregnancy.
- Glucose reabsorption does not increase during pregnancy, and the average renal threshold above which glycosuria is seen falls from about 200 mg/dL to 155 mg/dL. Therefore glycosuria can be a normal occurrence during pregnancy.
- The physiologic changes that occur during pregnancy are discussed in more detail in Chap. 4.

DIAGNOSTIC TESTS

- **Urinalysis** is the test most frequently utilized to evaluate the renal system during pregnancy. With the exception of urinary glucose, the test is interpreted just as it would be in a nonpregnant individual.
- Urinalysis is inadequate to screen for asymptomatic bacteriuria, and all pregnant women should undergo screening **urine culture** at the first prenatal visit (see Chap. 25).
- Assessment of a **24-h urine** collection for protein and creatinine clearance may be utilized to evaluate renal function. Total urinary protein values less than

150 mg/day are normal in nonpregnant individuals. Values in pregnant women may exceed this amount. However, values in excess of 300 mg/day are abnormal. The creatinine clearance rate normally is increased during pregnancy and may exceed 150 mL/min. Creatinine clearance is a much more sensitive indicator of renal function than serum creatinine. Blood urea nitrogen and serum creatinine levels may be normal until the creatinine clearance drops to 50 mL/min.

ACUTE RENAL DISEASES

- **Urinary tract infections** are discussed in Chap. 24.
- **Urolithiasis** is uncommon during pregnancy. It occurs at the same rate as in non-pregnant individuals, about 3 per 10,000.
  - The diagnosis should be suspected in the setting of renal colic and hematuria.
  - Ultrasound is now the test of choice for diagnosis of this condition, with intravenous pyelography reserved for cases in which the diagnosis cannot be made or excluded with ultrasound.
  - Laboratory evaluation should include serum calcium and phosphorus levels to evaluate for hyperparathyroidism.
  - Patients should be treated with intravenous hydration and narcotics, anticipating passage of the stone. Lithotripsy is contraindicated during gestation.
  - Staghorn calculi (composed of calcium phosphate) may develop in the renal pelves of patients with recurrent infections caused by urease-producing organisms, such as *Proteus* species. Such patients should undergo frequent urine cultures, and antibiotic suppression should be considered. Surgery to remove the calculi is best postponed until after pregnancy.
- **Acute renal failure** is defined as less than 400 mL of urine output in a 24-h period in the absence of urethral or bilateral ureteral obstruction.
  - It may occur in conjunction with hemorrhage due to placenta previa, placental abruption, or uterine atony; hypoperfusion due to sepsis; or volume constriction due to severe preeclampsia.
  - Renal ischemia occurs as a result of any condition leading to acute renal failure.
    - As the duration of ischemia increases, the risk of acute tubular necrosis increases. This condition is associated with a polyuric phase following the initial period of oliguria. With this condition, renal failure is reversible, as the glomeruli are not affected.
    - With continuing ischemia, cortical necrosis may result, leading to irreversible renal failure.
  - Treatment centers around elimination of the underlying cause. Regardless of the etiology, potassium

intake should be prohibited. Invasive hemodynamic monitoring yields objective data that can be used to guide treatment.

○ Hemodialysis may be needed in patients with hypernatremia, hyperkalemia, volume overload, severe uremia, or worsening acidosis.

- **Acute glomerulonephritis**, a rare complication of pregnancy, may be confused with preeclampsia.

  ○ Both conditions are associated with nondependent edema, hypertension, and proteinuria. Transient renal insufficiency can occur with both conditions.

  ○ Hematuria, red blood cell casts in the urine, and decreased serum complement levels are consistent with this disease. In the case of poststreptococcal glomerulonephritis, antistreptolysin O titers are elevated.

  ○ Treatment consists of blood pressure control and sodium and fluid restriction.

  ○ Rates of perinatal mortality, preterm delivery, and intrauterine growth restriction are higher than in the general population, and a minority of women have persistent renal insufficiency.

  ○ Preexisting hypertension, renal insufficiency, or nephrotic-range proteinuria herald a worse outcome for both mother and fetus.

  ○ The histologic type has little effect on pregnancy outcome. Therefore renal biopsy seldom is necessary.

- **Hemolytic uremic syndrome** is another rare condition that may be confused with preeclampsia.

  ○ This idiopathic condition is associated with a high mortality rate.

  ○ Initial symptoms may include nausea, vomiting, diarrhea, and malaise.

  ○ Hemolysis, renal failure, and disseminated intravascular coagulation occur.

  ○ Plasmapheresis is the treatment of choice.

CHRONIC RENAL FAILURE

- Patients with **chronic renal disease** should undergo preconception counseling (discussed in Chap. 1).

  ○ For women with baseline serum creatinine values less than 1.5 mg/dL, serious complications during pregnancy are uncommon.

  ○ For women with baseline serum creatinine values in excess of 2.5 mg/dL and/or preexisting hypertension, preeclampsia and preterm delivery occur in the majority of cases. Fetal growth restriction is also common in such patients, and serial growth ultrasounds and antenatal testing are indicated.

  ○ The degree of proteinuria usually worsens throughout gestation in these patients. Although worsening proteinuria does not generally increase the risk of

TABLE 7G-1   Relative Criteria for Timing Pregnancy in Patients with Renal Transplants

CRITERION	IDEAL STATUS
Time since transplant	At least 2 years
Immunosuppressive medications	Should be at baseline levels; continue throughout pregnancy
Plasma creatinine	Should be <1.5 mg/dL
Proteinuria	None or minimal
Evidence of rejection	No evidence of active rejection

maternal or fetal complications, it may complicate the diagnosis of preeclampsia in such patients.

○ Hypertension may develop in patients with chronic renal disease and can be quite severe.

○ Patients requiring chronic hemodialysis can have successful pregnancies. However, more frequent dialysis will be needed, and complications such as preterm delivery, fetal growth restriction, and preeclampsia are common.

- As for other patients with chronic renal disease, women with **renal transplants** should undergo preconception counseling. However, pregnancy can be successful in such patients.

  ○ Table 7G-1 lists criteria that may be used to guide counseling about when it is safest for such patients to conceive.

  ○ The risk of transplant rejection is greater than the risk of adverse fetal effects of immunosuppressive medications. Therefore such patients should continue their medications throughout pregnancy.

BIBLIOGRAPHY

Davison JM, Lindheimer MD. Renal disorders. In: Creasy RK, Resnik R, eds. *Maternal-Fetal Medicine*, 4th ed. Philadelphia: Saunders, 1999.

Lindheimer M, Katz A. Pregnancy in the renal transplant patient. *Am J Kidney Dis* 1992;19:173–176.

Samuels P, Colombo DF. Renal disease. In: Gabbe SG, Neibyl JR, Simpson JL, eds. *Obstetrics: Normal and Problem Pregnancies*, 4th ed. New York: Churchill Livingstone, 2002.

H   Substance Abuse

Patrick Duff

INTRODUCTION

- This chapter reviews the adverse effects associated with use of tobacco, marijuana, alcohol, cocaine, and narcotics during pregnancy.

TOBACCO

- Tobacco is the most commonly abused drug in pregnancy.
- Approximately one-third of pregnant women smoke.
- Use of smokeless tobacco products by women is uncommon.
- The major obstetric complications associated with smoking are as follows:
  ○ Increased frequency of low-birthweight infants
  ○ Increased frequency of preterm delivery
  ○ Increased frequency of placental abruption
- Tobacco does not cause a specific anatomic abnormality in the fetus.
- Pregnant women who smoke should be encouraged to quit entirely. If they cannot do so, they should reduce the number of cigarettes they smoke and try to smoke filtered cigarettes that are the lowest in tar and nicotine.
- The most effective interventions to help patients quit smoking are as follows:
  - **Psychologic counseling**
  - **Use of nicotine replacement systems** such as gum, nasal spray, and the patch
    □ The patch is the best-tolerated and most consistently effective nicotine substitute.
    □ Patients who smoke more than 10 cigarettes a day should begin treatment with a 21-mg patch applied daily. After 6 weeks, they should change to a 14-mg patch. After two additional weeks, they should use a 7-mg patch. After 2 more weeks, they should discontinue treatment.
    □ Patients who smoke less than 10 cigarettes a day may start with the 14-mg patch for 6 weeks and then change to the 7-mg patch for 2 additional weeks.
  - **Use of bupropion hydrochloride**
    □ This drug should be administered as a sustained-release tablet, 150 mg, orally twice daily.
    □ The drug should be discontinued when the patient feels she has successfully reduced her craving for tobacco.

MARIJUANA

- Marijuana is a commonly abused drug, especially among younger patients. In these individuals, marijuana is often the "starter or gateway drug" that then leads to multisubstance abuse.
- Marijuana is often used in conjunction with tobacco.
- The obstetric complications associated with use of marijuana are similar to those of tobacco.
- Marijuana does not cause a specific fetal anatomic malformation.

ALCOHOL

- Alcohol is the second most commonly abused drug in pregnancy.
- The most serious maternal complications associated with alcohol abuse in pregnancy are as follows:
  ○ Malnutrition
  ○ Pancreatitis
  ○ Hepatic injury
  ○ Injury during periods of intoxication
  ○ Abuse of other drugs, such as tobacco
- Fetuses chronically exposed to alcohol may develop one or several manifestations of the fetal alcohol syndrome:
  ○ Microcephaly, with resultant mental retardation
  ○ Facial dysmorphism
  ○ Intrauterine growth restriction
- Neonates of alcoholic women may display signs of withdrawal after delivery.
- Women who abuse alcohol should be encouraged to stop drinking. Effective interventions include the following:
  ○ Progressive withdrawal under close medical supervision
  ○ Psychologic counseling
  ○ Participation in support groups such as Alcoholics Anonymous

COCAINE

- Because crack cocaine is now so widely available and so inexpensive, cocaine has emerged as one of the major drugs of abuse in pregnancy.
- Controversy exists about the teratogenecity of cocaine. Some investigations have demonstrated an increased frequency of cardiac and genitourinary anomalies in infants exposed in utero to cocaine. Other studies have not confirmed these observations.
- However, cocaine abuse clearly is associated with increased risk for adverse consequences such as the following:
  ○ Preterm delivery
  ○ Intrauterine growth restriction
  ○ Placental abruption, a complication that is particularly likely in the setting of acute cocaine intoxication
  ○ Multisubstance abuse
  ○ Criminal behavior
  ○ Suicidal behavior
  ○ High-risk sexual behavior with the attendant risk of acquiring STDs such as gonorrhea, chlamydial infection, syphilis, hepatitis B and C, and HIV infection

- ◦ Malnutrition
- ◦ Complications of general anesthesia such as arrhythmias and hyperthermia
- Women who chronically abuse cocaine should be referred to drug treatment centers for intervention.
- Women who are acutely intoxicated with cocaine should be hospitalized, observed closely for cardiac arrhythmias and placental abruption, and given supportive therapy until they are stabilized.

NARCOTICS

- Patients may be addicted to intravenous narcotics such as heroin or to oral narcotics such as codeine, oxycodone, and hydrocodone.
- Narcotic addiction is not associated with specific fetal anatomic malformations.
- However, exposed infants are at risk for intrauterine growth restriction and neonatal withdrawal syndrome.
- Adverse maternal effects of narcotic addiction include the following:
  - ◦ Malnutrition
  - ◦ Multisubstance abuse
  - ◦ Criminal behavior
  - ◦ High-risk sexual behavior
  - ◦ Increased risk for bacterial endocarditis
  - ◦ Withdrawal syndrome
- Women who are addicted to narcotics should be referred to a drug treatment center. The most effective interventions include the following:
  - ◦ Psychologic counseling
  - ◦ Participation in a support group
  - ◦ Pharmacologic substitution with oral methadone
    - ▪ Use of this drug, even in pregnancy, is preferable to use of illicit drugs, particularly those administered parenterally.
    - ▪ Use of oral methadone eliminates the euphoria associated with other narcotics and reduces the need for criminal behavior to support the individual's drug habit.
    - ▪ Methadone also reduces the desire to inject narcotics, which decreases the risk of acquiring life-threatening infections from unsterile needles and syringes.

BIBLIOGRAPHY

American College of Obstetricians and Gynecologists. Substance abuse. *ACOG Tech Bull* No. 194, July 1994, pp. 1–7.

I   Thyroid Disease

Patrick Duff

THYROID PHYSIOLOGY

- The synthesis of thyroid hormone is controlled by thyrotropin-releasing hormone (TRH), produced by the hypothalamus, and thyroid-stimulating hormone (TSH), produced by the anterior pituitary gland.
- The principal thyroid hormones are thyroxine (T_4) and triiodothyronine (T_3).
- Both hormones exist in bound and unbound form. The unbound hormone is the biologically active form.
- The proteins that bind thyroid hormone are thyroid-binding globulin (TBG), albumin, and prealbumin. The serum concentration of TBG increases significantly in pregnancy.
- During a normal pregnancy, the serum concentrations of total T_4 and total T_3 increase, largely because of the increase in the concentration of TBG.
- The serum concentrations of free T_3, free T_4, and TSH remain normal during pregnancy.
- T_3, T_4, and TSH do not cross the placenta.

HYPOTHYROIDISM

ETIOLOGY

- The most common cause of hypothyroidism in pregnancy is *prior* treatment of hyperthyroidism.
- Hashimoto's thyroiditis is another important cause of hypothyroidism.

CLINICAL MANIFESTATIONS

- The most common manifestations of hypothyroidism are as follows:
  - ◦ Fatigue
  - ◦ Impaired concentration
  - ◦ Weight gain
  - ◦ Cold intolerance
  - ◦ Dry, coarse consistency of scalp hair
  - ◦ Deepening of the voice
  - ◦ Enlargement of the tongue
  - ◦ Constipation
  - ◦ Decreased deep tendon reflexes
  - ◦ Amenorrhea with resultant infertility
  - ◦ Galactorrhea
- **Myxedema coma,** characterized by profound mental status changes and low-output heart failure, is the most severe manifestation of hypothyroidism.

- Hypothyroidism may first become manifest in the postpartum period and must always be considered in the differential diagnosis of postpartum depression.

DIAGNOSIS

- Patients with hypothyroidism characteristically have an increased serum TSH concentration and a decreased free T_4 concentration.
- If the etiology of hypothyroidism is Hashimoto's thyroiditis, patients will also have an increased serum concentration of antithyroid antibodies.

MANAGEMENT

- Severely hypothyroid women are usually amenorrheic and hence infertile. Correction of the hypothyroid state typically restores ovulatory cycles and fertility.
- The most effective treatment for hypothyroidism is administration of levothyroxine.
  - The drug is administered orally, once daily, and is very well tolerated.
  - The usual dose range is 75 to 150 μg/day
  - The dose should be adjusted to maintain the TSH in the high range of normal.
- When hypothyroidism is well controlled, obstetric complications are rare.
- Infants delivered to hypothyroid mothers virtually always are euthyroid.
- In rare situations, infants of hypothyroid mothers may have a hereditary defect in their ability to synthesize thyroid hormone. Such infants require immediate treatment with thyroid hormone after birth.

HYPERTHYROIDISM

ETIOLOGY

- The most common cause of hyperthyroidism in pregnancy is Graves disease, an autoimmune disorder.

CLINICAL MANIFESTATIONS

- The principal clinical manifestations of hyperthyroidism are as follows:
  - Diffuse enlargement of the thyroid gland, with or without nodularity
  - Loss of scalp hair
  - Warm, moist velvety texture of skin

- Heat intolerance
- Excessive sweating
- Insomnia
- Emotional lability
- Tremor of the fingers and tongue
- Widened palpebral fissures, producing a characteristic stare
- Lid lag
- Exophthalmos
- Tachycardia
- Palpitations
- Weight loss despite a normal or increased appetite
- Increased deep tendon reflexes
- Proximal muscle weakness
- Severe thyroxtoxicosis may present as the life-threatening complication called **thyroid storm.** Affected patients have prominent neurologic symptoms and high-output congestive heart failure.
- Women with poorly controlled hyperthyroidism are at increased risk for spontaneous abortion and preeclampsia.

DIAGNOSIS

- Patients with thyrotoxicosis typically have a decreased serum TSH concentration, an increased free T_4 concentration, and an increased concentration of thyroid-stimulating antibodies (TSAb).
- In rare cases, patients with thyrotoxicosis have a normal free T_4 concentration but an increased free T_3 (T_3 *thyrotoxicosis*).

MANAGEMENT

- Radioiodine is contraindicated in pregnancy because this therapy may ablate the fetal thyroid gland and cause cretinism.
- Thyroidectomy is usually reserved for patients who fail to respond to medical management or who have thyroid storm. Complications of thyroid surgery in pregnancy include the following:
  - Hemorrhage
  - Recurrent laryngeal nerve injury
  - Removal of parathyroid tissue with resultant hypoparathyroidism
- The mainstay of therapy for hyperthyroidism in pregnancy is antithyroid medication.
  - Propylthiouracil (PTU)
  - Methimazole (Tapezol)
- Both PTU and methimazole cross the placenta and may impair synthesis of fetal thyroid hormone. However, fetal hypothyroidism is uncommon except

in patients who require very high doses of antithyroid medication.

- PTU is preferred for treatment because methimazole has been associated with an unusual defect of the fetal scalp—*aplasia cutis*.
  - The usual starting dose of PTU is 100 mg orally three times daily.
  - The dosage should be adjusted to maintain the serum free T_4 concentration in the upper range of normal.
- If the patient has a prominent tremor and tachycardia, she may be treated with a beta blocker such as propranolol. The dose should be adjusted to reduce the resting maternal heart rate to less than 100 beats per minute.
- Prior to surgery, patients with thyroid storm require treatment with high doses of PTU, propranolol, and potassium iodide. The last drug is used to prevent release of previously synthesized thyroid hormone.

BIBLIOGRAPHY

American College of Obstetricians and Gynecologists. Thyroid disease in pregnancy. *ACOG Tech Bull* No. 181, June 1993, pp. 1–6.

8   FETAL DEATH IN UTERO

Patrick Duff

DEFINITION

- A stillbirth is a fetal death after 20 weeks of gestation.
- Alternate terms for *stillbirth* are:
  - Intrauterine fetal demise (IUFD)
  - Fetal death in utero (FDIU)
- The stillbirth rate is expressed as number of fetal deaths per 1000 total births.

EPIDEMIOLOGY

- The incidence of stillbirth in the United States is 5 to 10 per 1000 total births.
- Possible etiologies of stillbirth include the following:
  - Anatomic abnormalities
  - Karyotype abnormalities
  - Umbilical cord accidents
  - Placental abnormalities
  - Intrauterine infection
  - Immunologic hydrops
  - Nonimmunologic hydrops
  - Fetal-to-maternal hemorrhage
  - Antiphospholipid syndrome
  - Medical complications of pregnancy, such as diabetes and hypertension, that lead to impaired perfusion of the fetoplacental unit
- In approximately one-third to one-half of stillbirths, a precise etiology cannot be determined.

CLINICAL MANIFESTATIONS

- A sudden increase in fetal movement followed by absence of movement
- A progressive decrease in fetal movement
- Abrupt cessation of fetal movement

DIAGNOSIS

- The fetal heart tones cannot be heard with a fetoscope or doptone.
- The fetal heart rate cannot be detected by electronic monitoring.
- Ultrasound findings may include:
  - Absence of fetal movement
  - Absence of cardiac activity
  - Decreased or absent amniotic fluid
  - Deformation of the fetal head
  - Angulation of the fetal spine
- Radiographic findings include:
  - Overlapping of the fetal skull bones
  - Gas in the fetal vascular system

MANAGEMENT

EXPECTANT MANAGEMENT

- Spontaneous labor typically begins within 2 to 4 weeks.
- If labor is delayed for ≥ 6 weeks, a consumption coagulopathy may develop in a small percentage of patients.
- From a psychologic perspective, expectant management is unacceptable to the majority of patients.

TERMINATION OF PREGNANCY

- The most uniformly effective, well-tolerated, and inexpensive method for evacuating the uterus is

administration of misoprostol, an analogue of prostaglandin E1.
- The drug is administered as a vaginal tablet in a dose of 200 µg every 6 h.
- The majority of patients will deliver within 18 to 24 h.
- Patients who fail to respond to misoprostol can be treated with high-dose infusions of oxytocin.
- The most ominous complication of medical evacuation of the uterus is uterine rupture. This complication is extremely rare, occurring in less than 0.5 percent of cases.
- If medical evacuation fails, a hysterotomy can be performed.

EVALUATION OF THE STILLBORN FETUS

- The following observations should be made of the umbilical cord:
  - Number of vessels
    - The cord should contain two umbilical arteries and one umbilical vein.
    - Approximately 1 percent of fetuses have a single umbilical artery.
    - Approximately 10 to 15 percent of these infants have other congenital anomalies.
  - Amount of connective tissue
  - Presence of a knot
  - Length
    - The mean length is 55 cm.
    - Cord entanglement may be more likely when the cord is unusually long.
    - Conversely, an extremely short cord may be associated with fetal complications.
  - Thrombosis
- The following observations should be made of the placenta:
  - Site of cord insertion
    - Eccentric insertion of the cord may be associated with an adverse fetal outcome.
  - Presence of an accessory lobe
  - Areas of infarction
  - Evidence of abruption
  - Meconium staining
  - Presence of a chorioangioma
    - May be associated with hydrops fetalis
- If possible, the fetal karyotype should be determined.
  - Approximately 5 to 10% of stillborn fetuses have a karyotype abnormality.
  - Possible tissue sites for karyotype assessment include the following:
    - Skin biopsy
    - Connective tissue biopsy
    - Placental biopsy
    - Amniotic fluid aspirate—most likely to be successful
  - A detailed examination of the fetus for anomalies should be performed, including a radiographic skeletal survey.

EVALUATION OF THE MOTHER

- Serologic tests for the following possible congenital infections should be performed:
  - Syphilis
  - Toxoplasmosis
  - Rubella
  - Cytomegalovirus
  - Parvovirus
- Blood type and antibody screen
- Thyroid-stimulating hormone determination
- Antinuclear antibody
- Screening test for diabetes
- Lupus anticoagulant
- Anticardiolipin antibody
- Tests for hereditary thrombophilias
  - Factor V Leiden assay
  - Antithrombin III deficiency
  - Prothrombin gene mutation
  - Elevated serum homocysteine concentration
- Kleihauer-Betke test to identify fetal-to-maternal hemorrage
- Genital tract cultures or nucleic acid determinations
  - *Neisseria gonorrhoeae*
  - *Chlamydia*
  - Group B streptococci
  - Herpes simplex virus
  - *Listeria monocytogenes*
  - Cytomegalovirus
- In addition to these tests, the mother and father should be offered appropriate supportive services, including psychologic counseling.

MANAGEMENT IN A SUBSEQUENT PREGNANCY

- The risk of recurrence depends on the etiology of the stillbirth.
- An early ultrasound should be performed to confirm fetal viability.
- Serum analyte screening should be performed at 15 to 16 weeks to assess for trisomy 18, trisomy 21, and a neural tube defect.
- A targeted ultrasound should be performed at approximately 20 weeks to assess for fetal anomalies.

- Antepartum surveillance (biophysical profile test or antepartum fetal heart rate testing) should be performed beginning approximately 2 weeks prior to the time of the previous stillbirth.
- As a matter of routine, delivery should be performed at term once fetal lung maturity has been assured.

BIBLIOGRAPHY

American College of Obstetricians and Gynecologists. Diagnosis and management of fetal death. *ACOG Tech Bull* No. 176, January 1993, pp. 1–8.

9   PRETERM DELIVERY

Rodney K. Edwards

DEFINITION AND SIGNIFICANCE

- A preterm delivery (PTD) is one that occurs at less than 37 and more than 20 weeks of gestational age. The PTD rate in the United States is currently 12 percent. Despite advances in obstetric care, the PTD rate is steadily rising (Fig. 9-1).
- PTD accounts for 70 percent of perinatal mortality and the majority of perinatal morbidity. Despite the fact that 40 to 50 percent of PTDs occur at 35 to 36 weeks of gestation, most of the morbidity and mortality is due to very early PTD ($<$ 32 weeks).

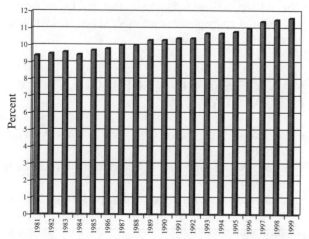

FIG. 9-1 Incidence of preterm delivery in the United States from 1981 to 1999. (National Center for Health Statistics, 2000.)

CAUSES

- Spontaneous preterm birth can be thought of as a multifactorial problem with multiple clinical presentations. These presentations include the following:
  - preterm labor (PTL)
  - preterm premature rupture of membranes (preterm PROM)
  - incompetent cervix (premature cervical effacement and dilation leading to membrane rupture and expulsion of the fetus)

These presentations are not clearly distinct from one another and may overlap.

- As shown in Fig. 9-2, approximately 80 percent of preterm births are "spontaneous"—that is, they occur after PTL or preterm PROM. The other 20 percent of preterm births are "indicated" by medical or obstetric complications that pose risks for the mother and/or fetus that outweigh the risks of prematurity. The most common causes of indicated PTD are preeclampsia (see Chap. 11) and intrauterine growth restriction (see Chap. 13).
- Without intervention, the majority of women with preterm PROM will labor spontaneously and deliver within a week. In contrast, half of the women with PTL deliver at term.

RISK FACTORS

- The most important risk factors for preterm birth are having had a prior preterm birth, being African American, being underweight, and having certain genital tract infections (eg, bacterial vaginosis, group B streptococcal urinary infection).
  - Depending on other factors, women with a prior PTD have a 15 to 80 percent chance of subsequent PTD.
  - African-American women have twice the risk of PTD as compared with women of other ethnicities. This increased risk persists after controlling for socioeconomic factors.

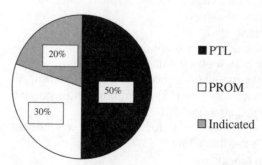

FIG. 9-2 Causes of preterm birth.

○ The presence of bacterial vaginosis doubles the risk of PTD. In addition, up to 80 percent of very early preterm births are associated with intrauterine inflammation.

• Other risk factors for PTD include low socioeconomic status, late or absent prenatal care, "stress," age < 18 or > 40 years, smoking, prior cervical injury, and uterine anomalies.

• Unfortunately, identification of these risk factors for PTD is not particularly useful in clinical practice. More than 50 percent of spontaneous preterm births occur in women who have no apparent risk factors. In addition, due to their high prevalence, the risk factors have limited predictive value.

PATHOPHYSIOLOGY

• The precise mechanism responsible for spontaneous PTD, whether via PTL with intact membranes or PROM, is unknown.

• However, the etiology is probably multifactorial. Factors such as volume of uterine contents, uterine contractions, microbial colonization of the genital tract, inadequate maternal resistance to infection, injury to the maternal-fetal interface, and defective cervical competence all act synergistically to cross a threshold that presents clinically as PTL, PROM, or incompetent cervix.

SCREENING AND PREDICTION

• Efforts to reduce the PTD rate through primary prevention have been unsuccessful. Approaches such as enhanced prenatal care and serial digital cervical examinations have been tested in clinical trials and shown to be of no benefit.

• In an attempt to improve the likelihood of successful treatment of PTL, the use of home monitoring of uterine activity has been proposed. Studies evaluating this approach have shown that such monitoring not only fails to improve outcome but also increases the cost of care.

• In "high-risk" patients (ie, those with a prior PTD or who are underweight), screening for bacterial vaginosis and treatment for same has been shown to decrease the rate of PTD. Unfortunately, such screening in the general population does not seem to have any effect on the PTD rate.

• A short cervix, measured on vaginal ultrasound examination, or the presence of fetal fibronectin in the vagina are two factors that show a strong correlation with risk of PTD. These two tests may have some utility in clinical management by limiting interventions in women who have normal/negative test results. However, their use as screening tests has not led to interventions that decrease the rate of PTD.

TREATMENT OF PRETERM LABOR

• Tocolytic medications (Table 9-1) are used to halt uterine contractions in patients with PTL. None of these medications has been shown to affect the ultimate rate of PTD; however, parenteral administration of these drugs can, on average, delay delivery for 24 to 48 h. Therefore the goal of treatment of PTL is to delay delivery in order to undertake interventions that reduce neonatal morbidity. These interventions include the following:
  ○ Transfer to or treatment in a hospital with a neonatal intensive care unit
  ○ Administration of glucocorticoids to the mother (betamethasone 12 mg IM q 24 h × 2 doses or dexamethasone 6 mg IM q 12 h × 4 doses) to decrease the likelihood of neonatal respiratory distress syndrome, intraventricular hemorrhage, and mortality
  ○ Administration of intrapartum antibiotic prophylaxis against early-onset neonatal infection with group B streptococcus (see Chap. 23)

TABLE 9-1 Commonly Used Tocolytic Medications

TOCOLYTIC	MECHANISM OF ACTION	SIDE EFFECTS
Magnesium sulfate	Compete with calcium at the muscle cell's plasma membrane and sarcoplasmic reticulum	Weakness Hypocalcemia
Beta-mimetics (eg, terbutaline)	Deplete intracellular calcium concentration	Cardiovascular (tachycardia, palpitations) Metabolic (hypokalemia, hyperglycemia)
Calcium channel blockers (eg, nifedipine)	Block the calcium channel on the muscle cell's plasma membrane	Hypotension
Nonsteroidal anti-inflammatory drugs (eg, indomethicin)	Inhibit prostaglandin synthesis	Constriction of the ductus arteriosus Oligohydramnios

- Extended administration of oral tocolytics after the initial treatment course provides little to no benefit.

TREATMENT OF PRETERM PREMATURE RUPTURE OF MEMBRANES

- The treatment of preterm PROM varies depending on the gestational age.
  - Beyond 34 weeks, the risks of continued pregnancy for both the mother and fetus generally are greater than the risk of prematurity complications, and delivery is indicated.
  - Prior to 32 weeks, most authorities agree that attempting to prolong the pregnancy is appropriate.
  - Treatment of preterm PROM at 32 to 33 weeks is controversial. Assessment of amniotic fluid measures of fetal lung maturity may be utilized to decide whether delivery or attempts to prolong the pregnancy is appropriate.
- Broad-spectrum antibiotics administered in the setting of preterm PROM effectively prolong the latency period (the duration of time between membrane rupture and delivery).
  - One antibiotic regimen of proven value is the combination of ampicillin (2 g IV q 6 h for 48 h) followed by amoxicillin (500 mg orally three times daily for 5 days) plus erythromycin (250 mg IV q 6 h for 48 h) followed by erythromycin base (333 mg orally three times daily for 5 days).
  - A reasonable substitute for erythromycin in this regimen is azithromycin (1000 mg orally as a single dose).
- Use of both tocolytic medications and corticosteroids in the setting of preterm PROM is controversial. The use of corticosteroids at gestational ages < 30 to 32 weeks is generally thought to be appropriate.
- Complications that may be encountered with attempts at prolonging the pregnancy of a patient with preterm PROM include chorioamnionitis, umbilical cord compression, and placental abruption.

TREATMENT OF INCOMPETENT CERVIX

- The treatment of incompetent cervix is usually surgical, consisting of placing a purse-string suture in the cervix in an attempt to bolster its strength. This procedure, called a **cerclage**, may be performed emergently in a patient presenting with cervical dilation. Alternatively, it may be performed prophylactically early in the second trimester in a patient with a prior pregnancy history consistent with incompetent cervix.

- Bleeding, uterine contractions, ruptured membranes, and chorioamnionitis are contraindications to cerclage placement.

BIBLIOGRAPHY

Association of Professors of Gynecology and Obstetrics: APGO Educational Series on Women's Health Issues. Prevention and management of preterm birth: The role of infection and inflammation. Washington, DC. December 1998.

Goldenberg RL. The management of preterm labor. *Obstet Gynecol* 2002;100:1020–1037.

Martin JA, Hamilton BE, Ventura SJ, et al. Births: Final data for 2000. *Natl Vital Stat Rep* 2002;50:1–101.

10 THIRD TRIMESTER BLEEDING

Patrick Duff

PLACENTA PREVIA

EPIDEMIOLOGY

- Placenta previa is characterized by implantation of the placenta over the internal cervical os.
- Placenta previa is usually characterized as **total** (central) or **partial** (Figs. 10-1 and 10-2).
- A placenta that extends close to, but not over, the cervical os is characterized as **low-lying**.
- In term patients, the frequency of placenta previa is approximately 0.5 percent. The frequency is slightly higher in patients with preterm gestations.
- The principal risk factors for placenta previa include the following:
  - Maternal age > 35 years
  - Multiparity
  - Prior uterine surgery, particularly cesarean delivery
  - Uterine malformations

CLINICAL MANIFESTATIONS

- The most common clinical presentation of placenta previa is *painless, bright-red vaginal bleeding.*
- If the bleeding is profuse, signs of hypovolemic shock (tachycardia, tachypnea, hypotension) and fetal compromise may be present.

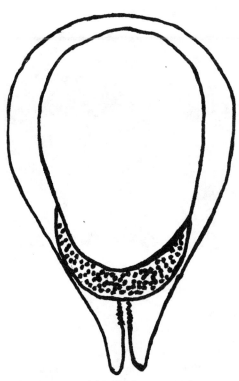

FIG. 10-1 Central (total) placenta previa.

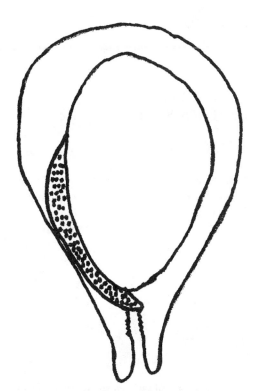

FIG. 10-2 Partial placenta previa.

DIAGNOSIS

- Placenta previa must be differentiated from abruptio placentae and "bloody show."
- In modern obstetric practice, the key diagnostic test for placenta previa is ultrasound (Fig. 10-3).

MANAGEMENT

- Term patients with placenta previa should be delivered immediately by cesarean. These patients may require resuscitation with isotonic crystalloid (normal saline or lactated Ringer's solution) or packed red blood cells if they are hemodynamically unstable.
- Preterm patients with placenta previa should initially be managed with fluid resuscitation (3 mL of isotonic crystalloid for each milliliter of estimated blood loss). If the mother and fetus can be stabilized, expectant management may be continued until fetal lung maturity is documented (usually at approximately 36 weeks). At that point, cesarean delivery is indicated.

COMPLICATIONS

- Patients with placenta previa may develop an adherent placenta.

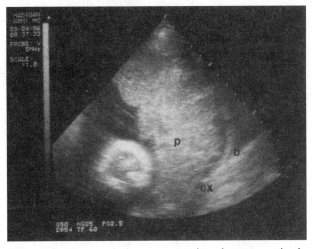

FIG. 10-3 Ultrasound shows an anterior placenta previa. b, bladder; cx, cervix; p, placenta.

- ○ **Placenta accreta**—the placenta is attached to the superficial layer of the myometrium.
- ○ **Placenta increta**—the placenta penetrates approximately halfway through the myometrium.
- ○ **Placenta percreta**—the placenta extends through the myometrium to the serosa.
  - An adherent placenta is a life-threatening emergency that can lead to profuse hemorrhage. Hysterectomy usually is necessary to control the hemorrhage.

• Patients with placenta previa are at increased risk for a recurrent previa in a subsequent pregnancy.

ABRUPTIO PLACENTAE

EPIDEMIOLOGY

• **Abruptio placentae** (placental abruption) is characterized by **premature separation of a normally implanted placenta.**
• The frequency of abruptio placentae is approximately 0.5 to 1.0 percent.
• The principal risk factors include the following:
  ○ Hypertension
  ○ Maternal age > 35 years
  ○ Multiparity
  ○ Cigarette smoking
  ○ Cocaine use
  ○ Uterine malformations
  ○ Trauma
  ○ Rapid decompression of an overdistended uterus (eg, from polyhydramnios or multiple gestation)

CLINICAL MANIFESTATIONS

• Abruptio placentae typically presents with heavy, dark-red vaginal bleeding and intense abdominal pain.
• Tetanic uterine contractions may occur, and fetal compromise is the norm.

DIAGNOSIS

• Abruptio placentae must be distinguished from placenta previa and "bloody show."
• The diagnosis is established almost entirely on the basis of clinical examination.
• In selected instances, ultrasound examination may identify a retroplacental blood clot (Fig. 10-4).

MANAGEMENT

• In the vast majority of cases of abruptio placentae, either the mother, the baby, or both are unstable and delivery is indicated.
• Similarly, in almost every case, the urgency of delivery is so great that cesarean is indicated.

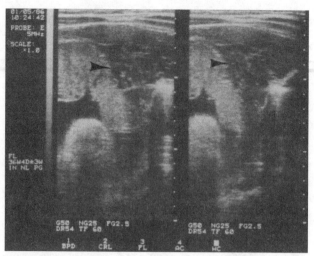

FIG. 10-4 Ultrasound shows an anterior placenta with a retroplacental blood clot (arrowheads).

COMPLICATIONS

• One of the most ominous complications of abruptio placentae is disseminated intravascular coagulation.
• Infants delivered to mothers with abruptio placentae may be hypovolemic, anemic, and hemodynamically unstable.
• Patients who have had abruptio placentae have a recurrence risk of at least 5 to 10 percent in a subsequent pregnancy.
• The recurrence risk is even higher when the abruption was so severe as to result in fetal or neonatal death.

POSTPARTUM HEMORRHAGE

EPIDEMIOLOGY

• Postpartum hemorrhage usually is defined as blood loss exceeding *500 mL* after a vaginal delivery and *1000 mL* after a cesarean delivery.
• The most common cause of postpartum hemorrhage is **uterine atony**. The principal factors that predispose to atony are:
  ○ Extended duration of labor
  ○ Intrapartum administration of magnesium sulfate
  ○ Overdistention of the uterus—eg, due to polyhydramnios or multiple gestation
  ○ Major uterine malformation—eg, a large intramural myoma
• Another important cause of postpartum hemorrhage is a cervical or vaginal laceration or vaginal wall hematoma.
  ○ Cervical lacerations typically occur as a result of precipitous labor.

- ○ Vaginal lacerations usually are associated with forceps delivery.
- ○ Vaginal wall hematomas usually occur in association with a precipitous delivery or instrumental delivery.
- A third important cause of postpartum hemorrhage is retained placental tissue. This condition is most likely to occur if the placenta has an abnormal configuration (eg, an accessory lobe) or if it has implanted in a relatively devascularized site in the uterus (eg, prior cesarean scar).
- A less common but potentially very serious cause of postpartum hemorrhage is disseminated intravascular coagulation. The principal factors that predispose to this disorder are:
  - ○ Abruptio placentae
  - ○ Severe preeclampsia
  - ○ Amniotic fluid embolism
  - ○ Fetal death in utero

CLINICAL MANIFESTATIONS

- Bright-red vaginal bleeding
- Tachycardia
- Tachypnea
- Hypotension
- Altered sensorium
- Cool, pale skin
- Decreased urine output

DIAGNOSIS

- The diagnosis of uterine atony, cervical or vaginal laceration, and vaginal wall hematoma is confirmed by physical examination.
- The diagnosis of retained placental tissue is best established by ultrasound examination.
- The following laboratory abnormalities confirm the diagnosis of disseminated intravascular coagulation:
  - ○ Thrombocytopenia
  - ○ Hypofibrinogenemia
  - ○ Increased serum concentration of fibrin degradation products

MANAGEMENT

- Uterine atony should be managed in a stepwise manner until the bleeding is controlled.
  - ○ Manual massage of the uterus
  - ○ Administration of intravenous pitocin (40 U in 1000 mL of Ringer's lactate at 250 mL/h)
  - ○ Administration of methergine, 0.2 mg IM

- ○ Administration of prostaglandin F-2 alpha, 250 μg IM or directly into the myometrium
- ○ Surgery
  - ▪ Ligation of uterine arteries
  - ▪ Ligation of ovarian arteries
  - ▪ Ligation of hypogastric arteries
  - ▪ Hysterectomy
- A cervical or vaginal laceration that is bleeding must be repaired surgically.
- A vaginal wall hematoma that is expanding must be opened, drained, and then packed.
- Retained placental fragments should be removed by uterine curettage under ultrasound guidance.
- Disseminated intravascular coagulation should be treated by administration of platelets, packed red blood cells, and fresh frozen plasma and/or cryoprecipitate.

COMPLICATIONS

- Immediate and serious nonfatal complications of postpartum hemorrhage include adult respiratory distress syndrome (usually due to excessive volume replacement) and acute tubular necrosis.
- A rare but very important long-term complication of severe postpartum hemorrhage is panhypopituitarism (**Sheehan syndrome**).

BIBLIOGRAPHY

American Congress of Obstetricians and Gynecologists. Hemorrhagic shock. *ACOG Educational Bulletin* No. 235, April 1997.

American Congress of Obstetricians and Gynecologists. Postpartum hemorrhage. *ACOG Educational Bulletin* No. 243, January 1998.

11 HYPERTENSIVE DISORDERS IN PREGNANCY

Patrick Duff

CHRONIC HYPERTENSION

EPIDEMIOLOGY

- Chronic hypertension is defined as a blood pressure greater than 140/90 mmHg prior to 20 weeks of gestation.

- It is one of the most common medical complications of pregnancy.
- Several clear risk factors for chronic hypertension have been identified:
  - African-American race
  - Age >35 years
  - Positive family history
  - Diabetes
  - Collagen vascular disease
  - Renal disease

ETIOLOGY

- Essential hypertension is the most common cause of chronic hypertension.
- Unusual but potentially curable causes of chronic hypertension include:
  - Renal artery stenosis
  - Hyperthyroidism
  - Hyperaldosteronism
  - Cushing's disease
  - Coarctation of the aorta
  - Pheochromocytoma

COMPLICATIONS DURING PREGNANCY

- Patients with long-standing, severe chronic hypertension may develop end-organ damage such as ischemic heart disease, stroke, retinopathy, and renal disease.
- The most likely maternal sequelae of chronic hypertension are superimposed preeclampsia, a complication experienced by at least one-third of hypertensive gravidas, and abruptio placentae.
- The major fetal complications of chronic hypertension are intrauterine growth restriction, changes in fetal heart rate due to uteroplacental insufficiency, and stillbirth.

MANAGEMENT

- Patients with mild, stable chronic hypertension may not require any therapy during pregnancy.
- If the patient's blood pressure increases to greater than 150 mmHg systolic or 100 mmHg diastolic, treatment should be instituted to prevent possible future damage to end organs. Unfortunately, treatment is not consistently effective in preventing superimposed preeclampsia.
- The principal drugs used for treating chronic hypertension in pregnancy are summarized in Table 11-1.
- As a general rule, diuretics should not be used in pregnancy for treatment of chronic hypertension. All diuretics can cause an undesired contraction of the patient's intravascular volume. Thiazide diuretics may also be associated with neonatal thrombocytopenia.
- As a general rule, pure beta blockers such as propranolol or atenolol should not be used in pregnancy because of their association with fetal growth restriction.
- Angiotensin-converting enzyme (ACE) inhibitors and angiotensin-II inhibitors should not be used in pregnancy because they may cause irreversible renal dysplasia in the fetus.
- Patients with chronic hypertension should have serial ultrasound examinations to assess fetal growth.
- Antepartum fetal heart testing should be used to assess for uteroplacental insufficiency. The onset of testing depends on the severity of the patient's hypertension but usually begins at 32 to 36 weeks of gestation.
- Delivery should be performed at approximately 38 to 39 weeks of gestation or sooner if fetal testing is not reassuring.

PREECLAMPSIA AND GESTATIONAL HYPERTENSION

EPIDEMIOLOGY

- **Preeclampsia** is defined by the following triad:
  - Blood pressure >140/90 mmHg beyond the first 20 weeks of pregnancy

TABLE 11-1 Principal Drugs for the Treatment of Chronic Hypertension in Pregnancy

DRUG	MECHANISM OF ACTION	USUAL ORAL DOSE RANGE	MAJOR ADVERSE EFFECT(S)
Alpha-methyldopa	Central alpha$_2$ agonist	500 mg to 2000 mg in 2 to 4 divided doses	Postural hypotension
Labetalol	Alpha and beta blocker	100 to 400 mg twice daily	Postural hypotension, headache
Long-acting nifedipine	Calcium channel blocker	30 mg once daily	Postural hypotension, headache

- Proteinuria >300 mg/24 h
- Edema
  - Face
  - Fingers
  - Feet
  - Presacral
- **Gestational hypertension** is defined by blood pressure >140/90 mmHg beyond the first 20 weeks of pregnancy without proteinuria and edema. Gestational hypertension should be evaluated and managed as described below for preeclampsia.
- Several well-established risk factors for gestational hypertension and preeclampsia have been identified:
  - Young age
  - First pregnancy
  - African-American race
  - Preexisting chronic hypertension
  - Diabetes
  - Collagen vascular disease
  - Renal disease
  - Multiple gestation
  - Molar pregnancy

ETIOLOGY

- The etiology of preeclampsia and gestational hypertension is unknown.

CLASSIFICATION

- Preeclampsia is classified as **mild** or **severe**.
- The criteria for **severe preeclampsia** include the following:
  - Blood pressure >160 mmHg systolic or >110 mmHg diastolic
  - Oliguria—urine output <400 mL/24 h
  - Pulmonary edema
  - Proteinuria >5 g/24 h
  - Central nervous system hyperexcitability
    - Headache
    - Increased deep tendon reflexes
  - Right-upper-quadrant or epigastric pain
  - Abnormal liver function tests
  - Thrombocytopenia
  - Intrauterine growth restriction
- A variant of severe preeclampsia is characterized by hemolysis, elevated liver enzymes (ALT, AST), and low platelet count (**HELLP syndrome**).

COMPLICATIONS OF PREECLAMPSIA

- Abruptio placentae
- Cerebrovascular accident
- Disseminated intravascular coagulation
- Hepatic hematoma
- Intrauterine growth restriction
- Stillbirth

MANAGEMENT

- Patients with mild preeclampsia or gestational hypertension who are preterm can be managed expectantly until they reach term or their disease worsens with the following:
  - Bed rest to control blood pressure
  - Ultrasound to assess fetal growth
  - Monitoring of the antepartum fetal heart rate to assess for compromised placental blood flow
- Patients with mild preeclampsia at term should be delivered.
- Patients with severe preeclampsia should usually be delivered regardless of gestational age. The principal reason to temporize is to administer corticosteroids to the very preterm patient.
- The mode of delivery should be based on:
  - Fetal presentation
  - Cervical examination
  - Assessment of the infant's ability to tolerate the stress of labor
- The patient should be treated intrapartum to prevent seizures. The drug of choice for this purpose is intravenous magnesium sulfate.
  - Loading dose—4 to 6 g over 30 min
  - Maintenance dose—2 to 4 g/h, titrated to keep the patient's deep tendon reflexes depressed
- Fluid balance should be monitored carefully to maintain urine output ≥30 mL/h and prevent pulmonary edema.
- Magnesium sulfate should be continued for 12 to 24 h postpartum until the patient's reflexes decrease and diuresis begins.
- Antihypertensive agents such as apresoline (5 to 10 mg IV) or labetalol (10 mg IV) should be administered as needed to keep the patient's blood pressure ≤150 mmHg systolic and ≤100 mmHg diastolic. Marked hypotension should be avoided because it may result in impaired placental blood flow.
- The neonate of the preeclamptic patient is at risk for neutropenia and thrombocytopenia and should be evaluated for these hematologic abnormalities.
- The patient with preeclampsia has an increased risk of preeclampsia in any subsequent pregnancy.

BIBLIOGRAPHY

American College of Obstetricians and Gynecologists. Chronic hypertension in pregnancy. *ACOG Practice Bulletin,* No. 29, July 2001, pp. 1–9.

American College of Obstetricians and Gynecologists. Diagnosis and management of preeclampsia and eclampsia. *ACOG Practice Bulletin,* No. 33, January 2002, pp. 1–9.

12 MULTIPLE GESTATION

Rodney K. Edwards

- The incidence of twins and higher-order multiple gestations has increased significantly over the past three decades. Almost 2 percent of pregnancies are now multifetal gestations. In considering only pregnancies resulting from the use of assisted reproductive technologies, 30 percent are multiple gestations, and triplets or higher-order gestations account for 5 percent.
- A host of maternal and fetal/neonatal complications are more likely with multiple gestations as compared with singleton gestations (Table 12-1). Perinatal mortality is approximately 10 times more likely for twins than singletons and twice as high for triplets than it is twins. Women undergoing treatment for infertility should be informed of these complications and the increased risk of multiple gestations with such treatment.
- Since the vast majority of multiple gestations are twin gestations, this chapter concentrates primarily on twins. The concepts presented also apply to triplet and higher-order multiple gestations.

TABLE 12-1   Complications That Are More Common with Multiple Gestations

MATERNAL	FETAL/NEONATAL
Preterm delivery (preterm labor and premature rupture of membranes)	Spontaneous abortion
	Prematurity/ low birth weight
Cesarean and other operative delivery	Birth injury
Anemia	Malpresentation
Hemorrhage	Growth restriction/discordant growth
Poly- or oligohydramnios	Congenital anomalies
Preeclampsia	Fetal death in utero
Hyperemesis gravidarum	Cord accidents/prolapse
Abruptio placentae	Twin-to-twin transfusion syndrome
Placenta previa	

EPIDEMIOLOGY

- Twins can result either from the fertilization of two separate ova by two separate sperm or from the splitting of a single conceptus. The former situation results in two genetically distinct or **dizygotic** twins, while the latter results in genetically identical or **monozygotic** twins.
- The frequency of monozygotic twins is relatively constant at 1 per 250 births. However, the rate of dizygotic twins depends on the ovulation of multiple oocytes and is positively correlated with African ancestry, increasing maternal age, increasing parity, family history of multiple gestation, and assisted reproductive technologies.
- Preterm delivery is the single most common complication encountered with multiple gestations. The average gestational age at delivery is 36 weeks for twins, 33 weeks for triplets, and 29 weeks for quadruplets. Therefore the risk of preterm delivery increases with increasing numbers of fetuses.

DIAGNOSIS

- The diagnosis of multiple gestation should be suspected any time there is a history of the use of fertility drugs, uterine size is larger than expected based on menstrual dates, or maternal serum screening tests (triple screen or quadruple screen) are abnormal.
- The test of choice for the diagnosis of twins is an obstetric ultrasound examination; this diagnosis should be made virtually 100 percent of the time by a competent ultrasonographer. Care should be taken to avoid the diagnosis of twins on first-trimester ultrasound examinations unless two viable embryos are seen. Misdiagnosis of an intrauterine blood clot or fluid collection as a nonviable twin may lead to unnecessary emotional trauma for the patient.
- With a careful ultrasound examination, one can not only make the diagnosis of twins but also describe the placentation.
  - All dizygotic twin pregnancies are **dichorionic**.
  - Approximately 25 percent of monozygotic twin pregnancies are dichorionic. The remainder are **monochorionic**. The type of placentation in monozygotic twin pregnancies depends on when in development splitting of the conceptus occurs (Table 12-2).
  - With monochorionic twin pregnancies, there may be one or two amniotic cavities.
  - Table 12-3 presents some of the ultrasound criteria that may be used to determine the number of chorions and amnions present.

TABLE 12-2 The Type of Placentation in Monozygotic Pregnancies Depends on the Day of Development When the Conceptus Splits[a]

TYPE OF TWINS	SPLITTING OCCURS
Dichorionic	Up to day 3
Monochorionic/diamniotic	Days 4–8
Monochorionic/monoamniotic	Days 9–12
Conjoined twins	Days 13–15
Obligate singleton (splitting no longer occurs)	After day 15

[a]Day of development is listed in the second column, with conception occurring on day 0.

TABLE 12-3 Ultrasound Criteria Used to Diagnose the Chorionicity and Amnionicity of Twin Gestations

ULTRASOUND SIGN	CONSISTENT WITH
Different fetal gender	Dichorionic/diamniotic (and dizygotic)
Separate placentas	Dichorionic/diamniotic
"Lambda" or "twin peak" sign	Dichorionic/diamniotic
Subjectively thick intervening membrane	Dichorionic/diamniotic
Subjectively thin intervening membrane	Monochorionic/diamniotic
No intervening membrane	Monochorionic/monoamniotic

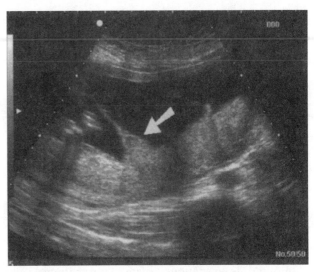

FIG. 12-1 The "lambda" or "twin peak" sign (denoted by the arrow) is consistent with a dichorionic/diamniotic placentation.

- ◦ The "lambda" or "twin peak" sign (Fig. 12-1) is seen on ultrasound as a triangular projection of placenta into the dividing membrane. As noted in Table 12-3, this sign is consistent with a dichorionic placentation.
- When ultrasound is used to establish the gestational age for a twin pregnancy and there is a small amount of discordance in the size of the two fetuses, the size of the larger twin should be used. As with singleton gestations, the utility of ultrasound for dating pregnancies in the third trimester is extremely limited due to the large range of physiologically normal fetal weight by that stage of development.

ANTEPARTUM MANAGEMENT

NUTRITION

- Women with multiple gestations should consume about 300 kcal per day more than women with singleton gestations.
- Although weight-gain recommendations for these women are not as well established as for women with singleton gestations, a prudent recommendation would be that women with multiple gestations should gain 35 to 45 lb during pregnancy.

PRENATAL DIAGNOSIS

- Because most twins are dizygotic and each conceptus has a risk of chromosomal abnormalities, the risk of aneuploidy in multiple gestations is increased at any given maternal age. The risk of Down's syndrome in at least one fetus in a woman 33 years of age is equal to the risk of a 35-year-old woman with a singleton. In a woman 31 years of age with a multiple gestation, the risk of any aneuploidy in at least one fetus is equal to the risk of a 35-year-old with a singleton. Because of this, some authors have advocated offering fetal karyotype assessment at younger maternal ages.
- Furthermore, although monozygotic twins are chromosomally identical, structural anomalies are more common in them than in dizygotic twins.
- The need to obtain tissue (amniotic fluid or chorionic villi) from both fetuses and the potential for discordant results increases both the technical difficulty and ethical challenge of prenatal diagnosis in the setting of twin gestations.
- The median value for maternal serum alphafetoprotein (MSAFP) is 2.5 times greater in twin than in singleton pregnancies. Therefore a cutoff value of 4.5 multiples of the median is commonly used for defining an increased risk of neural tube defects in one or both fetuses. Although use of MSAFP for screening for neural tube defects in twin pregnancies is fairly well standardized, the effectiveness of multiple-marker screening (triple or quadruple test) to detect aneuploid fetuses is not well defined.

PRENATAL CARE

- The frequency of prenatal visits should be greater for women with multiple gestations than for those with singletons. The timing of appointments should be individualized based on coexisting medical or obstetric problems, type of multiple gestation, and the course of the pregnancy.
- Although the value of bed rest for women with multiple gestations has not been definitely demonstrated, women with particularly strenuous occupations and/or lifestyles should be encouraged to decrease their activity in the second half of pregnancy.
- Because of the high rate of preterm delivery in multiple gestations, many interventions have been employed in an effort to make an early diagnosis of preterm labor and prevent preterm delivery. However, such measures as home monitoring of uterine activity, periodic cervical examination, prophylactic oral tocolytics, elective hospitalization, and prophylactic cerclage have no proven benefit.
- Ultrasound examinations to monitor fetal growth should be performed every 3 to 6 weeks. Antenatal testing (nonstress tests or biophysical profiles) should be performed weekly in the third trimester. The frequency of ultrasound examinations and timing of initiation of antenatal testing should be individualized.
- In cases of threatened or imminent preterm delivery prior to 34 weeks of gestation, administration of corticosteroids is beneficial in reducing the likelihood of neonatal respiratory distress syndrome and intraventricular hemorrhage.
- Because the rate of preterm delivery increases with increasing numbers of fetuses, **multifetal pregnancy reduction** can be considered in cases of higher-order multiple gestations.
  - This procedure is designed to increase the chances of delivering at a gestational age more consistent with intact neonatal survival by decreasing the number of fetuses in the uterus.
  - It is controversial in the setting of triplets but should be offered to women with quadruplets or higher-order gestations.
  - The procedure is performed only in selected centers, usually in the late first trimester.
  - In contrast to multifetal pregnancy reduction, **selective reduction** is performed on a specific fetus that has a structural or genetic abnormality. This procedure is more commonly performed in the second trimester.

DISORDERS SPECIFIC TO FETUSES OF MULTIPLE GESTATIONS

- The rate of complications in twin pregnancies is associated with the placentation. As placentation becomes increasingly shared, the rate of complications increases (dichorionic twins have the lowest and monochorionic/monoamniotic twins the highest rates of morbidity and mortality).
- As for singleton fetuses, **intrauterine growth restriction** is diagnosed when the estimated fetal weight is less than the 10th percentile for gestational age. In addition, **discordant growth** may be seen in twin pregnancies and is diagnosed when there is more than a 20 percent difference in estimated fetal weight between twins (expressed as a percentage of the larger twin's estimated weight). Either of these diagnoses should raise the possibility of uteroplacental insufficiency for the affected twin(s) and should result in increased antenatal surveillance and the consideration of delivery if the pregnancy has progressed to an appropriately advanced gestational age.
- **Twin-to-twin transfusion syndrome** is a complication unique to monochorionic twins.
  - Placental vascular connections are thought to exist in all monochorionic placentas. This problem results when there is unequal shunting of blood through these vascular connections.
  - Classically, this problem results in one growth-restricted twin with oligohydramnios and another twin with volume overload and polyhydramnios.
  - The perinatal mortality rate with this condition is approximately 50 percent, but it depends greatly on the gestational age at diagnosis (earlier is worse).
  - The standard treatment is serial reduction amniocentesis from the twin with polyhydramnios. An *experimental* therapy that is available is laser coagulation of the communicating vessels in the placenta.
- Monoamniotic twins have the additional risk of **umbilical cord entanglement**. These twins have a very high perinatal mortality rate, reported to be 40 to 60 percent.
- **Conjoined twins** are quite rare. The majority of these twins do not survive. Only where there is limited sharing of vital organs is survival possible.
- In utero death of one of a pair of monochorionic twins is a special problem that may result in complications for the remaining twin. Because of the above-described vascular communications in the placenta between such twins, acute hypotension may develop in the survivor and cause ischemic damage to the central nervous system in 20 to 25 percent. In addition,

the surviving twin is at very high risk of preterm delivery.

INTRAPARTUM MANAGEMENT

- The course of labor and/or delivery for women with multiple gestations can be unpredictable. Only clinicians experienced and skilled in such care should undertake these deliveries in a labor and delivery unit capable of continuous monitoring of the fetal heart rate and immediate cesarean delivery.
- Most authorities agree that the 40 percent of twins that are both in cephalic presentations should be delivered vaginally and that successful vaginal delivery of both fetuses may be expected to be highly likely.
- Likewise, most authorities agree that the 20 percent of twin births in which the presenting fetus is not in a cephalic presentation should be delivered by cesarean.
- The route of delivery for the remaining 40 percent of twins in which only the presenting baby is in a cephalic presentation is more controversial. Options in this setting include (1) vertex vaginal delivery of the first twin and breech vaginal delivery of the second twin, (2) vertex vaginal delivery of the first twin and attempted external cephalic version prior to delivery of the second twin, and (3) cesarean delivery. The available evidence supports the safety of option 1 as long as the estimated fetal weights are more than 1500 g. However, the experience of obstetricians in breech vaginal delivery is decreasing due to the now rare occurrence of breech vaginal delivery of singletons.
- Monoamniotic and conjoined twins should almost always be delivered by cesarean. In addition, cesarean delivery should almost always be recommended for triplets or higher-order multiple gestations.

BIBLIOGRAPHY

American College of Obstetricians and Gynecologists. Special problems of multiple gestation. *ACOG Educ Bull* Number 253, November 1998.

Newman RB. Multifetal gestations. In: Gilstrap LC III, Cunningham FG, VanDorsten JP, eds. *Operative Obstetrics*, 2nd ed. New York: McGraw-Hill, 2002.

Read JA. Multiple gestation. In: Ling FW, Duff P, eds. *Obstetrics & Gynecology: Principles for Practice*. New York: McGraw-Hill, 2001.

13 INTRAUTERINE GROWTH RESTRICTION

Patrick Duff

DEFINITION

- Intrauterine growth restriction (IUGR) is defined as fetal weight less than the 10th percentile for gestational age.
- Some infants who meet this criterion are completely normal but simply constitutionally small.
- Other infants are smaller than expected because of a pathologic process that adversely affects fetal growth. These infants are the subject of the following discussion.

ETIOLOGY

- Maternal vascular disease (eg, resulting from diabetes or hypertension) is one of the major causes of IUGR.
- Fetal genetic abnormalities and anatomic malformations also are important causes of IUGR
- Congenital infection (eg, cytomegalovirus, toxoplasmosis, rubella) is also a major cause of IUGR
- Other less common but still important causes of IUGR include:
  - Multiple gestation
  - Thrombophilic disorder
    - Antiphospholipid syndrome
    - Factor V Leiden mutation
    - Prothrombin gene mutation
    - Protein S deficiency
    - Protein C deficiency
    - Elevated serum homocysteine concentration
  - Drug exposure (eg, beta blockers, narcotics, tobacco, cocaine)
  - Severe malnutrition
  - Residence at high altitude
  - Abnormal placentation
    - Abruption
    - Previa
    - Circumvallate placenta
    - Chorioangioma

DIAGNOSIS

- Clinical examination alone is not particularly sensitive, specific, or predictive in making the diagnosis of IUGR.
- The best method to diagnose IUGR is an ultrasound examination. The following features of the examination are of particular importance:

- ○ Biparietal diameter
- ○ Head circumference
- ○ Abdominal circumference
- ○ Femoral length
- ○ Estimated fetal weight, based on the standard biometric measurements listed above
- ○ Complete anatomic survey
- ○ Amniotic fluid volume
  - ▪ Oligohydramnios is a particularly worrisome finding because it is strongly associated with decreased fetoplacental blood flow.
- ○ Doppler velocimetry of the umbilical artery
  - ▪ A markedly increased systolic-to-diastolic ratio and absent end-diastolic flow are key negative findings, indicating decreased fetoplacental blood flow.
- • Additional tests that may be of value in determining the etiology of IUGR are summarized in Table 13-1.

MANAGEMENT

- • A systematic effort should be made to identify the cause of IUGR.
- • The underlying cause should be corrected if possible eg, treatment of maternal hypertension or infection.
- • The well-being of the fetus should be assessed. Possible tests include:
  - ○ Nonstress test
  - ○ Contraction stress test
  - ○ Biophysical profile
  - ○ Doppler velocimetry
- • In a fetus with suspected IUGR, the following factors are a clear indication for delivery:
  - ○ No interval fetal growth over a period of 2 to 3 weeks
  - ○ Abnormal fetal assessment
  - ○ Oligohydramnios (amniotic fluid index <5 cm)

TABLE 13-1   Diagnostic Tests of Value in Determining the Etiology of Intrauterine Growth Restriction

ETIOLOGY OF IUGR	MOST APPROPRIATE DIAGNOSTIC TEST(S)
Maternal vascular disease	Clinical examination, antepartum heart rate testing, Doppler velocimetry
Anatomic malformation	Ultrasound
Karyotype abnormality	Amniocentesis or umbilical blood sampling
Congenital infection	Maternal serology, amniotic fluid for culture or PCR, umbilical blood sampling, ultrasound
Maternal thrombophilia	Serologic assays
Maternal drug use	History, urine or serum toxicology screen

- ○ Term gestation and cervix is favorable for induction of labor
- • Determinants of mode of delivery
  - ○ Fetal presentation
  - ○ Cervical examination
  - ○ Assessment of the ability of the fetus to tolerate labor

DETERMINANTS OF FETAL AND NEONATAL PROGNOSIS

- • Gestational age at delivery
  - ○ As a general rule, term infants with IUGR have a better prognosis than preterm infants.
- • Severity of growth restriction
  - ○ The less severe the growth restriction, the better the prognosis.
- • Etiology of IUGR
  - ○ The prognosis tends to be better when IUGR is due to maternal vascular disease and worse when the infant has an anatomic malformation or genetic abnormality.

BIBLIOGRAPHY

Resnik R. Intrauterine growth restriction. *Obstet Gynecol* 2002;99:490–496.

14   ISOIMMUNIZATION
Patrick Duff

DEFINITION

- • Isoimmunization occurs when a pregnant woman who is seronegative for certain red cell antigens develops antibodies against fetal red cell antigens that have been inherited from the baby's father.

PATHOPHYSIOLOGY

- • Isoimmunization affects less than 5 percent of all pregnancies.
- • Antibodies of the IgG class cross the placenta and may injure fetal red cells, leading to fetal anemia and then fetal hydrops.

- Antibodies of the IgM class do not cross the placenta. These are the antibodies that are formed against the major red cell antigens A and B. Therefore ABO incompatibility does not cause fetal isoimmunization.
- The two most common causes of isoimmunization are anti-D and anti-Kell.
  - Anti-D sensitization virtually always results from a prior pregnancy or abortion.
  - Anti-Kell sensitization typically results from a prior blood transfusion.
- Other important causes of isoimmunization include the following:
  - Anti-Kidd
  - Anti-Duffy
  - Anti-C or c
  - Anti-E or e
  - Anti-M, N, or S

CLINICAL MANIFESTATIONS

- Women who are isoimmunized are usually completely asymptomatic.
- When isoimmunization is mild (ie, the maternal antibody titers are low, ≤1:8) the fetus may show no sign of injury.
- When isoimmunization is severe (ie, the maternal antibody titers are high, >1:8), fetal anemia may lead to high-output congestive heart failure or **hydrops fetalis** (Fig. 14-1).

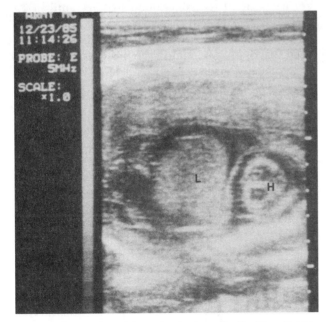

FIG. 14-1 Ultrasound illustrating hydrops fetalis. Note fluid in the fetal abdomen and chest. H, heart; L, liver.

DIAGNOSIS

- All pregnant women should have a blood-type determination and antibody screen at the time of their first prenatal appointments.
- If the patient's blood type is Rh-positive (D-positive) and the screen for antibodies other than anti-D is negative, no further testing is indicated.
- If the patient's blood type is Rh-negative (D-negative) and the antibody screen is negative, she should be retested at 28 weeks and postpartum.
- If the initial antibody screen is positive for an antibody known to cause isoimmunization, the father's blood type should be determined. If he is negative for the antigen in question, the fetus will not express the antigen and should not be at risk.
- If the father is positive for the antigen or he is not available for testing, the fetus should be considered at risk and serial antibody testing should be performed.
- Low maternal antibody titers (≤1:8) generally do not pose a serious risk to the fetus.
- Maternal antibody titers >1:8 may be associated with risk of serious fetal injury.

MANAGEMENT

- Once the antibody titer exceeds 1:8 and the fetus reaches 20 weeks of gestation, an ultrasound should be performed to assess for fetal hydrops, as well as an amniocentesis to assess the degree of fetal red cell hemolysis.
  - Hemolysis is estimated by measuring the concentration of bilirubin in amniotic fluid.
  - Bilirubin concentration is measured by spectrophotometry and is expressed as the optical density at 450 nm (delta OD450).
  - The delta OD450 is plotted on the Liley graph (Fig. 14-2). The higher the delta OD450, the greater the degree of fetal hemolysis and the more severe the fetal anemia.
- The Liley graph is usually divided into three zones.
  - **Zone I** ("safe zone"). A result in this zone indicates minimal risk of severe fetal injury, and the test should be repeated every 3 to 4 weeks.
  - **Zone II** ("intermediate zone"). A result in this zone indicates that the fetus may be at risk. The test should be repeated in approximately 7 to 10 days. If the result declines progressively, the fetus has a very good prognosis. If the result increases, the fetus is at great risk.
  - **Zone III** ("danger zone"). A result in this zone indicates the fetus is in imminent danger of death and that some form of intervention is mandatory.

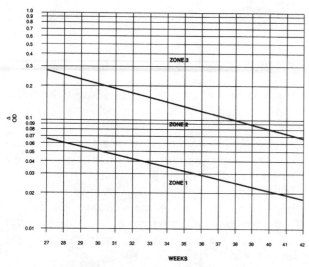

FIG. 14-2 The Liley graph, used to assess the severity of isoimmunization (see text). (Reprinted with permission from *ACOG Educl Bull* No. 227, August 1996. p. 4.)

- If the delta OD450 result is in high zone II or III and the gestational age is less than 34 weeks, cordocentesis should be performed to assess the fetal hematocrit. If severe anemia is present, an intravascular transfusion (via the fetal umbilical vein) should be performed immediately.
  - Sufficient red cells should be transfused to increase the fetal hematocrit into the range of 45 percent.
  - The component used for intrauterine transfusion consists of leukocyte-poor, cytomeglovirus-negative, Rh-negative red cells.
  - After the initial transfusion, the fetal hematocrit usually declines at a rate of about 1 percent per day. Therefore, depending on the gestational age, multiple transfusions may be necessary to prevent **hydrops fetalis**.
- If the delta OD450 is in a dangerous zone but the gestational age is ≥34 weeks, delivery usually is indicated.

PREVENTION

- In the late 1960s, Rh-immune globulin, an immunologic agent, was developed for prevention of Rh-isoimmunization.
- Rh-negative women should receive Rh-immune globulin following any event that could result in isoimmunization, such as:
  - Abortion
  - Ectopic pregnancy
  - Invasive prenatal diagnosis test—chronic villus sampling, amniocentesis, cordocentesis
  - Antenatal bleeding due to abruptio placentae or placenta previa

- Delivery
- In addition, Rh-negative women should receive Rh-immune globulin at approximately 28 weeks of gestation to prevent rare cases of antenatal isoimmunization.

BIBLIOGRAPHY

American College of Obstetricians and Gynecologists. Management of isoimmunization in pregnancy. *ACOG Educ Bull* No. 227, August 1996.

15 ALLOIMMUNE THROMBOCYTOPENIA

Rodney K. Edwards

DEFINITION AND CAUSE

- This disorder is analogous to red blood cell isoimmunization (discussed in Chap. 14). Maternal antibodies to antigens on the fetal platelets cause **alloimmune thrombocytopenia**. These fetal platelet antigens are inherited from the father and absent in the mother.
- The most common antigen, involved in three-quarters of cases, is PLA-1, or **human platelet antigen 1a** (HPA-1a). Other antigens that may be involved (HPA-2 through HPA-5, respectively) are KO, Bak, Pen/Yuk, and Br. All of these antigens are platelet-specific glycoproteins in the platelet membrane.

EPIDEMIOLOGY

- Approximately 1 in 40 women is PLA-1–negative. About 5 percent of the pregnancies in such women result in thrombocytopenic infants. Therefore the overall incidence of alloimmune thrombocytopenia is approximately 1 in 1000. Half of these infants are severely thrombocytopenic (platelet count < 10,000/mL) and half are mildly thrombocytopenic.
- Unlike red blood cell isoimmunization, alloimmune thrombocytopenia commonly occurs in the first pregnancy. In fact, the diagnosis is often not suspected until birth, when the neonate may have petechiae, ecchymoses, or intracranial hemorrhage.

- The recurrence rate is high. If the father is a heterozygote for the offending antigen, the recurrence rate is 50 percent; if he is a homozygote, recurrence is almost certain.

FETAL/NEONATAL EFFECTS

- Nearly three-quarters of affected infants have platelet counts below 50,000/mL, and half have counts below 20,000/mL.
- The worst complication is intracranial hemorrhage.
  - Approximately 20 percent of infants with alloimmune thrombocytopenia have this complication.
  - Half of the hemorrhages occur prior to labor, and some have been reported as early as 20 weeks of gestation.
  - The risk is inversely proportional to the platelet count.
  - The risk is increased in siblings of affected infants.
  - Figure 15-1 shows the gross pathologic appearance of an intracranial hemorrhage.
  - Figure 15-2 shows an ultrasound image of a fetus with a porencephalic cyst that resulted from an intracranial hemorrhage.

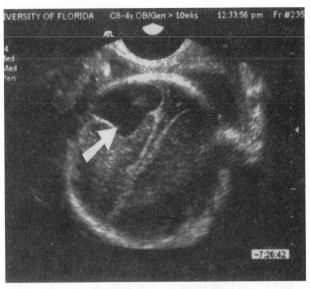

FIG. 15-2 Obstetric ultrasound image showing a fetus with a porencephalic cyst (denoted by the arrow) that resulted from an intracranial hemorrhage. (Courtesy of Douglas S. Richards, MD, Department of Obstetrics and Gynecology, University of Florida College of Medicine, Gainesville.)

DIAGNOSIS

- Because typing of platelet antigens and screening for alloimmune platelet antibodies are not readily available, diagnosis is usually not made until an affected infant is born.
- When a woman has a history of a previously affected child or there is a prenatal ultrasound finding consistent with a fetal intracranial hemorrhage, screening for platelet alloantibodies and typing for platelet antigens are indicated.

MONITORING AND THERAPY

- Since half of the intracranial hemorrhages in these infants occur prior to labor, cesarean delivery prior to labor is not an effective therapy.
- Fetal platelet antigen status can be determined from a sample obtained by amniocentesis.
- Beginning at about 20 weeks of gestation, it is technically possible to perform a cordocentesis, or **percutaneous umbilical blood sampling** (PUBS), and obtain fetal blood from the umbilical vein. If the fetus is antigen-positive, the fetal platelet count can then be determined.
- In cases where the fetal platelet count is below 100,000/mL, weekly maternal administration of **intravenous immunoglobulin** (IVIG) is the most widely used therapy. The mechanism of action of this therapy is uncertain but may be related to blockade of placental transfer of platelet antigen-specific antibodies.

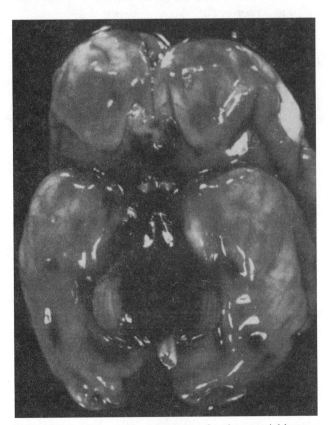

FIG. 15-1 Gross anatomic appearance of an intracranial hemorrhage.

- Daily maternal administration of prednisone has also been advocated in cases refractory to IVIG.
- Serial cordocenteses should be performed to monitor response to therapy and/or plan for delivery route. In addition, maternal (antigen-negative) platelets can be transfused into the fetus's umbilical vein. However, fetal death rates with PUBS are as high as 2 percent, and fetuses with thrombocytopenia are at greatest risk with this procedure owing to the possibility of exsanguination from the puncture site.
- Because of the rarity of alloimmune thrombocytopenia, there are no well-designed studies comparing outcomes of infants stratified by delivery route. However, unless the platelet count is known to be > 50,000/mL, cesarean prior to labor is the preferred method of delivery. Also due to the rarity of this condition, the optimal management of cases of alloimmune thrombocytopenia is uncertain.
- In all cases of known alloimmune thrombocytopenia, maternal platelets should be available for transfusion to the neonate after delivery.
- Antenatally, cases of alloimmune thrombocytopenia should be managed by specialists in maternal-fetal medicine who are capable of performing cordocentesis and intrauterine transfusion. Delivery should occur in a hospital where neonatologists are capable of managing a neonate with severe thrombocytopenia.

BIBLIOGRAPHY

American College of Obstetricians and Gynecologists. Thrombocytopenia in pregnancy. *ACOG Pract Bull* Number 6, September 1999.

Jackson M, Branch DW. Alloimmunization in pregnancy. In: Gabbe SG, Niebyl JR, Simpson JL, eds. *Obstetrics: Normal and Problem Pregnancies,* 4th ed. New York: Churchill Livingstone, 2002.

O'Shaughnessy R, Kennedy M. Isoimmunization. In: Ling FW, Duff P, eds. *Obstetrics & Gynecology: Principles for Practice.* New York: McGraw-Hill, 2001.

16   POSTTERM PREGNANCY

Patrick Duff

DEFINITION

- A pregnancy that extends beyond 42 weeks is considered postterm.

FREQUENCY

- The frequency of postterm pregnancies among those that are accurately dated is approximately 3 to 5 percent.

COMPLICATIONS

- **Postmaturity syndrome** is one of the most serious complications of postterm pregnancies. Fortunately it occurs in fewer than 25 percent of cases. Clinical manifestations in the postmature fetus include:
  - Weight loss near the end of pregnancy
  - Wrinkled skin
  - Long nails
  - Polycythemia
  - Small umbilical cord with decreased Wharton's jelly
  - Small placenta with extensive fibrinoid change in the vascular system
- **Fetal macrosomia** (weight > 4000 g) occurs in up to 20 percent of postterm pregnancies. Macrosomia, in turn, is associated with an increased risk for cesarean delivery and shoulder dystocia.
- **Meconium-stained amniotic fluid** may complicate 10 to 20 percent of postterm pregnancies.
- **Fetal death in utero** may occur as a result of diminished perfusion of the fetoplacental unit. The odds ratio (OR) for fetal mortality is 1.8 at 42 weeks and 2.9 at 43 weeks. However, this complication occurs in < 1:1000 cases if the fetus is monitored appropriately.

MANAGEMENT

- At 41 weeks of gestation, the patient should have a cervical examination to assess the Bishop score. If the score is favorable (≥6) and the patient is an appropriate candidate for vaginal delivery, labor should be induced.
- If the cervical examination is unfavorable at 41 weeks, the patient should be scheduled within the next 7 days for a nonstress test or contraction stress test plus an ultrasound examination for assessment of amniotic fluid volume. Alternatively, a biophysical profile may be performed.
- If antepartum monitoring is not reassuring or oligohydramnios is present, delivery is indicated. The mode of delivery should be based on the cervical examination and assessment of the ability of the fetus to tolerate the stress of labor.
- If a favorable cervical Bishop score is present at 42 weeks, labor should be induced.

- If the cervical status is unfavorable at 42 weeks but antepartum testing is reassuring and the amniotic fluid volume is normal, two management options are acceptable:
  ○ Ripening of the cervix with prostaglandin agents, followed by induction of labor with oxytocin
  ○ Expectant management for an additional week until spontaneous labor ensues or the cervix becomes favorable for induction of labor
- Because patient anxiety typically increases dramatically in the postterm period, most clinicians are reluctant to allow a pregnancy to progress beyond 43 weeks.
- Continuous electronic fetal heart rate monitoring during labor is advisable in postterm patients because of the relatively high frequency of abnormal fetal heart rate tracings.
- Patients with meconium-stained amniotic fluid should receive an amnioinfusion intrapartum to reduce the fetal risk for meconium aspiration syndrome.
- If fetal macrosomia is suspected, the clinician should be alert to the possibility of prolonged labor and shoulder dystocia. Cesarean delivery is clearly preferable to a complicated operative vaginal delivery.

BIBLIOGRAPHY

American College of Obstetricians and Gynecologists. Management of posterm pregnancy. *ACOG Practice Patterns* No. 6, October 1997, pp 1–5.

17 ANTEPARTUM FETAL ASSESSMENT

Patrick Duff

PURPOSE

- The principal purpose of antepartum fetal assessment is to identify the fetus that is in imminent danger of dying in utero because of a compromised blood supply due to impaired perfusion of the placenta or umbilical cord compression.

INDICATIONS

- The most common indications for antepartum fetal assessment are:
  ○ Decreased fetal movement
  ○ Insulin-dependent diabetes
  ○ Hypertension (chronic hypertension, gestational hypertension, preeclampsia)
  ○ Suspected intrauterine growth restriction
  ○ Postterm pregnancy
- Other important indications for antepartum fetal assessment include but are not limited to:
  ○ Preterm premature rupture of membranes
  ○ Prior history of stillbirth
  ○ Prior history of abruptio placentae
  ○ Fetal anomaly
  ○ Sickle cell disease
  ○ Connective tissue disease
  ○ Multiple gestation
  ○ Oligohydramnios

TIMING OF ANTEPARTUM FETAL ASSESSMENT

- The timing of antepartum assessment must be individualized. As a general rule, the more high-risk the pregnancy, the earlier and more frequent the assessment.
- Antepartum assessment is usually not performed until delivery is considered a viable option (minimum of 24 weeks gestation).
- The usual interval of testing is 1 week.

COUNTING OF FETAL MOVEMENT

- Counting of fetal movement is simple and incurs no expense.
- Several different methods of accomplishing this have been described in published reports.
- One of the most common methods requires the mother to choose a quiet period of the day or evening and to monitor the length of time necessary to feel 10 fetal movements. If this period exceeds 2 h, the mother is directed to the hospital or office for additional testing.

NONSTRESS TEST (NST)

- The NST is the simplest and least expensive of the formal antepartum fetal assessment tests.
- It may be performed in the physician's office or in the labor and delivery suite.
- The test is based on the principle that a healthy, well-oxygenated fetus should have frequent accelerations in its heart rate, which are typically associated with movement.

- The patient should be positioned with the head of the bed elevated approximately 45 degrees. The external fetal heart rate monitor (Doppler) should be applied to the maternal abdomen so that a clear, uninterrupted fetal heart rate tracing is recorded for 20 min.
- The tracing is then interpreted in one of three ways:
  - **Reactive** (Fig. 17-1)
    - Two accelerations of the fetal heart rate are noted.
    - Each acceleration is at least 15 s in duration and at least 15 beats per minute above the baseline. (At gestational ages <32 weeks, the criteria for reactivity are two accelerations of 10 beats per minute for 10 s.)
    - The baseline fetal heart rate is normal (120 to 160 beats per minute) and no variable decelerations are present.
  - **Nonreactive** (Fig. 17-2)
    - Fewer than two accelerations are present or

- The accelerations are not 15 beats per minute above the baseline or 15 s in duration (10 beats per minute x 10 s if gestational age is <32 weeks).
  - **Suspicious** (Fig. 17-3)
    - Baseline bradycardia (<120 beats per minute) or tachycardia (>160 beats per minute) is present.
    - Variable decelerations are evident.
- A reactive NST is usually repeated within 3 to 7 days, depending on the severity of the patient's medical complication. A nonreactive or suspicious test requires either additional testing or delivery.

CONTRACTION STRESS TEST (CST)

- The CST exposes the fetus to the "stress" of a uterine contraction and then evaluates the response of the fetal heart. When the vascular supply to the fetus is

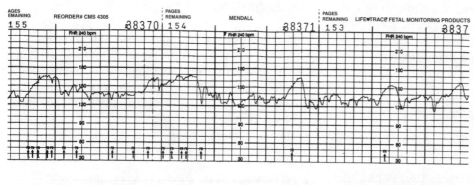
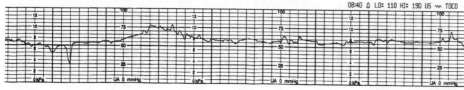

FIG. 17-1 Reactive nonstress test.

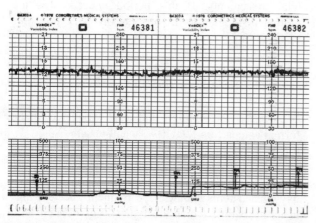

FIG. 17-2 Nonreactive nonstress test.

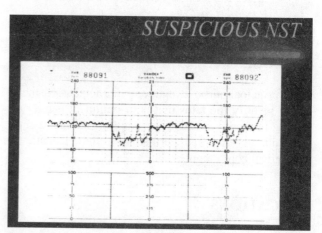

FIG. 17-3 Suspicious nonstress test. Note variable decelerations.

sufficiently compromised, the stress of a contraction may cause transient hypoxia, which will be manifest as a late deceleration.
- Contractions may be induced by administering oxytocin (**oxytocin challenge test**). Alternatively, the mother can stimulate her breast for approximately 30 s, thus triggering release of endogenous oxytocin (**nipple stimulation test**).
- The patient should be positioned as for the NST. Both the external fetal heart rate monitor and the tocodynamometer (contraction monitor) should be applied.
- The goal of testing is to induce three contractions within a 10-min period.
- The CST is interpreted in one of four ways:
  - **Negative-reactive** (Fig. 17-4)
    - No late decelerations occur.
    - At least one acceleration of 15 beats per minute x 15 s is present.
  - **Negative-nonreactive** (Fig. 17-5)
    - No late decelerations occur but no accelerations are present.
  - **Suspicious**
    - One of the contractions is associated with a late deceleration.
  - **Positive** (Fig. 17-6)
    - Two or three of the contractions are associated with late decelerations.

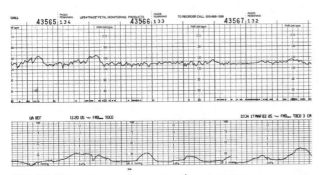
FIG. 17-4 Negative-reactive contraction stress test.

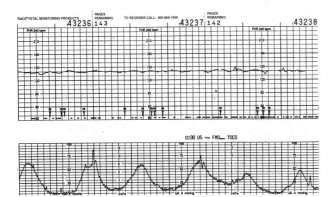
FIG. 17-5 Negative-nonreactive contraction stress test.

- A negative-reactive test is typically repeated in 1 week.
- A negative-nonreactive test should be repeated within 24 h.
- A suspicious or positive test is usually an indication for delivery.

BIOPHYSICAL PROFILE

- This test provides the most comprehensive assessment of fetal well-being.
- It is the most time-consuming and expensive of the antepartum assessment tests.
- The biophysical profile assesses the fetal heart rate tracing, fetal movement, fetal breathing, fetal tone, and volume of amniotic fluid (Table 17-1).
- A biophysical score of 8 or 10 is considered reassuring, and the test usually is repeated in 3 to 7 days.
- A biophysical score of 6 is indeterminate, and the test should be repeated within 24 h.
- A biophysical score of 0, 2, or 4 is omnious and almost always an indication for delivery.

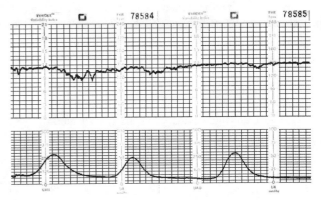
FIG. 17-6 Positive contraction stress test.

TABLE 17-1 The Biophysical Profile Score

VARIABLE	SCORE	
	2	0
NST	Reactive	Nonreactive
Fetal breathing movements	At least one breathing episode of >30 s in 30 min	Absent
Fetal movements	At least three discrete body or limb movements in 30 min	Less than three movements
Fetal tone	At least one episode of active flexion and extension of limb or trunk	Fetus is in a state of passive extension of limbs
Amniotic fluid volume	At least one vertical pocket of fluid >2 cm or Amniotic fluid index >5 cm	No vertical pocket of fluid >2 cm or Amniotic fluid index <5 cm

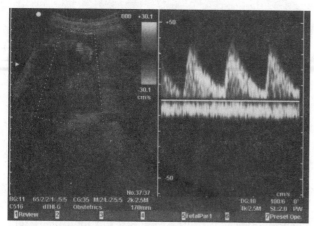

FIG. 17-7 Umbilical artery Doppler velocimetry—normal S/D.

UMBILICAL ARTERY DOPPLER VELOCIMETRY

- This test assesses the velocity of blood flow in the umbilical artery. It is of particular value in evaluating infants with suspected intrauterine growth restriction.
- A high resistance to blood flow in the umbilical artery circulation may be indicative of severe uteroplacental insufficiency.
- Under normal circumstances, blood flow in the umbilical artery still is present although decreased during diastole. In the latter part of third trimester, the usual systolic:diastolic ratio (S/D) is <3:1 (Fig. 17-7).
- If the S/D exceeds 3:1 and any other assessment test is nonreassuring, delivery is usually indicated.
- If Doppler velocimetry shows absent or reverse end-diastolic flow, delivery is virtually always indicated.

BIBLIOGRAPHY

American College of Obstetricians and Gynecologists. Antepartum fetal surveillance. *ACOG Pract Bull* No. 9, October 1999, pp. 1–11.

18   INTRAPARTUM FETAL ASSESSMENT

Patrick Duff

PURPOSE

- The purpose of intrapartum assessment is to identify the "stressed" or "compromised" fetus who is in imminent danger of death or severe brain injury due to asphyxia and who, therefore, will benefit from immediate delivery.

TYPES OF INTRAPARTUM ASSESSMENT

- Intermittent auscultation
- Continuous electronic assessment

INTERMITTENT AUSCULTATION

- Intermittent auscultation is a labor-intensive process that requires virtual one-on-one nursing support. Nevertheless, it can produce neonatal outcomes equivalent to those achieved with continuous electronic assessment, particularly in low-risk patients.
- The fetal heart tones may be ausculted with a doptone or fetoscope.
- Fetal heart tones should be assessed every 15 min during the first stage of labor and after every contraction during the second stage.

CONTINUOUS ELECTRONIC ASSESSMENT

- If the fetal heart rate is not reassuring, continuous electronic assessment should be performed.

METHODOLOGY OF ELECTRONIC FETAL HEART RATE ASSESSMENT

- The **external assessment** system employs a doptone to assess fetal heart rate and a tocodynamometer to detect uterine contractions (Fig. 18-1).

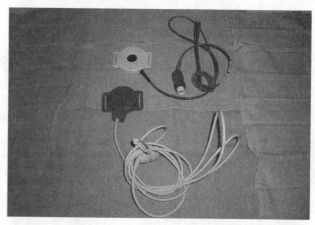

FIG. 18-1 External assessment devices: doptone and tocodynamometer.

- ○ The new Doppler instrumentation is remarkably sophisticated and can produce a clear, consistent heart rate tracing in virtually all patients except those who are morbidly obese.
- ○ The tocodynamometer provides an accurate record of frequency and duration of contractions. However, it cannot quantitate the magnitude of individual contractions.
- The **internal assessment** system employs a scalp electrode to record fetal heart rate and an intrauterine pressure catheter to document the frequency, duration, and magnitude of uterine contractions (Fig. 18-2).

COMPLICATIONS OF ELECTRONIC FETAL HEART RATE ASSESSMENT

- Essentially no complications are associated with the external assessment system.
- Approximately 0.5 percent of infants will develop a localized infection at the site of attachment of the scalp electrode. In very rare circumstances, bacteremia or viremia results from such an infection.
- The intrauterine pressure catheter slightly increases the risk of chorioamnionitis.

INTERPRETATION OF ELECTRONIC FETAL HEART RATE PATTERNS

BASELINE HEART RATE

- The normal baseline heart rate is 120 to 160 beats per minute (bpm)

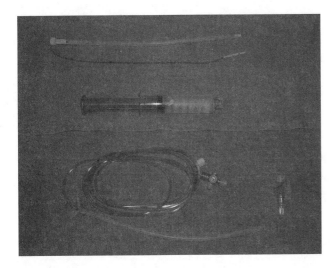

FIG. 18-2 Internal assessment devices: fetal scalp electrode and intrauterine pressure catheter.

- The principal causes of **fetal tachycardia** ($>$160 bpm) (Fig. 18-3) are as follows:
  - ○ Maternal fever
  - ○ Hypoxia
  - ○ Maternal hyperthyroidism
  - ○ Fetal arrhythmia (supraventricular tachycardia)
  - ○ Maternal drugs (eg, betamimetics)
- The principal causes of **fetal bradycardia** ($<$120 bpm) (Fig. 18-4) are as follows:
  - ○ Hypoxia
  - ○ Fetal arrhythmia (heart block)
  - ○ Maternal drugs (e.g. beta blockers)

FETAL HEART RATE VARIABILITY

- Normally, the fetal heart rate varies by approximately 5 to 15 bpm.
- Variability in the heart rate results from a fine interplay between the sympathetic and parasympathetic nervous systems.
- The principal causes of **diminished or absent variability** (Fig. 18-5) are as follows:
  - ○ Fetal sleep
  - ○ Hypoxia
  - ○ Tachycardia
  - ○ Maternal drugs (eg, analgesics and sedatives)

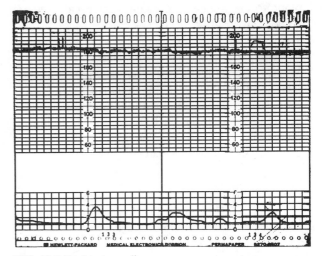

FIG. 18-3 Fetal tachycardia.

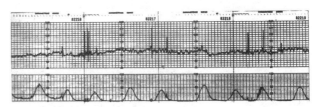

FIG. 18-4 Fetal bradycardia.

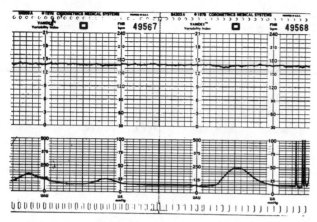

FIG. 18-5 Decreased fetal heart rate variability.

- The principal cause of **exaggerated variability** is transient hypoxia. This type of pattern is typically seen during the second stage of labor, coincident with maternal Valsalva maneuvers (Fig. 18-6).

PERIODIC DECELERATIONS

EARLY DECELERATIONS (FIG. 18-7)
- Early decelerations result from pressure on the fetal head, leading to activation of the vagus nerve and a reflex slowing of the heart rate.
- Early decelerations are not typically associated with other fetal heart rate abnormalities and usually require no corrective action.

VARIABLE DECELERATIONS (FIG. 18-8)
- Variable decelerations result from compression of the fetal umbilical cord, resulting in transient hypoxia.
  - Severe variable decelerations are particularly omnious and are defined by any of the following criteria:
    - Deceleration to less than 60 bpm

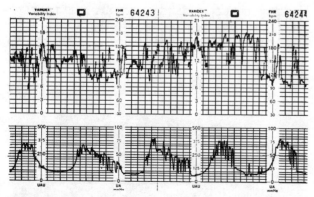

FIG. 18-6 Increased fetal heart rate variability (saltatory or "leaping" pattern).

- Deceleration more than 60 bpm below baseline
- Duration of the deceleration is >60 seconds.
  - Initial management of variable decelerations:
    - Rotate mother to left or right side in an attempt to relieve cord compression.
    - Administer oxygen by face mask.
    - Perform amnioinfusion (infusion of normal saline into the uterine cavity via the pressure catheter).
  - If the variable decelerations persist, either scalp pH assessment or delivery is indicated, depending on the patient's progress in labor.

LATE DECELERATIONS (FIG. 18-9)
- Late decelerations result from impaired perfusion of the fetoplacental unit during a uterine contraction (uteroplacental insufficiency, or UPI).
- Classification of late decelerations:
  - **Mild** deceleration is <15 bpm below baseline.
  - **Moderate** deceleration is 15 to 45 bpm below baseline.

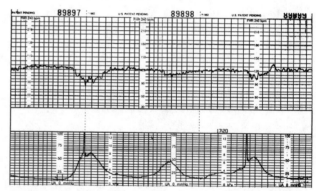

FIG. 18-7 Early decelerations.

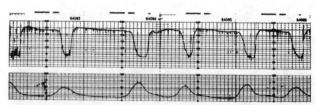

FIG. 18-8 Severe variable decelerations.

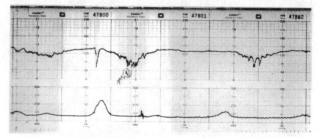

FIG. 18-9 Late decelerations.

○ **Severe** deceleration is >45 bpm below baseline.
- Management of late decelerations:
  ○ Position mother on her left side.
  ○ Administer oxygen by face mask.
  ○ Correct maternal hypotension, if present.
  ○ Perform fetal scalp pH assessment or deliver the patient, depending upon progress in labor.

SINUSOIDAL FETAL HEART RATE PATTERN (FIG. 18-10)

- The etiologies of the sinusoidal wave form include:
  ○ Fetal anemia
  ○ Hypoxia
  ○ Chorioamnionitis
  ○ Maternal narcotics
- Management
  ○ Position mother on her left side.
  ○ Administer oxygen by face mask
  ○ Perform fetal scalp pH assessment or deliver the patient, depending upon progress in labor.

SCALP PH ASSESSMENT

- Scalp pH assessment is appropriate in highly select circumstances:
  ○ If the fetal heart rate is nonreassuring but not ominous and the patient is progressing rapidly in labor.
- A sample of capillary blood is obtained by puncturing the superficial layer of the scalp with a small scalpel. The blood is collected into a long thin capillary tube and then processed through a microanalyzer.
- The interpretation and management of scalp pH determinations is summarized in Table 18-1.
- An alternative to fetal scalp sampling is fetal scalp stimulation. The fetal scalp can be stimulated with

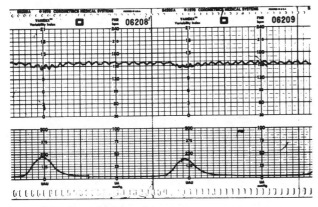

FIG. 18-10 Sinusoidal waveform.

TABLE 18-1   Interpretation of Scalp pH Determinations

pH	INTERPRETATION	MANAGEMENT
>7.25	Reassuring	Manage expectantly
7.20–7.25	Problematic	Attempt to correct fetal heart rate abnormalities Repeat in 20–30 min
<7.20 or declining from prior value of 7.20–7.25		Deliver immediately

the blunt end of an amniohook or the tip of the examiner's finger. A fetal heart rate acceleration of greater than or equal to 15 bpm after stimulation usually correlates closely with a reassuring fetal scalp pH.

BIBLIOGRAPHY

American College of Obstetricians and Gynecologists. Fetal heart rate patterns: Monitoring, interpretation, and management. *ACOG Tech Bull* No. 207, July 1995, pp 1–6.

19 LABOR AND DELIVERY

Rodney K. Edwards

- **Labor** is the process by which uterine contractions cause effacement and dilation of the cervix. This process results in expulsion of the fetus from the uterus (delivery or **parturition**). When labor and delivery occur at term (37.0 to 41.9 weeks of gestation), they represent a normal physiologic event.
- Labor (term or preterm) is diagnosed clinically in the presence of regular uterine contractions and progressive cervical effacement and dilation. Neither contractions nor cervical change alone meet the definition. The precise onset of labor is often difficult to determine, as women may have episodic contractions in the weeks prior to labor. In addition, the cervix may begin to soften, efface, and dilate weeks or even months prior to the onset of labor.

MECHANISM OF LABOR

- The factors that initiate spontaneous labor in humans are unknown.
  ○ The process probably involves a multitude of endocrine and inflammatory mediators and has inherent redundancy.

○ The final common pathway is characterized by increased concentrations of prostaglandins E_2 and $F_{2\alpha}$ in the decidua and uteroplacental circulation.

- As pregnancy progresses, the number of gap junctions between myometrial cells increase. These intercellular electrical communications result in coordinated uterine contractions.

PROGRESSION OF LABOR

- The course of labor is divided into three functional stages.
  - ○ The **first stage** of labor is the interval between the onset of labor and complete cervical dilation. The first stage is further divided into two phases. The **latent phase** occurs first and is associated with relatively slow cervical dilation. The **active phase** usually begins at a cervical dilation of 3 to 5 cm and is associated with more rapid cervical dilation.
  - ○ The **second stage** of labor begins with full cervical dilation and ends with delivery of the infant.
  - ○ The **third stage** encompasses the time between delivery of the infant and delivery of the placenta.
  - ○ The normal durations of the stages of labor vary by parity and are presented in Table 19-1. For all patients, the normal duration of the third stage of labor should be less than 30 min.
- For the 95 percent of fetuses at term that are in vertex presentations, passage through the birth canal occurs with seven **cardinal movements of labor**, directed by the force of uterine contractions. These movements should be thought of as a continuum, not a series of distinct steps.
  - ○ **Engagement** occurs when the biparietal diameter of the fetus descends below the pelvic inlet. Clinically, this condition may be diagnosed when the presenting vertex is palpated at or below the ischial spines (0 station). Particularly in nulliparas, engagement may occur prior to the onset of labor.
  - ○ **Descent** through the birth canal occurs primarily during the latter parts of the first stage and during the second stage of labor.
  - ○ **Flexion** of the fetal head allows the smallest diameter of the fetal head to present to the maternal pelvis.
  - ○ **Internal rotation** of the head into the hollow of the sacrum occurs to maintain presentation of the smallest diameter of the fetal head to the maternal pelvis as further descent occurs. This movement is necessary because the birth canal at the midpelvis is wider in its anteroposterior diameter than in its transverse diameter. The opposite relationship is true for the pelvic inlet.
  - ○ **Extension** of the fetal head occurs as it traverses the introitus.
  - ○ **External rotation** of the fetal head occurs after delivery of the head to return to neutral position relative to the shoulders, which are located in an anteroposterior orientation.
  - ○ **Expulsion** is the final delivery of the fetus from the birth canal. Once delivery of the shoulders is achieved, the remainder of the infant readily is expelled.

LABOR INDUCTION

- When an indication exists that warrants delivery prior to spontaneous labor, methods aimed at medical induction of labor may be undertaken. Assessment of the cervix prior to labor induction aids in decisions regarding whether labor induction is prudent and what method to choose. In 1964, Bishop described a system for evaluating the cervix. This scoring system is presented in Table 19-2. Although the scoring system was originally developed for parous women, many clinicians extrapolate use of the **Bishop score** to nulliparous women undergoing labor induction.
- **Clinical pelvimetry** is the process whereby the diameters of the pelvic inlet, midpelvis, and pelvic outlet are estimated by palpation. Four prototypes of pelvic shape have been described. The gynecoid pelvis is the

TABLE 19-1 Mean and Upper/Lower Limit of Normal for Stages and Phases of Labor

GROUP	LATENT PHASE (HOURS)	ACTIVE PHASE (CM/HOUR)	SECOND STAGE (HOURS)
Nulliparous			
Mean	6	3	1
Limit	20	1.2	2[a]
Parous			
Mean	5	6	0.4
Limit	14	1.5	1[a]

[a]Add one hour if the patient is receiving epidural analgesia.

TABLE 19-2 Bishop Score for Assessing the Cervix Prior to Labor Induction[a]

FACTOR	SCORE			
	0	1	2	3
Dilation (cm)	Closed	1–2	3–4	≥5
Effacement (%)	0–30	40–50	60–70	≥80
Station (−3 to +3 scale)	−3	−2	−1 or 0	+1 or lower
Consistency	Firm	Medium	Soft	—
Position	Posterior	Mid	Anterior	—

[a]A score of 6 or more is considered favorable.

most common and most conducive to vaginal delivery. Other types include anthropoid, android, and platypelloid (Fig. 19-1A-D).

- **Oxytocin** is an octapeptide that is released from the posterior pituitary. It has traditionally been the most common agent used to induce or augment labor.
  - Oxytocin is administered in a dilute intravenous infusion and has a half-life in the circulation of 5 to 10 min.
  - Uterine hyperstimulation is the most common side effect. Since oxytocin is structurally similar to antidiuretic hormone, another posterior pituitary product, water retention may occur with prolonged or high-dose administration.
  - For labor induction, oxytocin is most useful when the patient has a favorable cervix.
  - Oxytocin is also used to augment labor in patients who have dysfunctional labor patterns.
- Owing to their place in the final common pathway of spontaneous labor, **prostaglandins** (PGs) have been investigated as agents of labor induction. These agents are most useful in undertaking labor induction in a woman with an unfavorable cervix.
  - Multiple formulations of PGE_2 are available (gel, pessary, tablet).
  - Misoprostol, a synthetic PGE_1 analogue, was originally developed to treat gastrointestinal ulcers. This agent is comparable to or better than PGE_2 in terms of efficacy, safety, and side-effect profile. In addition, misoprostol is markedly less expensive than PGE_2 preparations. Misoprostol may be administered orally or vaginally. The most common dose is 25 µg vaginally. This dosage may be repeated in 3 to 4 h, depending on the patient's contraction pattern.
  - Like oxytocin, prostaglandins may cause uterine hyperstimulation. These agents should not be used for labor induction at or near term in patients with a prior uterine incision, as the likelihood of uterine rupture is increased.
- Amniotomy (artificial rupture of the membranes) was the first method used to facilitate labor. Today, it is rarely used in isolation for labor induction. However, amniotomy increases the likelihood of successful induction in patients who are receiving oxytocin.

LABOR ABNORMALITIES

- Plotting a labor curve aids the management of labor by facilitating the diagnosis of labor abnormalities. Figure 19-2 displays the graph used for this purpose at our center.
- A **prolonged latent phase** occurs when the duration of this phase exceeds the upper limit of normal, as

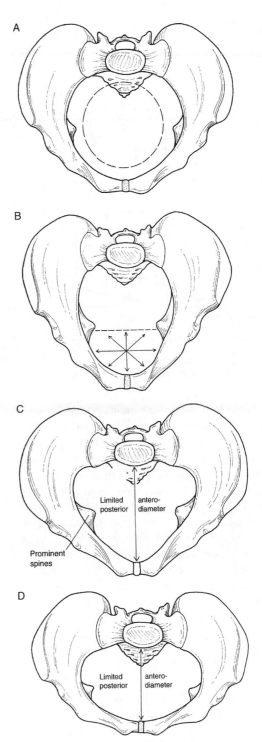

FIG. 19-1 The four basic types of pelves are illustrated. The gynecoid pelvis (A) is the most common type. It has a rounded inlet and generous anteroposterior and transverse diameters. The anthropoid pelvis (B) has a limited capacity anteriorly and often predisposes to a persistent occiput posterior position. The android pelvis (C), like the anthropoid pelvis, has convergent side walls and prominent spines. However, it also has a limited anteroposterior diameter. Finally, the most striking characteristic of the platypelloid pelvis (D) is its contracted anteroposterior dimension. This type of pelvis predisposes to occiput transverse positions.

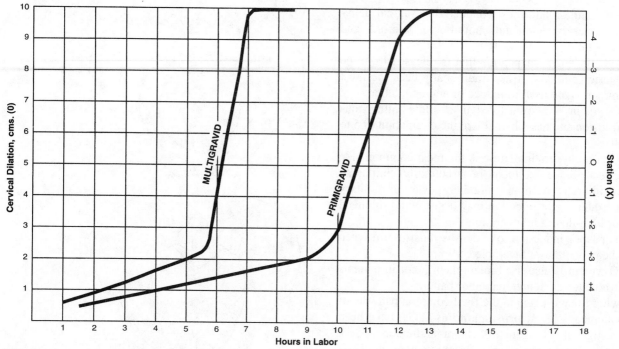

FIG. 19-2 Labor curve of cervical dilation over time.

shown in Table 19-1. Because patients presenting with this labor abnormality are usually exhausted, either expectant management or labor augmentation may be ill-fated. The best course of action is usually induction of therapeutic rest with narcotics (eg, morphine sulfate 4 mg intravenously and 12 mg intramuscularly). Women will usually awaken from such sedation either without contractions or in the active phase of labor. Either way, the gravida will be better rested than when she presented to the labor and delivery unit.

• A **protracted active phase** occurs when the rate of cervical dilation in the active phase is less than the lower limit of normal shown in Table 19-1. Since digitial cervical examination is rather imprecise, this clinical diagnosis should be made when, in the active phase, there is less than 2 cm of cervical dilation over 2 h. Figure 19-3 shows a labor curve for a patient with a protracted active phase.

• **Arrest of dilation in the active phase** is defined as the absence of further cervical dilation over 2 h in the active phase. Figure 19-4 shows a labor curve for a patient with an arrest of dilation. If arrest of dilation persists in the presence of adequate contractions achieved with oxytocin augmentation, cesarean delivery should be undertaken.

• Labor abnormalities also may occur in the second stage of labor. A **prolonged second stage** occurs when the duration of the second stage exceeds the upper limit of normal, as presented in Table 19-1. This abnormality does not necessarily require treatment.

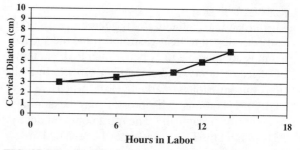

FIG. 19-3 Protracted active phase.

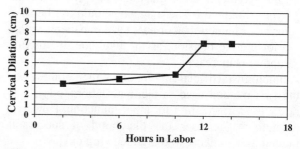

FIG. 19-4 Arrest of active phase.

However, it is associated with an increased likelihood of operative vaginal delivery or cesarean delivery.

• If no descent of the presenting part occurs over 1 h during the second stage, an **arrest of descent** has occurred. In this situation, operative vaginal delivery or cesarean delivery may be prudent.

• If the third stage of labor exceeds 30 min in duration, the patient has a **prolonged third stage**. Prolongation of the third stage is associated with increased blood loss, need for uterine curettage, and placenta accreta.

SPONTANEOUS VAGINAL DELIVERY

- At all deliveries, the attendants should be prepared not only to assist in the delivery but also to provide immediate neonatal cardiorespiratory support if needed.
- As the fetal head undergoes extension, support of the perineal body by the birth attendant helps to prevent or minimize perineal lacerations. Avoiding rapid expulsion at all points during the delivery also minimizes vaginal and perineal lacerations.
- Once the head delivers, the nasopharynx and oropharynx are cleared of amniotic fluid and mucus with a suction bulb (or catheter if meconium is present). The head undergoes external rotation, and the neck should be palpated to detect a nuchal cord, which should be either reduced or clamped and transected.
- With hands on the fetal parietal bones, the attendant should apply gentle downward pressure to achieve delivery of the anterior shoulder. After delivery of the anterior shoulder, pressure should be redirected upward to achieve delivery of the posterior shoulder. Once the shoulders traverse the introitus, the rest of the infant delivers easily.

SHOULDER DYSTOCIA

- When the fetal head delivers but the remainder of the fetus does not readily deliver with standard maneuvers, a **shoulder dystocia** has occurred. This situation often is diagnosed by recognition of the "turtle sign," where the fetal head retracts against the mother's vulva and perineum.
- The majority of cases of shoulder dystocia can be relieved with McRobert's maneuver (hyperflexion of the maternal hips) and suprapubic pressure. In more difficult cases of shoulder dystocia, rotational maneuvers, delivery of the posterior arm, or cephalic replacement and cesarean delivery may be required.
- Overly aggressive downward traction on the fetal head should be avoided. Such action may stretch the superior portion of the brachial plexus of the anterior shoulder and cause the infant to have an Erb's palsy. Most but not all cases of Erb's palsy resolve within 3 months of delivery.
- As discussed in Chap. 7C, infants born to diabetic mothers are at increased risk of macrosomia and shoulder dystocia.

UTERINE INVERSION

- **Uterine inversion** is an uncommon complication of the third stage of labor. It can result in massive hemorrhage and shock.
- Risk factors for uterine inversion include fundal implantation of the placenta, excessive traction on the umbilical cord during the third stage of labor, and excessive use of uterine relaxing agents. However, this complication may occur in the absence of any risk factor.
- If uterine inversion occurs, the placenta should be left in place and gentle force applied with the operator's hand to replace the inverted uterine fundus. If uterine relaxation is necessary to allow replacement of the inverted fundus, nitroglycerin, 0.4 to 0.8 mg sublingually or 50 to 200 µg intravenously, or a 4-g intravenous bolus of magnesium sulfate may achieve enough uterine relaxation to allow replacement.
- Once the uterine fundus has been returned to its original position, the placenta should be extracted manually provided that the patient is hemodynamically stable. Since placenta accreta may be present, the delivery team should be prepared to proceed with hysterectomy if necessary.

REPAIR OF VAGINAL LACERATIONS AND EPISIOTOMY

- An **episiotomy** is a relaxing incision in the perineum. The two types are the **median** (in the midline from the perineum toward the anus) and **mediolateral** (directed obliquely from the posterior fourchette). In the prior century, these incisions were advocated as a way to minimize perineal trauma associated with vaginal delivery.
- In actuality, episiotomy is associated with an increased likelihood of third- and fourth-degree lacerations (involving the rectal sphincter or rectal sphincter and rectal mucosa, respectively). Therefore, episiotomy is currently used in more selective situations today. Examples of indications would be hastening delivery in the setting of a nonreassuring fetal heart rate tracing or when maternal expulsive efforts are insufficient to achieve delivery of the fetal head.
- Repair of a median episiotomy or second-degree laceration (involving the vaginal mucosa and/or perineal skin and the underlying muscular tissue) may be accomplished in multiple ways. Typically, a #3-0 absorbable suture (eg, polyglactin, polyglycolic acid, or chromic) is used to reapproximate the subcutaneous vaginal tissue and the vaginal mucosa and per-

ineal skin. The goal of the repair is to restore normal anatomy of the perineum and hymen.

- Repair of more significant perineal lacerations or episiotomy extensions is similar. In the case of a fourth-degree laceration, the rectal mucosa is reapproximated with #4-0 absorbable suture. One or two submucosal layers of #3-0 absorbable sutures are then placed. Three to four interrupted #0 absorbable sutures are used to reapproximate the rectal sphincter. The repair then proceeds as a second-degree closure. Improper repair of a third-or fourth-degree laceration may lead to wound breakdown, infection, rectovaginal fistula, or fecal incontinence.

BIBLIOGRAPHY

Chow GE, Yancey MK. Labor and delivery: Normal and abnormal. In: Ling FW, Duff P, eds. *Obstetrics & Gynecology: Principles for Practice.* New York: McGraw-Hill, 2001.

Norwitz ER, Robinson JN, Repke JT. Labor and delivery. In: Gabbe SG, Niebyl JR, Simpson JL, eds. *Obstetrics: Normal and Problem Pregnancies,* 4th ed. New York: Churchill Livingstone, 2002.

20   OPERATIVE VAGINAL DELIVERY

Rodney K. Edwards

BACKGROUND

- Obstetric forceps are paired metal instruments designed to hasten vaginal delivery by applying direct traction on the fetal skull. Vacuum extractors are suction cup–like devices that indirectly produce traction on the skull by applying traction to the fetal scalp. Figure 20-1 shows some commonly used obstetric forceps and a type of vacuum extractor.
- The choice between obstetric forceps and a vacuum extractor for accomplishing an operative vaginal delivery is largely based on operator experience and preference; the indications, prerequisites, and classification of operations are similar. Use of the vacuum extractor is contraindicated for delivery of an infant of less than 36 weeks' gestation and is not appropriate for deliveries requiring rotation of the fetal head to achieve delivery.

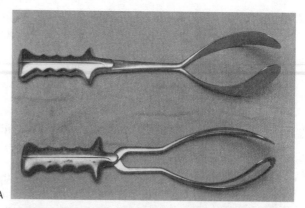

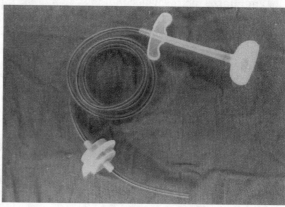

FIG. 20-1 Commonly used obstetric forceps and a type of vacuum extractor. *A.* Tucker-McLane (top) and Simpson (bottom) forceps. *B.* Mityvac "M cup."

- Any operative vaginal delivery may be inappropriate in certain circumstances. An example is the fetus with a bleeding disorder.

INDICATIONS

- The most common indications for operative vaginal delivery are summarized in Table 20-1.
- No indication for operative vaginal delivery is absolute. The option of cesarean delivery should be considered and should be available if attempts at operative vaginal delivery are unsuccessful.

PREREQUISITES

- All of the following prerequisites must be met before attempting an operative vaginal delivery:
  ○ The fetal head is engaged.
  ○ The cervix is fully dilated.
  ○ The position of the fetal head is known with certainty.
  ○ The membranes are ruptured.
  ○ The operator has deemed that cephalopelvic disproportion is not present.

TABLE 20-1   Indications for Operative Vaginal Delivery

INDICATION	EXAMPLES
Fetal	Nonreassuring heart rate tracing
	Aftercoming head of a breech
Maternal	Exhaustion
	Bleeding
	Contraindication to Valsalva maneuver (eg, cardiac disease)
Combined fetal and maternal	Arrest of descent at a low station
	Prolonged second stage of labor

- ○ The maternal bladder has been emptied.
- ○ An experienced operator is present.
- ○ Finally and most importantly, there must be a willingness to abandon attempts if the delivery does not proceed readily.
- Prior to an operative vaginal delivery, the patient should have appropriate anesthesia. At a minimum, a pudendal block should be placed prior to a low or outlet delivery. Midpelvic deliveries and deliveries requiring significant rotation of the fetal head should be attempted only in patients who have received a regional anesthetic, such as an epidural or spinal block.

CLASSIFYING OPERATIONS

- Operative vaginal deliveries should be classified according to the 1988 American College of Obstetricians and Gynecologists (ACOG) classification. This system was designed to describe forceps deliveries, but the categories (except for rotation >45 degrees) apply equally well to vacuum extractions. The 1988 ACOG classification is shown in Table 20-2. Note that "high" forceps or vacuum deliveries of fetuses that are not engaged in the pelvis are not included in the classification. These operations should not be performed because they may cause severe fetal and maternal injury.
- The likelihood of adverse maternal or neonatal outcome is directly related to the station of the fetal head and the amount of rotation involved. It is important to consider that the maternal laceration rate with cesarean delivery is 100 percent and that maternal transfusion and infection rates are both higher with cesarean compared to operative vaginal delivery.

TECHNIQUE

- A detailed discussion of the technique used to perform operative vaginal deliveries is beyond the scope of this book.
- Attempts at forceps delivery should be abandoned when moderate traction force does not result in any gain in station.

TABLE 20-2   Classification of Forceps Deliveries According to Station and Rotation

TYPE OF DELIVERY	CHARACTERISTICS
Outlet forceps	The scalp is visible between contractions without separating the labia
	The fetal skull has reached the pelvic floor
	Position of the fetal head is ≤45 degrees from direct occiput anterior or posterior
Low forceps	Leading point of the fetal skull is at station +2 cm or lower but the delivery does not qualify as outlet
	Separated into deliveries requiring ≤45 degrees rotation and those requiring >45 degrees rotation
Midforceps	Station above +2 cm but the head is engaged (at or below the ischial spines)

- Multiple (more than three) "pop offs" with a vacuum extractor should lead the operator to abandon the attempt at vaginal delivery. Prolonged application (greater than a total of 15 min of suction) of the vacuum extractor to the fetal scalp should be avoided. The pressure in the vacuum cup should be released between contractions.

CHOOSING AN INSTRUMENT

- The choice between forceps and vacuum is largely based on operator experience and preference. Choice of type of forceps is based on the condition of the fetal head.
- Forceps with a longer, more tapered cephalic curve are desired for the delivery of fetuses with molded heads. This situation exists more commonly when the mother is nulliparous. Examples of appropriate forceps in this situation would be a Simpson type with or without the Luikart modification.
- When minimal molding is present (the usual situation with multiparas), forceps with a shorter, more rounded cephalic curve are appropriate. Examples of these instruments are Elliot or Tucker-McLane forceps.
- When rotation in excess of about 60 degrees is required, Kielland forceps (which are unique in that there is no pelvic curve) are the most common choice.
- Instruments such as Bill's traction handle (Fig. 20-2) can provide assistance with axis traction.

COMPLICATIONS

- Both forceps and vacuum extraction deliveries are associated with lacerations of the maternal lower gen-

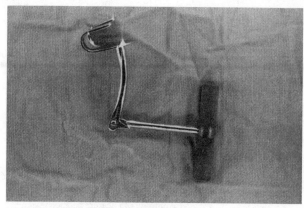

FIG. 20-2 Bill's traction handle, a device designed to assist with correct axis traction for forceps deliveries.

ital tract. These injuries are more common with forceps deliveries, particularly with decreasing operator experience.

• Compared with forceps delivery, the vacuum extractor is associated with an increased incidence of neonatal cephalohematoma, retinal hemorrhages, and jaundice. Although rare, fetal skull fractures and facial nerve palsies are more common with forceps than with vacuum extraction deliveries.

• Shoulder dystocia is more common with operative than spontaneous vaginal deliveries.

BIBLIOGRAPHY

American College of Obstetricians and Gynecologists. Operative vaginal delivery. *ACOG Pract Bull* No. 17, June 2000.

Bofill JA. Operative delivery by vacuum. In: Gilstrap LC III, Cunningham FG, VanDorsten JP, eds. *Operative Obstetrics,* 2d ed. New York: McGraw-Hill, 2002.

Gilstrap LC III. Forceps delivery. In: Gilstrap LC III, Cunningham FG, VanDorsten JP, eds. *Operative Obstetrics,* 2d ed. New York: McGraw-Hill, 2002.

21 MALPRESENTATION AND SHOULDER DYSTOCIA

Patrick Duff

INTRODUCTION

• This chapter focuses on four major malpresentations—breech, face, brow, and transverse lie—and shoulder dystocia.

BREECH PRESENTATION

FREQUENCY

• The frequency of breech presentation at term is 3 to 4 percent.
• The frequency is higher in preterm gestations.

CLASSIFICATION

FRANK BREECH
• The thighs are flexed, the lower legs are extended, and the buttocks are presenting ("jack-knife" position) (Fig. 21-1).
• This is the most common type of breech presentation.

COMPLETE BREECH
• The thighs are flexed, the lower legs are flexed, and the buttocks and heels are presenting ("cross-legged" sitting position) (Fig. 21-2).
• This type of breech presentation usually converts to an incomplete breech during labor.

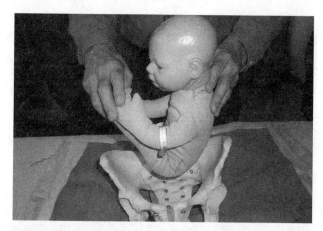

FIG. 21-1 Frank breech presentation.

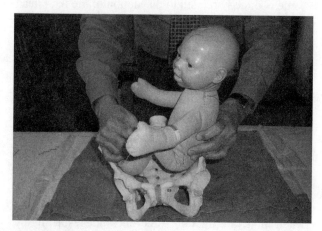

FIG. 21-2 Complete breech presentation.

INCOMPLETE BREECH

- Both the thigh and lower leg are extended.
- The presentation may be either a **single footling** (Fig. 21-3) or **double footling** (Fig. 21-4).

PREDISPOSING FACTORS

- Prematurity
- Multiple gestation
- Uterine anomaly
- Fetal anomaly—eg, anencephaly, hydrocephalus, neck mass
- Polyhydramnios
- Placenta previa

DIAGNOSIS

- On abdominal examination (Leopold's maneuvers), the fetal head is palpated in the upper portion of the uterus

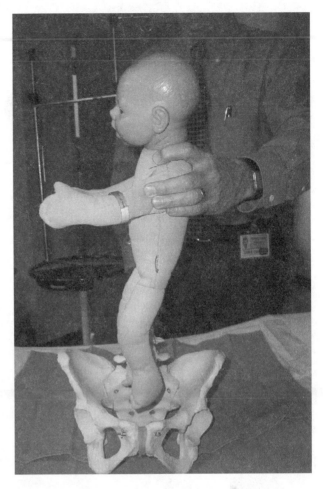

FIG. 21-4 Incomplete breech presentation—double footling.

and the fetal heart tones are heard in one of the upper quadrants, usually on the same side as the fetal back.
- On vaginal examination, "soft parts" (the fetal buttocks and genitalia) are palpated through the cervix.
- The diagnosis is confirmed by ultrasound examination.

MANAGEMENT

- When the diagnosis is made at ≥37 weeks of gestation, an **external cephalic version** should be attempted if there is no contraindication to the procedure or contraindication to subsequent vaginal delivery.
  - This maneuver should be performed in the labor and delivery suite.
  - A nonstress test (NST) should be performed prior to the version to assess fetal well-being.
  - The procedure is usually performed after administration of a tocolytic, such as terbutaline or magnesium sulfate. Alternatively, it can be performed under epidural anesthesia.

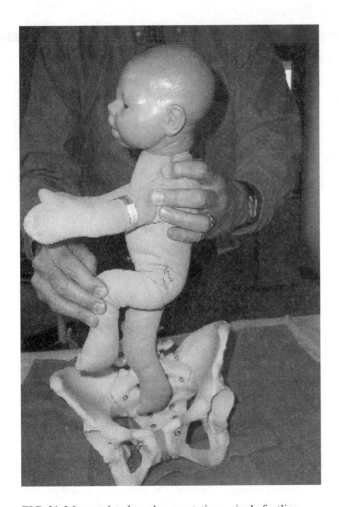

FIG. 21-3 Incomplete breech presentation—single footling.

○ The maneuvers used for the version are either a "forward roll" or "back flip."

○ The probability of success is 50 to 70 percent.

○ Contraindications to version include the following:

- Fetal macrosomia
- Nonreassuring fetal heart rate tracing
- Oligohydramnios
- Uterine anomaly
- Fetal anomaly
- Placenta previa
- Advanced labor

• As a general rule, external cephalic version should not be performed prior to 37 weeks because of the high probability of spontaneous version.

• If version is unsuccessful or the patient presents in advanced labor, a cesarean delivery should be performed.

• A recent multicenter, randomized, controlled trial demonstrated that term breech infants delivered by cesarean had fewer adverse outcomes than those delivered vaginally (see "Bibliography," below).

• Multiple retrospective investigations have demonstrated greater fetal safety with cesarean delivery in preterm gestations.

FACE PRESENTATION

FREQUENCY

• The frequency of face presentation is 1:300 to 1:600 deliveries.

CLASSIFICATION

• **Mentum anterior**—the chin points anteriorly (Fig. 21-5).

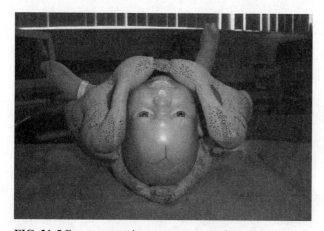

FIG. 21-5 Face presentation, mentum—anterior.

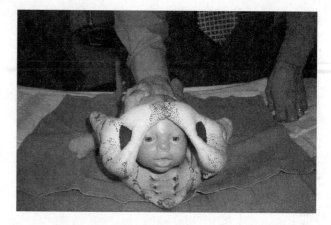

FIG. 21-6 Face presentation, mentum—posterior.

• **Mentum posterior**—the chin points posteriorly (Fig. 21-6).

PREDISPOSING FACTORS

• Prematurity
• Macrosomia
• Anencephaly
• Grand multiparity
• Cephalopelvic disproportion

DIAGNOSIS

• The diagnosis should be suspected when "soft parts" are palpated through the cervix.

• Face presentation must be differentiated from brow presentation, breech presentation, and anencephaly.

• The diagnosis can usually be confirmed by ultrasound examination.

• If the ultrasound examination is indeterminate, an x-ray should be obtained to confirm the diagnosis.

MANAGEMENT

• Once the diagnosis is confirmed, a detailed ultrasound examination should be performed to exclude anatomic anomalies such as anencephaly.

• The prognosis for vaginal delivery is excellent if the mentum is anterior.

• Rotation from mentum posterior to mentum anterior may be delayed until late in labor. Therefore, if labor is progressing, a plan of expectant management should be followed.

• The goal of management is to achieve a spontaneous vaginal delivery. Operative vaginal delivery should not be attempted because of the risk of injury to the fetus.

- If labor fails to progress or rotation from mentum posterior to mentum anterior does not occur, cesarean delivery should be performed.
- A pediatrician should attend the delivery, because some infants may have laryngeal edema (resulting from hyperextension of the fetal head during labor) and may require airway support. In addition, some infants may have such extensive facial bruising that hyperbilirubinema develops.

BROW PRESENTATION

FREQUENCY

- The frequency of brow presentation is approximately 1:1500 deliveries.

CLASSIFICATION

- **Frontum anterior**—the brow points anteriorly (Fig. 21-7).
- **Frontum posterior**—the brow points posteriorly (Fig. 21-8).

PREDISPOSING FACTORS

- Prematurity
- Grand multiparity
- Cephalopelvic disproportion

DIAGNOSIS

- The diagnosis may be suspected on vaginal examination.

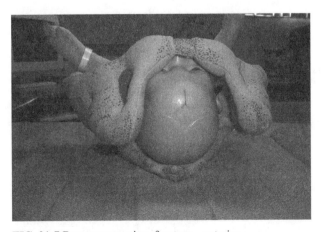

FIG. 21-7 Brow presentation, frontum—anterior.

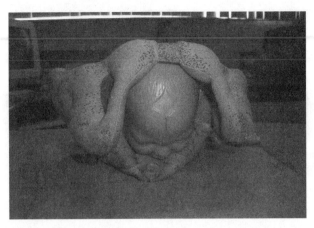

FIG. 21-8 Brow presentation, frontum—posterior.

- The diagnosis usually can be confirmed by ultrasound examination. If the ultrasound is indeterminate, an x-ray should be obtained.

MANAGEMENT

- Vaginal delivery with a persistent brow presentation is very unlikely unless the pelvis is unusually large or the infant unusually small.
- Fortunately, most brow presentations will spontaneously convert to either a face presentation or vertex.
- If the brow presentation persists, cesarean delivery should be performed. Operative vaginal delivery is contraindicated.

TRANSVERSE LIE

FREQUENCY

- The frequency of transverse lie is approximately 1:300.

CLASSIFICATION

- **Fetal back up** (Fig. 21-9)
- **Fetal back down** (Fig. 21-10)

PREDISPOSING FACTORS

- Grand multiparity
- Multiple gestation
- Polyhydramnios
- Prematurity
- Uterine anomaly
- Fetal anomaly

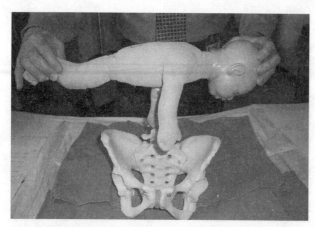

FIG. 21-9 Transverse lie, fetal back up.

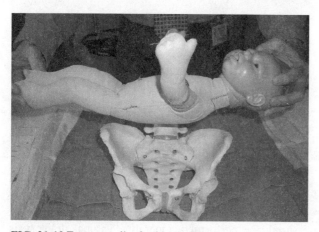

FIG. 21-10 Transverse lie, fetal back down.

- Placenta previa
- Cephalopelvic disproportion

DIAGNOSIS

- The diagnosis should be suspected on physical examination.
  - The uterus seems unusually wide.
  - No presenting part is palpated above the pubic symphysis.
- The diagnosis is confirmed by ultrasound examination.

MANAGEMENT

- If the diagnosis is made at ≥37 weeks of gestation and the patient is not in labor, an external version may be scheduled.
- If the diagnosis is made in labor (term or preterm) and delivery is likely, version can be attempted under epidural anesthesia.

- If version is unsuccessful, cesarean delivery must be performed.
  - If the fetal back is up, a low transverse uterine incision is acceptable.
  - If the fetal back is down, a classical uterine incision is indicated.

SHOULDER DYSTOCIA

DEFINITION

- **Shoulder dystocia** is defined as an unusual delay in delivery of the fetal shoulders.
- This complication results from impaction of the anterior shoulder behind the pubic symphysis.

FREQUENCY

- Shoulder dystocia occurs in approximately 1 to 2 percent of deliveries.

RISK FACTORS

- The principal risk factors for shoulder dystocia are those known to be associated with an increased frequency of fetal macrosomia.
  - Diabetes
  - Postterm pregnancy
  - Maternal obesity
  - Excessive maternal weight gain
- Other risk factors for shoulder dystocia are
  - Prolonged second stage of labor, particularly in a multiparous patient.
  - Instrumental delivery of the fetal head from the midpelvis.

PREVENTION

- A patient with a well-documented history of shoulder dystocia should be offered cesarean delivery in a subsequent pregnancy.
- When labor has been prolonged, especially the second stage, an operative vaginal delivery from the midpelvis should not be performed.
- When the estimated fetal weight by ultrasound exceeds 4500 g (4250 g if the mother has diabetes), a primary cesarean delivery should be strongly considered.

- Unfortunately, however, only about one-third of shoulder dystocias are suspected on the basis of clinical risk factors.
- Therefore the majority of shoulder dystocias can not be prevented. For this reason, the obstetric practitioner must be skilled in the recognition and management of this ominous complication.

DIAGNOSIS

- The typical manifestation of an imminent shoulder dystocia is the "turtle sign." This is characterized by delivery of the fetal head and then almost immediate retraction of the head back against the vaginal introitus and perineum (Fig. 21-11).
- The diagnosis is confirmed when simple downward traction on the fetal head fails to deliver the anterior shoulder beneath the pubic symphisis.

MANAGEMENT

- Shoulder dystocia is an acute obstetric emergency; the practitioner must be able to implement a sequence of interventions in a calm, deliberate manner.
  - The clinician should immediately call for assistance from both another obstetric provider and an anesthesiologist or nurse-anesthetist.
  - Gentle, sustained downward traction should be placed on the fetal head.
  - The mother's thighs should be flexed onto her abdomen (**McRoberts maneuver**). This maneuver widens the pelvic outlet slightly.
  - A large midline episiotomy should be made.
  - Suprapubic (not fundal) pressure should be applied. Fundal pressure will worsen the impaction of the anterior shoulder.

- If the dystocia does not resolve, an effort should be made to rotate the shoulders to an oblique plane. If rotation occurs, the anterior shoulder often drops beneath the pubic symphysis and delivery then is possible.
- If rotation into an oblique diameter of the pelvis is ineffective, the operator should place his or her hand into the vagina alongside the fetal back and try to rotate the baby 180 degrees, so that the anterior shoulder falls below the pubic symphysis into the posterior pelvis (**Wood's screw maneuver**) (Fig. 21-12).
- Alternatively, the operator can place a hand into the vagina alongside the fetal chest and attempt to deliver the posterior arm (Fig. 21-13). If successful, this maneuver permits the impacted anterior shoulder to drop beneath the pubic symphysis.
- If the measures outlined above fail, cephalic replacement (**Zavanelli maneuver**) should be attempted.
- If cephalic replacement is unsuccessful, the final intervention is to perform a laparotomy, open the

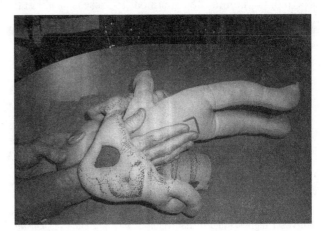

FIG. 21-12 Wood's screw maneuver.

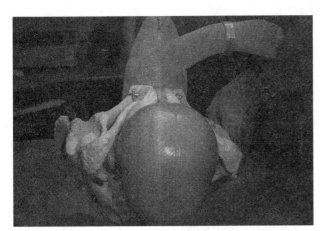

FIG. 21-11 "Turtle sign" indicative of impending shoulder dystocia.

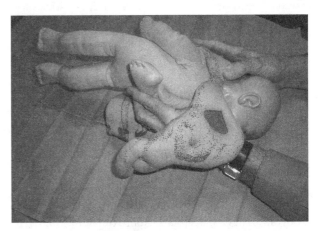

FIG. 21-13 Delivery of the posterior arm.

uterus, and then force the anterior shoulder beneath the pubic symphysis. The delivery is then completed vaginally.

○ After completion of the delivery, the obstetrician should prepare a detailed and accurate record of the exact sequence of maneuvers used to effect delivery and the time allotted to each one. The record should also contain a precise description of any fetal injuries or cardiopulmonary depression obvious at the time of delivery.

▪ **Brachial plexus injury**—This injury usually results from excessive lateral traction on the fetal head and neck. Fortunately, the majority of brachial plexus injuries are transient.

▪ **Fractured clavicle**—This injury usually occurs as the anterior shoulder negotiates beneath the pubic symphysis.

▪ **Fractured humerus**—The humerus is usually injured during efforts to deliver the posterior arm.

○ The Apgar scores at 1 and 5 min should be recorded.

○ Umbilical arterial and venous blood-gas measurements should be obtained to assess for fetal hypoxia.

BIBLIOGRAPHY

American College of Obstetricians and Gynecologists. External cephalic version. *ACOG Pract Bull* No. 13, February 2000, pp. 1–6.

American College of Obstetricians and Gynecologists. Shoulder dystocia. *ACOG Pract Bull* No. 40, November 2002, pp. 1–5.

Duff P. Diagnosis and management of face presentation. *Obstet Gynecol* 1981;57:105–112.

Hannah ME, Hannah WJ, Hewson SA, et al. Planned cesarean section versus planned vaginal birth for breech presentation at term: A randomized multicentre trial. *Lancet* 2000;356: 1375–1383.

22   CESAREAN DELIVERY

Patrick Duff

EPIDEMIOLOGY

• Cesarean delivery is the most frequently performed operation in U.S. hospitals. Approximately 800,000 to 1 million cesareans are performed annually.

TABLE 22-1   Principal Indications for Cesarean Delivery in the United States

INDICATION	APPROXIMATE PERCENTAGE OF ALL CESAREANS
Repeat cesarean	30
Labor abnormalities (dystocia)	30
Nonreassuring fetal status	15
Malpresentation	10
Placental abruption or previa	10
Other	5
TOTAL	100

• The two most common indications for cesarean delivery in the United States are abnormal labor (dystocia) and repeat cesarean (Table 22-1).

TYPES OF CESAREAN DELIVERY

• The most common type of cesarean is the low transverse (Kerr) procedure (Fig. 21-1). Approximately 95 percent of all cesareans are performed in this manner. The incision is in the noncontractile portion of the uterus and usually heals very well, posing minimal risk of dehiscence during a subsequent delivery.

• The low vertical (Kronig) procedure (Fig. 22-2) is performed in fewer than 3 percent of cases. The most common indication is a poorly developed lower uterine segment, particularly in association with a noncephalic fetal presentation.

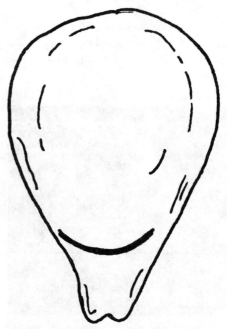

FIG. 22-1 Low transverse (Kerr) uterine incision.

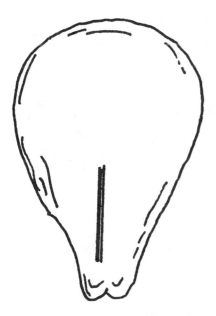

FIG. 22-2 Low vertical (Kronig) uterine incision.

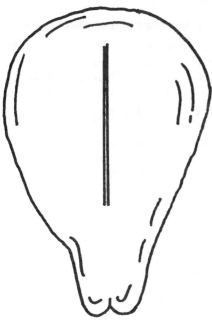

FIG. 22-3 Classic uterine incision.

• The classic uterine incision (Fig. 22-3) is also performed in fewer than 3 percent of cases. The most common indications are transverse lie/fetal back down, anterior placenta previa, higher order multiple gestation (three or more fetuses), major fetal anomalies (eg, severe hydrocephalus, large sacrococcygeal teratoma), and obstruction of the lower uterine segment by a leiomyoma.

COMPLICATIONS OF CESAREAN DELIVERY

• The most common complication of cesarean delivery is infection. The most common infection is endometritis, followed by urinary tract infection, bacteremia, and wound infection. The frequency of infection increases if the patient is in labor prior to surgery, has multiple vaginal examinations, and is indigent. Prophylactic antibiotics decrease the risk of infection.
• The second most common complication is hemorrhage. The following factors increase the likelihood of perioperative hemorrhage: placenta previa, placental abruption, severe preeclampsia, coagulation disorders, and uterine atony.
• Other less likely complications include injury to the bowel, bladder, and ureter.
• The risk of maternal mortality associated with cesarean delivery is <1:1000. However, the relative risk of maternal mortality associated with cesarean delivery is increased two- to fourfold over a vaginal delivery.

ANESTHESIA FOR CESAREAN DELIVERY

• Cesarean delivery is most frequently performed under regional anesthesia (spinal or epidural). Regional anesthesia reduces the risk of serious complications, such as aspiration pneumonitis or faulty intubation, and allows the mother and father to share more fully in the birth experience.
• General anesthesia is typically used when emergency delivery is required: eg, maternal hemorrhage, an ominous fetal heart rate tracing, or prolapse of the umbilical cord. General anesthesia also may be used when the patient has a contraindication to regional anesthesia: eg, previous spinal injury or a coagulopathy.
• In an extreme emergency when an anesthesiologist or nurse-anesthetist is unavailable, cesarean delivery can be performed under local anesthesia.

VAGINAL BIRTH AFTER CESAREAN

• Each type of uterine scar has a different risk for dehiscence in a subsequent pregnancy (Table 22-2).
• When any of the vertical incisions disrupt, the results are usually catastrophic maternal hemorrhage and severe fetal distress.
• Most disruptions of low transverse incisions are small and asymptomatic.
• Patients who have had a single prior low transverse uterine incision have approximately a 70 percent probability of successful vaginal delivery if allowed to labor.

TABLE 22-2 Risk of Uterine Scar Dehiscence with Different Types of Previous Cesarean Incision

TYPE OF UTERINE INCISION	APPROXIMATE RISK OF DEHISCENCE IN A SUBSEQUENT PREGNANCY
Low transverse	0.2–1.5%
Low vertical	1–7%
T-incision (low transverse incision that requires a vertical extension into contractile portion of uterus)	4–9%
Classic	4–9%

- The principal advantages of vaginal birth after cesarean (VBAC) include decreased risk of maternal mortality and morbidity, decreased hospital expense, and more rapid recovery time for the mother.
- Contraindications to VBAC include patient refusal, recurring or new indication, vertical or T-shaped incision, and lack of appropriate anesthesia and blood bank services.
- Patients undergoing VBAC may safely receive pitocin for induction or augmentation of labor. However, use of prostaglandins in such patients is contraindicated because of an unacceptably high risk of uterine scar dehiscence.
- If there is a suspicion of uterine scar dehiscence either during labor or immediately after delivery, urgent laparotomy is indicated. Most dehiscences can be repaired by reapproximating the edges of the uterine incision. In some situations, hysterectomy may be necessary.

BIBLIOGRAPHY

American College of Obstetricians and Gynecologists. Vaginal birth after previous cesarean delivery. *ACOG Pract Bull No. 5, July 1999,* pp. 1–8.

Duff P. Cesarean delivery and cesarean hysterectomy. In: Ling FW, Duff P. *Obstetrics and Gynecology. Principles for Practice.* New York: McGraw-Hill, 2001.

23 OBSTETRIC ANESTHESIA
Patrick Duff

OBJECTIVE

- The purpose of obstetric analgesia and anesthesia is to effectively relieve the pain of childbirth without causing harm to the mother or fetus.

INTRAVENOUS ANALGESICS

- The simplest way to provide pain relief during childbirth is to administer parenteral narcotics and sedatives intermittently during labor.
- Meperidine hydrocholoride and morphine sulfate are the two most commonly used narcotics. Typical dosing regimens for these drugs are listed in Table 23-1.
- Because narcotics often cause nausea and vomiting, they are usually administered in combination with a sedative/antiemetic such as promethazine (12.5 mg IV every 4 to 6 h).
- Nalbuphine and butorphanol are narcotic agonists-antagonists that have become increasingly popular for obstetric analgesia. Typical dosing regimens for these drugs are listed in Table 23-1.

LOCAL ANESTHETICS

- Local anesthetics act directly on the nerve membrane to block the propagation of nerve impulses.
- Local anesthetics are of two types:
  - Amides
  - Esters
- The three most commonly used local anesthetics are lidocaine (amide, intermediate duration of action), bupivicaine (amide, long duration of action), and chloroprocaine (ester, short duration of action).
- Local anesthetics may be administered in one of four ways:
  - Direct infiltration of the perineum
  - Pudendal block
  - Epidural block
  - Subarachnoid block

PERINEAL INFILTRATION

- Perineal infiltration provides satisfactory anesthesia for performance and repair of an episiotomy and/or repair of a vaginal or perineal laceration.
- Complications associated with direct perineal infiltration are extremely rare.
- Perineal infiltration does not provide acceptable anesthesia for an instrumental vaginal delivery.

TABLE 23-1 Common Dosage Regimens of Narcotics and Narcotic Agonists-Antagonists for Obstetric Anesthesia

DRUG	DOSE	DOSE INTERVAL
Meperidine hydrochloride	25–50 mg IV	Every 3–4 h
Morphine sulfate	4–10 mg IV	Every 3–4 h
Nalbuphine	10 mg IV	Every 3 h
Butorphanol	1–2 mg IV	Every 3–4 h

- Perineal infiltration does not provide any pain relief during the actual process of labor.

PUDENDAL BLOCK

- The lower half of the vagina and perineum are innervated by the pudendal nerve, which is derived from fibers emanating from S2-4.
- The pudendal nerve can be blocked as it passes in close proximity to the ischial spines.
- Pudendal block anesthesia provides no pain relief during the course of labor. However, it does provide effective anesthesia for an uncomplicated low or outlet forceps delivery or vacuum extraction. It is also an acceptable anesthetic technique for performance and repair of an episiotomy or repair of a vaginal or perineal laceration.
- The potential adverse effects of a pudendal block include the following:
  - Uneven anesthetic effect
  - Laceration of the pudendal artery or vein, resulting in a paravaginal hematoma
  - Intravascular injection with resultant seizure or cardiac arrhythmia

EPIDURAL ANESTHESIA

- With this type of anesthetic, local anesthesia, often combined with narcotics such as morphine or fentanyl, is injected into the epidural space via a small indwelling catheter.
- The catheter is usually inserted at the L3-4 or L4-5 interspace.
- Epidural anesthesia provides the most consistently effective pain relief for *both* labor and delivery (vaginal or cesarean).
- For pain relief during labor, an anesthetic level at approximately T10 is desirable. For anesthesia during cesarean delivery, a level at approximately T6 is necessary.
- Potential adverse effects of epidural anesthesia include the following:
  - Uneven distribution of anesthesia
  - Intravascular injection with resultant seizure or cardiac arrhythmia
  - Maternal hypotension, leading to impaired uterine perfusion and fetal hypoxia
  - Laceration of an epidural vein with resultant epidural hematoma

SPINAL ANESTHESIA

- With spinal anesthesia, a local anesthetic—with or without a narcotic—is injected directly into the subarachnoid space, usually at the level of L3-4 or L4-5.
- Spinal anesthesia is not usually administered for pain relief during labor. Rather, it is typically used for a complicated instrumental vaginal delivery (eg, a midforceps extraction or rotation) or cesarean delivery.
- Potential adverse effects of spinal anesthesia include the following:
  - Intravascular injection with resultant seizure or cardiac arrhythmia
  - Maternal hypotension, which may lead to impaired uterine perfusion and fetal hypoxia
  - Laceration of a blood vessel with a resultant intrathecal hematoma
  - "High spinal," with resultant paralysis of the muscles of respiration
  - Spinal headache

GENERAL ANESTHESIA

- General anesthesia is used primarily for emergency operative deliveries, particularly cesarean delivery.
- The agents typically used for **balanced general anesthesia** include the following:
  - A **muscle relaxant,** such as succinylcholine—used primarily to facilitate intubation
  - A **narcotic,** such as fentanyl
  - **Nitrous oxide**
  - A **sedative/amnesic,** such as midazolam or diazepam
- When immediate uterine relaxation is needed, an anesthetic such as halothane is indicated.
- Whenever a pregnant woman receives general anesthesia, an endotracheal tube must be in place to secure the airway and prevent aspiration.
- Potential adverse effects of general anesthesia include the following:
  - Neonatal apnea and bradycardia
  - Aspiration pneumonitis
  - Injury to the teeth, pharynx, or larynx
  - Intubation of the esophagus rather than trachea, with resultant hypoxic brain injury in the mother

BIBLIOGRAPHY

James CF. Obstetric analgesia and anesthesia. In: Ling FW, Duff P, eds. *Obstetrics and Gynecology*. Principles for Practice. New York: McGraw-Hill, 2001.

24 PUERPERAL INFECTION: CHORIOAMNIONITIS, ENDOMETRITIS, GROUP B STREPTOCOCCAL INFECTION

Patrick Duff

CHORIOAMNIONITIS

DEFINITION

- The term **chorioamnionitis** refers to the clinical syndrome of infection of the placenta, placental membranes, amniotic fluid, and fetus.
- Alternative terms include **amnionitis** and **intraamnionitic infection** (IAI).

EPIDEMIOLOGY

- Clinically evident chorioamnionitis occurs in approximately 3 to 5 percent of term patients and up to 25 percent of patients who deliver preterm.
- The most common microorganisms are group B streptococci, *Escherichia coli,* anaerobes, and mycoplasmas. The first two organisms pose the greatest risk to the neonate.
- Most affected patients have multiple organisms isolated from the amniotic fluid.
- The most important risk factors for chorioamnionitis are low socioeconomic status, nulliparity, extended duration of labor and ruptured membranes, multiple vaginal examinations, and pre-existing lower genital tract infection (bacterial vaginosis, group B streptococcal infection).

CLINICAL MANIFESTATIONS

- The most common clinical manifestations of chorioamnionitis are fever, maternal and fetal tachycardia, and uterine tenderness.

FETAL/NEONATAL COMPLICATIONS

- The most common neonatal complications of chorioamnionitis are pneumonia and bacteremia.
- Neonatal meningitis is a much less common but potentially very serious, complication.
- In rare instances, chorioamnionitis results in a severe **fetal sepsis syndrome** that leads to fetal brain injury and cerebral palsy.

DIAGNOSIS

- In term patients, the diagnosis of chorioamnionitis is made almost entirely on the basis of clinical findings.
- In patients with preterm labor, amniocentesis may be of value in confirming or excluding the diagnosis of chorioamnionitis. Amniotic fluid should be cultured and assessed for Gram's stain and glucose concentration. A positive Gram's stain and low concentration of glucose (less than 15 mg/dL) are indicative of bacterial colonization.

TREATMENT

- Delivery is an essential part of the management of all patients with chorioamnionitis.
- Intrapartum, patients should be treated with a combination of penicillin (5 million U IV every 6 h) or ampicillin (2 g IV every 6 h) plus gentamicin (1.5 mg/kg IV every 8 h).
- If a patient has an allergy to beta-lactam antibiotics, clindamycin (900 mg IV every 8 h) may be substituted for penicillin or ampicillin.
- If a patient requires cesarean delivery, an antibiotic with excellent anaerobic coverage should be added to the regimen. Alternatives include clindamycin (900 mg IV every 8 h) or metronidazole (500 mg IV every 12 h).
- Intravenous antibiotics should be continued until the patient has been afebrile for approximately 24 h. An extended course of oral antibiotics is usually not necessary.

ENDOMETRITIS

EPIDEMIOLOGY

- Puerperal endometritis occurs in approximately 1 to 3 percent of patients who deliver vaginally.
- Endometritis is many times more common in women who require cesarean delivery.
- The most important risk factors for postcesarean endometritis are the following:
  - Low socioeconomic status
  - Extended duration of labor
  - Extended duration of ruptured membranes
  - Multiple vaginal examinations
  - Internal fetal monitoring
  - Preexisting lower genital tract infection (bacterial vaginosis and group B streptococcal infection)
- Puerperal endometritis is a polymicrobial mixed aerobic-anaerobic infection caused by bacteria that are part of the normal vaginal flora.

CLINICAL MANIFESTATIONS

- The most common manifestations of endometritis are fever, tachycardia, pelvic pain, and uterine and adnexal tenderness.
- On average, approximately 5 to 10 percent of women with endometritis are bacteremic. In addition, about 3 to 5 percent have a concurrent urinary tract infection and about 3 percent have a wound infection.

DIAGNOSIS

- The diagnosis is usually made on the basis of clinical examination.
- A urine culture or chest x-ray should be obtained only if pyelonephritis or pneumonia is suspected.
- Blood cultures should be obtained in the following situations:
  ○ Patient is immunocompromised
  ○ Patient is at increased risk for bacterial endocarditis
  ○ Patient has had a poor response to initial treatment

TREATMENT

- There are several extended-spectrum cephalosporins, penicillins, and carbapenems that provide excellent coverage against a broad range of pelvic pathogens (Table 24-1).
- Although these agents are acceptable for the treatment of puerperal endometritis, they are more expensive than the generic combination regimens presented in Table 24-2.

TABLE 24-1 Single Agents Effective for the Treatment of Puerperal Endometritis

CEPHALOSPORINS	PENICILLINS	CARBAPENEMS
Cefipime	Ampicillin-sulbactam	Imipenem-cilastain
Cefotaxime	Mezlocillin	Ertapenem
Cefotetan	Piperacillin	Meropenem
Cefoxitin	Piperacillin-tazobactam	
Ceftizoxime	Ticarcillin-clavulanic acid	

TABLE 24-2 Combination Regimens for Treatment of Puerperal Endometritis

DRUGS	DOSE
Clindamycin	900 mg IV every 8 h
plus gentamicin	7 mg/kg IBW[a] IV every 24 h
OR	
Penicillin	5 million U IV every 6 h
plus metronidazole	500 mg IV every 12 h
plus gentamicin	7 mg/kg IBW IV every 24 h

[a]Ideal body weight.

- Antibiotics should be continued until the patient has been afebrile for 24 h.
- The two most common causes of a poor response to treatment are resistant organism and wound infection. The management of these conditions is summarized in Table 24-3.

GROUP B STREPTOCOCCAL INFECTION

EPIDEMIOLOGY

- *Streptococcus agalactiae* (group B streptococcus) is part of the normal flora of the genital tract and rectum. The organism can be recovered from 20 to 30 percent of women at some time during pregnancy.
- When this organism is present in the lower genital tract and rectum at the time of labor, the mother is at increased risk for chorioamnionitis and puerperal endometritis. In addition, the neonate is at increased risk for pneumonia, bacteremia, and meningitis.
- Mortality from early-onset neonatal group B streptococcal infection is less than 5 percent in term infants but may be severalfold higher in preterm infants.

CLINICAL MANIFESTATIONS

- The vast majority of women with group B streptococcal colonization are completely asymptomatic.
- The organism can cause both asymptomatic bacteriuria and acute cystitis in colonized patients.
- The organism also can be part of the polymicrobial flora that causes chorioamnionitis and puerperal endometritis.

DIAGNOSIS

- Group B streptococci are most readily identified by culture. The specimen for culture should be obtained

TABLE 24-3 Management of Patients With a Poor Initial Response to Treatment for Puerperal Endometritis

CONDITION	MANAGEMENT
Resistant organism	If patient is receiving a single agent, convert to combination therapy with clindamycin or metronidazole plus penicillin or ampicillin plus gentamicin. If patient is receiving clindamycin plus gentamicin, add penicillin or ampicillin.
Wound infection	Incise and drain wound. Add antibiotic with specific antistaphylococcal coverage, such as nafcillin.

by swabbing the lower third of the vagina, perineum, and perianal area with a cotton applicator and inoculating the applicator into a nutrient broth. The result of the culture is usually available in 24 to 48 h.

- The organism also can be detected by a newly developed polymerase chain reaction (PCR) test. The result of the test can be available within 1 h.

MANAGEMENT

- The current guidelines for management were published by the Centers for Disease Control and Prevention in 2002.
- All pregnant women should be cultured for group B streptococci at 35 to 37 weeks.
- All colonized women should be treated *intrapartum* with penicillin, 5 million U IV initially, then 2.5 million U every 4 h until delivery.
- If penicillin is unavailable, patients may be treated with ampicillin, 2 g IV initially, then 1 g every 4 h until delivery.
- If the patient has a history of a mild allergic reaction to penicillin, she should be treated with cefazolin, 1 g IV every 8 h until delivery.
- If the patient has a history of an anaphylactic reaction to penicillin, she should be treated with vancomycin, 1 g IV every 12 h, or clindamycin, 900 mg IV every 8h.
- If the result of the culture is unknown, the patient should be treated intrapartum if she has any of the following risk factors:
  ◦ Rupture of membranes greater than 18 h
  ◦ Prior history of a child with neonatal group B streptococcal infection
  ◦ History of group B streptococcal infection
  ◦ History of group B streptococcal bacteriuria in the present pregnancy
  ◦ Intrapartum fever (chorioamnionitis)
- If the new PCR test is available 24 h/day, the antepartum culture can be omitted in favor of testing at the time of admission for labor. Women who have a positive PCR test require intrapartum antibiotic prophylaxis.

BIBLIOGRAPHY

Duff P. Maternal and perinatal infection. In: Gabbe SG, Niebyl JR, Simpson JL, eds. *Obstetrics. Normal and Problem Pregnancies,* 4th ed. New York: Churchill Livingstone, 2002.
Prevention of perinatal group B streptococcal disease. *MMWR* 2002;51:1–24.

25 URINARY TRACT INFECTIONS IN PREGNANCY

Patrick Duff

Urinary tract infections (UTIs) are among the most common medical complications of pregnancy. They may be classified into four types: urethritis, asymptomatic bacteriuria, cystitis, and pyelonephritis.

ACUTE URETHRITIS

EPIDEMIOLOGY

- Acute urethritis is most commonly caused by *Chlamydia trachomatis* or *Neisseria gonorrhoeae*. Low concentrations of coliform organisms such as *Escherichia coli, Klebsiella pneumoniae,* and *Proteus* species may also cause urethritis.
- Chlamydial infection may be present in 3 to 5 percent of prenatal patients. Gonorrhea is usually less common, affecting approximately 1 percent.

CLINICAL MANIFESTATIONS

- The usual clinical manifestations of urethritis include:
  ◦ Frequency
  ◦ Urgency
  ◦ Dysuria
  ◦ Hesitancy
  ◦ Dribbling
  ◦ Purulent urethral discharge
- The urethral discharge is particularly helpful in distinguishing urethritis (discharge is present) from cystitis (discharge is absent).

DIAGNOSIS

- Patients with urethritis typically have many white cells in their microscopic urinalysis.
- *C. trachomatis* and *N. gonorrhoeae* are most rapidly identified by PCR. Samples for testing may be obtained from a urine sample or a cervical swab.

POSSIBLE SEQUELAE

- Since urethritis usually is due to chlamydial infection or gonorrhea, the patient may transmit infection to her sexual partner.

- Pregnant women with untreated chlamydial or gonococcal infection are at increased risk for preterm labor, preterm premature rupture of membranes, chorioamnionitis, and puerperal endometritis. Their neonates are at risk for potentially serious eye infections caused by either of these organisms and pneumonia caused by *Chlamydia*.

TREATMENT

- The most cost-effective treatment in pregnancy for chlamydial urethritis is azithromycin powder, 1 g in a single dose.
- For gonococcal urethritis in pregnancy, the most cost-effective treatment is ceftriaxone, 125 mg IM in a single dose. For the patient who is allergic to beta-lactam antibiotics, the drug of choice is spectinomycin, 2 g IM in a single dose.

ASYMPTOMATIC BACTERIURIA

EPIDEMIOLOGY

- Asymptomatic bacteriuria (ASB) is present in 5 to 10 percent of sexually active women, including pregnant women.
- The dominant pathogen is *E. coli*, which is responsible for approximately 75 percent of all cases. Two other aerobic gram-negative bacilli, *Klebsiella pneumoniae* and *Proteus species,* are each responsible for 5 to 10 percent of cases. Gram-positive organisms such as group B streptococci, enterococci, and staphylococci are responsible for most of the remaining cases.

DIAGNOSIS

- ASB is identified by documenting $> 10^5$ colonies per milliliter in a midstream clean-catch urine culture.
- Because this infection is so prevalent, all pregnant women should have a urine culture at the time of their first prenatal appointment. ASB typically antedates the pregnancy. Therefore, if the initial culture is negative, ASB is unlikely to develop later in pregnancy.

POSSIBLE SEQUELAE

- If not properly treated, ASB will evolve into pyelonephritis in 20 to 30 percent of those infected.
- Ascending infection is more common in pregnant than in nonpregnant women because of urinary stasis.

Stasis, in turn, results from the inhibitory effect of progesterone on ureteral peristalsis and compression of the ureter by the gravid uterus.

TREATMENT

- Nitrofurantoin monohydrate macrocrystals (Macrobid) is an excellent drug for the treatment of ASB. For the initial infection, it should be administered in a dose of 100 mg orally twice daily for 3 days. Recurrent infections should be treated for 7 to 10 days.
- The combination of trimethoprim/sulfamethoxazole (Bactrim and Septra) also is an excellent choice for the treatment of ASB. It is not quite as effective as nitrofurantoin against *E. coli*. However, it has superb activity against *Proteus* species, whereas nitrofurantoin is not effective against these organisms. Trimethoprim/sulfamethoxazole (double-strength tablets) should be administered orally twice daily for 3 days for the initial infection and for 7 to 10 days for recurrent infections.
- Ampicillin (250 mg orally four times daily) or amoxicillin (250 mg orally three times daily) should be administered *only* if the infection is caused by *Enterococcus*. At least one-third of strains of *E. coli* and more than half of the strains of *Klebsiella pneumoniae* are resistant to ampicillin or amoxicillin, so these drugs are not good choices for the empiric treatment of UTIs.
- The combination of amoxicillin/clavulanic acid (Augmentin), 875 mg orally twice daily for 7 to 10 days, is an excellent drug for the treatment of recurrent infections caused by resistant microorganisms. However, this drug is very expensive and should not be used when less expensive antibiotics would work as well.

CYSTITIS

EPIDEMIOLOGY

- Acute cystitis occurs in 2 to 3 percent of pregnant women, typically in patients who have unidentified or inadequately treated ASB.
- Cystitis is caused by the same bacteria that are responsible for ASB.

CLINICAL MANIFESTATIONS

- The usual clinical manifestations of acute cystitis are as follows

- ○ Frequency
- ○ Urgency
- ○ Dysuria
- ○ Hematuria
- ○ Pyuria
- ○ Suprapubic pain
- ○ Low-grade fever
- A purulent urethral exudate is not typically present, whereas it is very common in women with acute urethritis.

DIAGNOSIS

- Patients with symptoms suggestive of cystitis should have a sample of urine obtained by sterile catheterization. This sample should be divided into two aliquots.
- One urine aliquot should be submitted for culture and sensitivity. In a symptomatic patient in whom urine is obtained by catheterization, a colony count of greater than or equal to 10^2 colonies/ml confirms the diagnosis of cystitis.
- A second urine aliquot should be tested by dipstick for nitrites and leukocyte esterase. If either test is positive, the diagnosis of cystitis is likely.
- If the urine pH is greater than or equal to 8, *Proteus* is the most likely pathogen.

POSSIBLE SEQUELAE

- As noted above for ASB, cystitis may evolve into ascending pyelonephritis if it is not treated properly.

TREATMENT

- Patients with cystitis should be treated as outlined above for ASB.

PYELONEPHRITIS

EPIDEMIOLOGY

- Pyelonephritis affects 0.5 to 2 percent of pregnant women.
- It usually occurs in patients with undiagnosed or inadequately treated lower UTIs.
- The infection is usually caused by aerobic gram-negative bacilli, primarily *E. coli*, *Klebsiella pneumoniae*, and *Proteus* species.

- Approximately 75 percent of cases affect the right kidney, because the right ureter is more subject to compression by the gravid uterus.

CLINICAL MANIFESTATIONS

- Patients with pyelonephritis may have the signs and symptoms of UTI previously mentioned.
- In addition, they also typically have a high fever (greater than 38°C), chills, flank pain and tenderness, and nausea and vomiting.

DIAGNOSIS

- Patients with suspected pyelonephritis should be tested as outlined above for cystitis.
- In addition, blood cultures should be obtained in the following situations:
  - ○ The patient is immunocompromised.
  - ○ The patient has a risk factor for bacterial endocarditis.
  - ○ The patient has had a poor response to initial therapy.

POSSIBLE SEQUELAE

- ○ Patients with acute pyelonephritis are at increased risk for preterm labor.
- ○ Approximately 5 to 10 percent of affected patients will be bacteremic.
- ○ Less than 1 percent of affected patients will develop adult respiratory distress syndrome.

TREATMENT

- Stable, compliant patients in the first half of pregnancy may be treated as outpatients. The most appropriate drugs for treatment are trimethoprim/ sulfamethoxazole, double strength (one tablet orally twice daily for 10 days), and amoxicillin/ clavulanic acid (875 mg orally twice daily for 10 days).
- Unstable or noncompliant patients and those in the second half of pregnancy (where the risk of serious sequelae is greater) should be hospitalized and treated with intravenous antibiotics. Table 25-1 lists possible treatment regimens. Patients should receive intravenous medications until they are afebrile and asymptomatic. They can then be continued on an oral

TABLE 25-1 Intravenous Antibiotics for Treatment of Acute Pyelonephritis in Pregnancy

CONDITION OF PATIENT	DRUG	DOSE
Initial episode Immune competent Hemodynamically stable	Cefazolin	1 g IV every 8 h
Recurrent episode or immunocompromised or hemodynamically unstable	Cefazolin plus gentamicin or aztreonam	1 g IV every 8 h 1.5 mg/kg/actual body weight IV every 8 h 1 g IV every 8 h

TABLE 25-2 Evaluation of Patients with a Poor Response to Treatment for Pyelonephritis

POSSIBLE CAUSE OF POOR RESPONSE	DIAGNOSTIC TEST	MANAGEMENT
Resistant organism	Urine culture and sensitivity	Modify antibiotic therapy
Obstruction due to ureteral stone	Renal ultrasound or intravenous pyelogram in problematic cases	Diuresis Surgery to remove stone
Obstruction due to compression of ureter by uterus	Renal ultrasound	Percutaneous nephrostomy or placement of ureteral stent

antibiotic to which the organism is sensitive for a total of 10 to 14 days of treatment.

- Within 72 h of the start of treatment, approximately 95 percent of patients will be substantially improved. The two most common causes of poor response to treatment are resistant organism and urinary tract obstruction. Patients with persistent fever and symptoms should be evaluated and treated as outlined in Table 25-2.
- Patients who have had a single episode of acute pyelonephritis in pregnancy have approximately a 20 percent possibility of developing a recurrent UTI later in gestation.
- Recurrent infection is most effectively prevented by administering prophylactic antibiotics for the duration of pregnancy. Possible choices for prophylaxis include:
  - Nitrofurantoin monohydrate macrocrystals, 100 mg orally daily
  - Trimethoprim-sulfamethoxazole, one double-strength tablet daily

BIBLIOGRAPHY

Duff P. Urinary tract infections in women. *Primary Care Update OB/GYNs* 1994;1:12–16.

Duff P. Infections in pregnancy. In: Ling FW, Duff P, eds. *Obstetrics and Gynecology. Principles for Practice.* New York: McGraw-Hill, 2001.

Stamm WE, Hooton TM. Management of urinary tract infections in adults. *N Engl J Med* 1993;329:1328–1334.

26 ROUTINE POSTPARTUM CARE
Patrick Duff

INTRODUCTION

- Some aspects of postpartum care depend on the method of delivery. Others are the same regardless of method of delivery.
- The first portion of this chapter discusses the differences in the clinical evaluation for women who have had a vaginal delivery compared to those who have had a cesarean.
- The second portion of the chapter reviews aspects of medical care common to all postpartum women.

CLINICAL EVALUATION

WOMEN HAVING VAGINAL DELIVERY

- In most instances, the patient should be allowed to room in with her infant.
- As a general rule, she should have unrestricted activity and an unrestricted diet.
- The patient should be allowed to bathe or shower at her discretion.
- Patients who experience perineal pain from an episiotomy or laceration may find that sitzbaths provide symptomatic relief.
- Vital signs should be checked every 8 to 12 h. Postpartum fever should be evaluated promptly, as outlined in Chap. 24.
- The patient should be evaluated for excessive bleeding, uterine cramping, perineal pain, perineal or vaginal hematoma (particularly if an instrumental delivery was performed), difficulty voiding, and leg pain and edema.
- An analgesic should be prescribed if indicated to control the patient's pain. Reasonable choices for inex-

pensive, safe, and effective analgesics include ibuprofen, 600 mg orally every 6 to 8 h, or acetaminophen, 325 mg, plus codeine, 30 mg, every 4 to 6 h.

- Most patients who have had a vaginal delivery can be discharged home 24 to 48 h after delivery.

WOMEN HAVING CESAREAN DELIVERY

- Most women who have had an operative delivery still are able to room in with their infants.
- A Foley catheter usually is left in place for 6 to 12 h after surgery.
- The patient's activity should gradually be increased as her pain is controlled. Within 24 h, most patients can ambulate reasonably well.
- The patient's diet can be advanced rapidly. Within 6 h of delivery, most patients will be able to consume liquids. Within 12 h, most patients are able to consume a regular diet without experiencing nausea or vomiting. Until the patient is able to tolerate solid food, she should receive intravenous fluids, such as glucose and lactated Ringer's solution or glucose and normal saline administered at a rate of 125 to 150 mL/hr.
- Once the patient is taking liquids and solid food, her intravenous infusion can be discontinued and she can shower or bathe.
- Vital signs should be assessed every 6 to 8 h. Fever is particularly likely to denote infection, usually endometritis, and the patient should be evaluated promptly, as outlined in Chap. 24.
- Initially, the patient will require intravenous or epidural narcotics to control her incisional pain. Within 24 to 36 h, she should be transitioned to oral analgesics.
- Some patients who have had an uncomplicated cesarean delivery will feel well enough to leave the hospital on the second postoperative day. Most patients will be ready for discharge on the third postoperative day. Patients who develop endometritis or a wound infection may require hospitalization for 4 to 5 days.

DISCHARGE PLANNING

- The patient should be encouraged to breastfeed and receive counseling from a lactation consultant.
- The patient should receive instruction in bathing and care of her infant.
- Nursing and medical personnel should ensure that the patient has an approved car seat in which to transport her baby.
- The patient should be counseled about contraception.
- She should be advised that if she breastfeeds, she will probably not resume ovulatory cycles for at least 3 to

4 months. If she bottle feeds her baby, ovulatory cycles usually begin in about 2 months.

- The patient should be instructed to continue her prenatal vitamin or another multivitamin supplement.
- The patient's immunizations should be reviewed. If she is not immune to rubella, measles, and mumps, she should receive the trivalent measles-mumps-rubella vaccine (MMR). If she is not immune to chickenpox, she should receive the first dose of the varicella vaccine. The second dose should be administered in approximately 6 weeks. If she is susceptible to hepatitis B, she should receive the first dose of hepatitis B vaccine. The second and third doses should be administered in 1 and 6 months, respectively.
- The patient should be given a postpartum appointment in 4 to 6 weeks. At this appointment, special attention should be directed to the following:
  ○ Difficulties in breastfeeding
  ○ Difficulties in care of the infant
  ○ Possible signs and symptoms of depression
  ○ Method of contraception

BIBLIOGRAPHY

Boardman A. The puerperium. In: Ling FW, Duff P, eds. *Obstetrics & Gynecology. Principles for Practice.* New York: McGraw-Hill; 2001:545–575.

27 POSTPARTUM STERILIZATION PROCEDURES

Patrick Duff

INTRODUCTION

- Sterilization now is the single most common method of birth control in the United States.
- Many sterilization procedures in women are performed at the time of cesarean delivery or within 12 to 48 hours of a vaginal delivery.

SURGICAL TECHNIQUE

- The two most common types of postpartum tubal interruption are the Pomeroy (Fig. 27-1) and Parkland (Fig. 27-2) procedures.

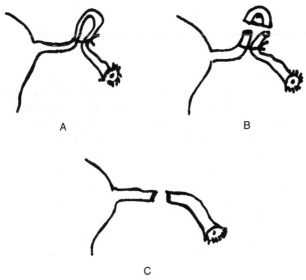

FIG. 27-1 Pomeroy procedure. The fallopian tube is ligated in its midportion (A), and a portion of the isthmus is excised (B). When the suture resorbs, the two ends of the tube are separated from one another (C).

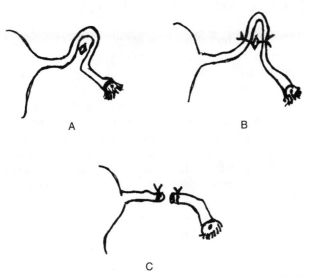

FIG. 27-2 Parkland procedure. A small window is created in the mesosalpinx below the midportion of the tube (A). The proximal and distal ends of the tube are ligated (B) and a segment of the isthmus is excised (C).

- Both procedures are easily and quickly performed at the time of cesarean delivery or through a small infraumbilical incision after a vaginal delivery.
- Both procedures have comparable rates of complication and failure.
- The Uchida (Fig. 27-3) and Irving (Fig. 27-4) procedures are more complex operations. The former can be performed at the time of cesarean delivery or through a small infraumbilical incision. The latter is usually performed only at the time of cesarean delivery.

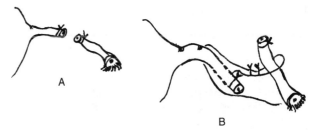

FIG. 27-3 Uchida procedure. The serosa of the tube is excised and the muscularis is exposed. The midportion of the tube is doubly ligated (A) and a segment of the isthmus is removed. The distal end of the tube is exteriorized, and the proximal end is inverted between the leaves of the broad ligament (B).

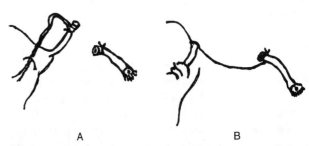

FIG. 27-4 Irving procedure. The distal end of the tube is excised (A) and the proximal end is embedded into a tunnel created in the anterior uterine wall (B).

- The Uchida and Irving procedures have a lower failure rate than the Pomeroy and Parkland operations. They are usually reserved for patients who have had a previous failed tubal interruption.
- The suture used for the actual ligation of the fallopian tubes is usually 0-plain or chromic. For fascial closure, a delayed resorbable suture such as 0 gauge polyglycolic acid or polydioxanone is preferred. For skin closure, a 4-0 gauge of the same material should be used.
- Puerperal sterilizations are best performed under regional (epidural or spinal) or general anesthesia.

COMPLICATIONS

- Concurrent sterilization does not significantly increase the rate of postcesarean complications.
- The risk of hemorrhage associated with a postpartum tubal sterilization is less than 1 percent.
- Similarly, the risk of a wound infection or soft tissue pelvic infection following a puerperal sterilization procedure is less than 1 percent.
- The long-term risk of method failure after a Pomeroy or Parkland procedure is approximately 0.5 to 1.0 percent.
- The long-term risk of method failure after a Uchida or Irving procedure is less than 0.5 percent.

POSTOPERATIVE CARE

- Postoperative ileus is very uncommon after a puerperal sterilization procedure. Most patients can be fed a regular diet and can ambulate within 6 h of surgery.
- Postoperative pain can usually be controlled with oral analgesics such as the combination of acetaminophen and codeine.
- Puerperal sterilization should not prolong the patient's hospital stay beyond that usually required for recovery from delivery.

SELECTION OF PATIENTS FOR STERILIZATION

- Unfortunately, a small number of women express regret after having puerperal sterilization.
- The two most common reasons for an unfavorable psychologic reaction to sterilization are change in marital partner and death of a child.
- Therefore physicians should be wary of performing sterilization procedures in women who are both young (below 30 years of age) and of low parity (only one or two children) or who are in unstable social/marital situations at the time of surgery.

BIBLIOGRAPHY

Boardman A. The puerperium. In: Ling FW, Duff P, eds. *Obstetrics and Gynecology. Principles for Practice.* New York: McGraw-Hill, 2001.

28 MEDICAL AND SURGICAL ABORTION TECHNIQUES

Rodney K. Edwards

GENERAL CONCEPTS

- Terminations of pregnancy are commonly performed in the United States. More than 300 abortions per 1000 live births are reported annually. Many of these are due to the fact that half of all pregnancies in this country each year are unintended, and half of these unintended pregnancies end in induced abortion.
- Legalization of abortion in 1973 has been associated with greater access to abortion services, lower fatality rates, and refinement of techniques. Case fatality rates are currently less than 1 per 100,000 induced abortions; this number is lower than the mortality rate associated with a continuing pregnancy (5 to 10 per 100,000).
- Although mortality associated with induced abortions is rare, the rate varies by gestational age, anesthetic used, and procedure performed. Both morbidity and mortality rates are higher with second-trimester than with first-trimester abortions, with general than with local anesthesia, and with medical than with surgical abortions (at similar gestational ages).
- The majority of abortions are accomplished by first-trimester cervical dilation and suction curettage. However, there has been a recent expansion in the availability and interest in pharmacologic agents that effect abortion.
- Women who are Rh-negative and unsensitized should receive Rh immune globulin in conjunction with either medically or surgically induced abortion.

INDICATIONS FOR ABORTION

- Certain **maternal medical conditions** are associated with such high rates of morbidity and mortality during pregnancy that termination of pregnancy should be *recommended*. Examples of such conditions include certain cardiac diseases (eg, primary pulmonary hypertension, Eisenmenger's syndrome, Marfan's syndrome with a dilated aortic root), severe renal insufficiency, and invasive carcinoma of the cervix. However, there are no uniformly accepted guidelines on which to base such a recommendation. Furthermore, the risk/benefit ratio for continuing the pregnancy will vary based on the woman's personal beliefs and motivation for currently being pregnant.
- Structural and genetic **abnormalities of the fetus** complicate 3 to 5 percent of pregnancies, and these conditions may be indications for pregnancy termination.
- Finally, so-called **elective** abortion may be sought simply because of a desire to not continue with the current pregnancy.

MEDICAL ABORTION

FIRST TRIMESTER

- Until recently, essentially all first-trimester abortions were performed surgically. However, the current availability of medications that induce abortion effectively and safely have increased access to legal abortion and expanded women's choices.

- **Mifepristone (RU 486)** is an agent that antagonizes the action of progesterone. Such antagonism results in increased prostaglandin synthesis, decreased prostaglandin metabolism, decidual necrosis, and endometrial sloughing.
  - This agent has some utility as a single agent for inducing abortion, but only in very early pregnancies. It is 75 to 85 percent effective in terminating pregnancies within 10 days of missed menses.
  - When followed 2 days later with 400 μg of misoprostol, a 200- or 600-mg dose of mifepristone successfully induces abortion in over 90 percent of pregnancies at 49 days gestation or less (7 weeks from the last menstrual period).
  - Side effects associated with the use of mifepristone include nausea, vomiting, fatigue, abdominal pain, anorexia, light-headedness, headache, and breast tenderness. Addition of a prostaglandin increases the likelihood of gastrointestinal side effects. In cases of failed medical abortion, the teratogenic potential of mifepristone is unknown.
- **Methotrexate** is cytotoxic to trophoblast cells. An intramuscular dose of 50 mg/m^2 of body surface area is used for the medical treatment of ectopic pregnancies.
  - This dose is associated with few side effects and is also effective for inducing abortion of intrauterine pregnancies of less than 42 days' gestation.
  - When combined with misoprostol, efficacy remains high until 56 days' gestation.
  - Time to completion of the abortion is longer with methotrexate-based regimens than with mifepristone-based regimens and can take as long as 2 weeks. One advantage of this slower onset of action is that uterine cramping and hemorrhage may be less severe.
  - Side effects of methotrexate include nausea, vomiting, diarrhea, headache, light-headedness, fever, and stomatitis. This medication is a known teratogen. However, its teratogenic potential in the setting of a failed medical abortion is uncertain.
- More than 30 years ago, **prostaglandins** were recommended as single agents for medical induction of first-trimester abortion. However, doses required to achieve satisfactory success rates are associated with a high incidence of side effects (nausea, vomiting, diarrhea, and abdominal pain).
  - Use of these agents in combination with mifepristone or methotrexate allows increased efficacy with lower doses, thereby reducing the incidence of side effects.
  - **Misoprostol** is a prostaglandin E$_1$ analogue that is marketed as an oral agent to combat peptic ulcer disease. This agent is inexpensive, readily available in the United States, and stable at room temperature.

- In women with an anembryonic gestation or embryonic death, misoprostol as a single agent is effective in causing pregnancy termination.
- The optimal dose of misoprostol in combination with mifepristone or methotrexate for induction of first trimester abortion, seems to be 800 μg vaginally.
- Table 28-1 lists recommended regimens for medical termination of pregnancy in the first trimester.

SECOND TRIMESTER

- Medical induction of abortion in the second trimester is achieved either by instilling hypertonic agents into the amniotic cavity or administering uterotonic agents.
- **Instillation of hypertonic saline or urea** requires amniocentesis and is currently rarely used.
  - This method is associated with a relatively long time to abortion.
  - Disseminated intravascular coagulation is an uncommon complication of this procedure.
  - In addition, inadvertent intravascular instillation of hypertonic saline has been associated with cardiovascular collapse, pulmonary and cerebral edema, and renal failure.
- **Instillation of a prostaglandin** into the amniotic cavity is occasionally utilized. The preparation available commercially is carboprost tromethamine (Hemabate).
  - If used, 1 mg should be given very slowly via amniocentesis.
  - Time to abortion and cervical trauma are reduced when preceded by the use of osmotic cervical dilators.
- **Systemic administration of prostaglandins** can achieve uterotonic effects and effect abortion.
  - Vaginal, as opposed to oral or parenteral, administration of these agents seems to combine the greatest efficacy with the lowest incidence of side effects.

TABLE 28-1 Recommended Regimens for Medical Termination of Pregnancy in the First Trimester[a]

REGIMEN	MEDICATION DOSES
Methotrexate and misoprostol	Methotrexate, 50 mg/m^2 intramuscularly, followed 7 days later with misoprostol, 800 μg vaginally
Mifepristone and misoprostol	Mifepristone (RU 486), 200 or 600 mg orally, followed in 48 h by misoprostol, 800 μg vaginally

[a]These regimens have significantly decreased efficacy beyond 49 days of gestation.

- The agents that have been most widely evaluated include **dinoprostone** (prostaglandin E_2) suppositories, **misoprostol** tablets, and **gemeprost** (another prostaglandin E_1 analogue) suppositories. Of these agents, misoprostol is the least expensive and best tolerated and has similar efficacy.
- The optimal regimen for inducing abortion in the second trimester with any of these agents is yet to be determined. We favor misoprostol, 400 µg vaginally every 6 h. In cases of fetal demise, we adjust this dose to 200 µg every 6 h.
- Administration of **concentrated solutions of oxytocin** may induce labor in the second trimester. The doses of oxytocin used are orders of magnitude higher than those used for labor induction or augmentation at term.

COMPLICATIONS OF MEDICAL ABORTION

- Compared with surgical abortion techniques, all methods of medical abortion are associated with relatively high rates of incomplete expulsion of the pregnancy, either failed abortion or retained products of conception. Incomplete expulsion of the embryo or fetus and/or placenta can result in excessive blood loss and infection. Furthermore, a surgical approach is required to complete the abortion.
- Uterine rupture may occur as a result of a medically induced abortion. Risk factors for uterine rupture include prior uterine surgery (such as myomectomy or cesarean delivery), multiparity, and polyhydramnios. Any of these factors should be considered a relative contraindication to medically induced abortion.

SURGICAL ABORTION

FIRST TRIMESTER

- In the mid-1990s, essentially all first-trimester abortions were performed by uterine curettage. **Cervical dilation and suction curettage** (D&C) is still the most common method used for abortion in the first trimester.
  - Choices of anesthesia include conscious sedation with a combination of a narcotic and benzodiazepine, paracervical block with a local anesthetic, and general anesthesia.
  - This procedure should be limited to pregnancies between 7 and 13 weeks of gestation. Intrauterine gestation should be confirmed preoperatively with an ultrasound examination.
  - The vagina and cervix should be prepared with an antiseptic solution.
  - A single-toothed tenaculum should be placed vertically (not horizontally) on the anterior lip of the cervix and used for countertension while graduated cervical dilators are used to dilate the cervix. In order to decrease the risk of applying excessive force to the cervix, the dilator should be held like a pencil, and the fourth and fifth fingers of the hand holding the dilator should rest against the patient's perineum while the dilator is advanced.
  - Preoperative use of osmotic dilators (laminaria tents or Dilapan), mifepristone, or prostaglandins can soften the cervix and decrease the force required to dilate it, thus reducing the risk of cervical trauma and uterine perforation. Misoprostol, administered the evening before surgery, is probably the most cost-effective option and poses the lowest risk of side effects.
  - Rigid cannulas used for suction curettage range from 6 to 14 mm in diameter and are either straight or curved. The appropriate choice for size of cannula is equal to the gestational age or 1 mm less.
  - The cannula should be advanced, unattached to suction, close to the fundus. Suction should be applied with a pump pressure of 50 to 70 mmHg and the cannula rotated and slowly withdrawn.
  - A sharp curette is used to confirm completeness of the evacuation. A gritty, rather than slick, feel of the endometrium suggests complete removal of the products of conception.
  - Upon completion of the procedure, the uterus should be firm, contracted, and bleeding minimally from the cervix.
  - Aspirated tissue should be sent for pathologic examination or inspected carefully by the surgeon. Villi can be identified by floating the tissue in water.
- A modification of D&C is termed **minisuction** or **menstrual regulation**.
  - This technique employs a flexible cannula connected to a 60-mL self-locking syringe.
  - Care should be taken to ensure that the gestational age is no greater than 7 weeks and that the patient is indeed pregnant (via use of a sensitive test for β-human chorionic gonadotropin).
  - The same principles as for D&C apply. The primary risks are incomplete uterine evacuation and misdiagnosis of an ectopic gestation.

SECOND TRIMESTER

- Fetuses beyond 13 to 14 weeks of gestation cannot be evacuated by suction cannulas. After cervical dilation, they can be removed from the uterus manually with grasping forceps. This procedure is termed **dilation and evacuation** (D&E).

○ Prior to 16 to 18 weeks, morbidity and mortality rates for D&E are lower than those for medically induced abortion in the second trimester. However, second-trimester abortion by whatever means carries higher rates of morbidity and mortality than abortions performed in the first trimester.

○ Other advantages of D&E include shorter times to abortion and less expense.

○ Performance of D&E requires a high degree of operator experience and skill and specialized instruments.

○ A greater degree of cervical dilation is required, up to 20 mm if the procedure is performed at or beyond 18 weeks. Achieving this degree of cervical dilation may require a multistage process with osmotic dilators.

○ Intraoperatively, uterotonic agents (eg, intravenous oxytocin) should be administered.

○ Generally, the intraoperative steps include rupturing the membranes, aspirating the amniotic fluid, removing the fetus from the uterus, and removing the placenta.

COMPLICATIONS OF SURGICAL ABORTION

- **Cervical laceration** probably is the most common complication of surgical abortion. If external and caused by the tenaculum, these lacertions are readily repaired with suture. Vertical placement of the tenaculum in the midline of the cervix and preoperative use of cervical ripening agents can decrease the incidence and severity of lacerations.
- **Hemorrhage** may occur as a result of uterine atony, retained products of conception, uterine trauma, or a coagulopathy.
  ○ **Uterine atony** can be confirmed on bimanual examination by a soft uterine fundus. Atony is treated with bimanual uterine compression and administration of uterotonic agents (Table 28-2).
  ○ **Retained products of conception** should be suspected when there is immediate or delayed hemorrhage or postabortal infection. The treatment is reaspiration with the largest cannula that will fit through the cervix.
- The most common site of **uterine perforation** is the midportion of the fundus and is usually due to failure to identify a retroverted and/or retroflexed uterus before dilating the cervix.
  ○ When fundal perforations during a first-trimester D&C are recognized prior to beginning uterine

TABLE 28-2 Uterotonic Agents Commonly Employed for Treating Uterine Atony

DRUG	ROUTE OF ADMINISTATION	DOSE
Oxytocin (Pitocin)	Intravenous	40 U in 1000 mL of isotonic crystalloid solution
Methylergonovine (Methergine)	Intramuscular	0.2 mg (200 μg)
Carboprost tromethamine (Hemabate)	Intramuscular	0.25 mg (250 μg)

evacuation, the procedure can usually can be completed under ultrasound guidance.

○ More hazardous are perforations of the lower uterine segment or cervix, especially if lateral and in proximity to branches of the uterine arteries. Uterine perforation occurring during D&E or accompanied by hemorrhage should prompt laparotomy.

- **Syncopal episodes** may occur due to vagal stimulation with placement of a paracervical block or with cervical manipulation. A vasovagal response should be distinguished from local anesthetic toxicity. The former responds to placing the patient in Trendelenburg's position and the administration of atropine.
- **Postabortal endometritis** usually occurs due to retained products of conception.
  ○ As in the case of postpartum endometritis or pelvic inflammatory disease, the infection is polymicrobial in etiology, and antibiotic therapy is indicated (see Table 28-3).
  ○ In more severe cases, hospitalization, intravenous antibiotics, and reaspiration are needed.
  ○ Prophylactic antibiotic therapy decreases the risk of postabortal infection. Doxycycline is the antibiotic most commonly recommended. Two regimens with proven efficacy are 400 mg of doxycycline given orally as a single preoperative dose or 100 mg preoperatively and 200 mg 30 min after completion of the procedure.

TABLE 28-3 Recommended Antibiotic Therapy for Postabortal Infection

DRUG(S)	ROUTE	DOSE
Mild infection: amoxicillin/clavulanate (Augmentin)	Oral	875 mg twice daily for 7–10 days
More severe infection: gentamicin plus clindamycin	Intravenous	7 mg/kg IBW[a] daily, until afebrile for 48 h
	Intravenous	900 mg every 8 h, until afebrile for 48 h

[a]Ideal body weight.

BIBLIOGRAPHY

Locksmith GJ. Pregnancy termination. In: Ling FW, Duff P, eds. *Obstetrics & Gynecology: Principles for Practice.* New York: McGraw-Hill, 2001.

Owen J. Pregnancy termination: First and second trimesters. In Gilstrap LC III, Cunningham FG, VanDorsten JP, eds. *Operative Obstetrics,* 2d ed. New York: McGraw-Hill, 2002.

Spitz IM, Bardin CW, Benton L, Robbins A. Early pregnancy termination with mifepristone and misoprostol in the United States. *N Engl J Med* 1998;338:1241–1247.

29 ECTOPIC PREGNANCY

John D. Davis

DEFINITION

- An ectopic pregnancy is a pregnancy that develops following implantation of the blastocyst in a location other than the endometrium lining the uterus. An unruptured tubal pregnancy is shown in Fig. 29-1.

EPIDEMIOLOGY

- In the United States, 1 in every 50 conceptions results in an ectopic pregnancy.
- The incidence of ectopic pregnancy has increased fourfold since 1970, primarily due to the increased incidence of salpingitis, improved diagnostic techniques, and increased use of assisted reproductive technologies (eg, in vitro fertilization).
- While the incidence of ectopic pregnancy has increased dramatically over the last three decades, the overall death-to-case rate of ectopic pregnancy has decreased 10-fold over the same time period. This decreased death rate is due to earlier detection of ectopic gestations and subsequent treatment prior to tubal rupture.
- Despite a declining death rate, ectopic pregnancy remains the third most common cause of maternal death in pregnancy, accounting for 9 percent of all pregnancy-related deaths.

ETIOLOGY

- The most important risk factor for ectopic pregnancy is previous salpingitis (pelvic inflammatory disease).

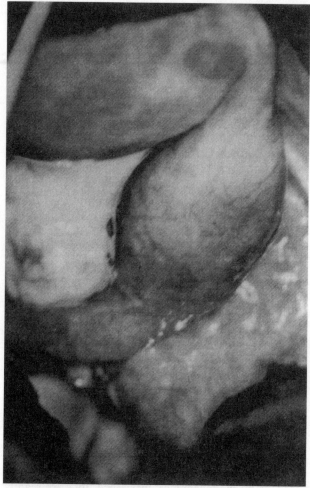

FIG. 29-1 Ectopic pregnancy located in the midportion of the right fallopian tube. (From Davis JD. Ectopic pregnancy. *Current Probl Surg* 2001;38(4):243. With permission.)

- Other risk factors for ectopic pregnancy include previous tubal surgery (such as a tubal reanastomosis), previous ectopic pregnancy, history of infertility, and current use of Progestasert, a progesterone-containing intrauterine device (IUD).

LOCATION

- The majority of ectopic pregnancies are located in the fallopian tube; 80 percent of ectopic pregnancies in the oviduct are located in the ampulla.
- Table 29-1 shows the relative frequency of ectopic gestation in various locations.

DIAGNOSIS

- Abdominal pain is the most common symptom experienced by women with an ectopic pregnancy.

TABLE 29-1 Relative Frequency of Ectopic Gestations in Various Locations

LOCATION	APPROXIMATE PERCENTAGE OF ALL ECTOPIC PREGNANCIES
Fallopian tube	98%
Abdomen	1.4%
Cervix	<1%
Ovary	<1%

Abnormal bleeding is the second most common symptom.

- In patients suspected of having an ectopic pregnancy, transvaginal ultrasound (TVUS), serum measurements of human chorionic gonadotropin (hCG), and serum progesterone levels can be used as diagnostic tests.
- TVUS findings consistent with an ectopic gestation include a fetal pole or gestational sac outside the uterine cavity, a complex adnexal mass, normal pelvic anatomy in a patient with a serum hCG level greater than 1500 mIU/mL, and blood in the posterior cul-de-sac.
- A serum hCG value of 1500 mIU/mL is the discriminatory level for TVUS in diagnosing ectopic pregnancy—ie, 1500 mIU/mL is the hCG level above which an intrauterine pregnancy should be seen if one is present.
- Patients suspected of having an ectopic pregnancy who have a nondiagnostic TVUS and are clinically stable should have serum hCG levels checked 48 h apart to help determine whether their pregnancy is ectopic or intrauterine.
- In early gestation, 85 percent of patients with normal intrauterine pregnancies will have an increase of at least 66 percent in their serum hCG level over 48 h.
- In early gestation, 87 percent of patients with ectopic pregnancies will have less than a 66 percent increase in their serum hCG level over 48 h.
- Serum progesterone concentrations can be used in the first trimester to distinguish viable from nonviable pregnancies. Patients with progesterone values greater than 20 ng/mL will have a viable intrauterine pregnancy 97.4 percent of the time, while patients with progesterone values below 5 ng/mL will have a non-viable pregnancy 99.7 percent of the time.

NONSURGICAL THERAPY

- With improved diagnostic techniques and earlier detection of ectopic pregnancies, many patients are candidates for nonsurgical therapy. The most frequently used medication to treat ectopic pregnancy is intramuscularly injected methotrexate.

- Methotrexate inhibits dihydrofolic reductase, the enzyme that converts dihydrofolate to tetrahydrofolate. Without tetrahydrofolate, rapidly dividing cells, such as fetal cells, are unable to replicate.
- Contraindications to methotrexate treatment for ectopic pregnancy are listed in Table 29-2. Many obstetrician/gynecologists also consider the presence of fetal cardiac activity and undesired future fertility contraindications to methotrexate treatment.
- In well-chosen patients, methotrexate is approximately 90 percent successful in treating an ectopic pregnancy.
- The dose of methotrexate is calculated using a body-surface-area nomogram and equals 50 mg/m^2 (the majority of patients receive between 75 and 100 mg of methotrexate).
- Patients treated with methotrexate should have serum hCG concentrations drawn weekly to ensure resolution of the ectopic pregnancy. Less than 5 percent of patients will require a second dose of medication.
- Side effects of methotrexate—such as ulcerative stomatitis, nausea, leukopenia, elevated liver function tests, and blood dyscrasias—are possible but occur very rarely with single-dose therapy.

SURGICAL THERAPY

- Patients with an ectopic pregnancy who are not candidates for medical therapy or who refuse it may be treated with surgery.
- Patients with small, unruptured ampullary ectopic pregnancies who desire future fertility are best treated with a linear salpingostomy. During this procedure, which may be performed laparoscopically or via laparotomy, the fallopian tube is opened and the pregnancy tissue removed. The tube will heal spontaneously and does not require closure with sutures.
- In some situations, removal of the affected tube (salpingectomy) may be required. Indications for salpingectomy include tubal rupture or extensive damage to the affected tube, a previous ectopic pregnancy in the affected tube, and undesired fertility.

TABLE 29-2 Contraindications to Methotrexate Treatment for Ectopic Pregnancy

Hemodynamic instability
Mass >3.5–4.0 cm
Serum hCG >15,000 mIU/mL
Liver disease
Renal disease
Bleeding dyscrasia
Unreliable patient
Coexistent intrauterine pregnancy

SUBSEQUENT FERTILITY

- After treatment with either intramuscular methotrexate or linear salpingostomy, patients have a tubal patency rate of approximately 80 percent and a subsequent intrauterine pregnancy rate of approximately 60 percent.
- Women who have had one ectopic pregnancy have approximately a 15 percent risk of having another ectopic pregnancy in the future.

BIBLIOGRAPHY

Davis JD. Ectopic pregnancy. *Current Probl Surg* 2001;38(4):243.

Mishell DR Jr. Ectopic pregnancy: Etiology, pathology, diagnosis, management, fertility prognosis. In: Stenchever MA, Droegemueller W, Herbst AL, Mishell DR Jr, eds. *Comprehensive Gynecology.* St. Louis: Mosby, 2001, chap 17.

30 GENERAL COUNSELING: LIFESTYLE MODIFICATIONS

John D. Davis

HEALTHY DIET

- Dietary factors contribute to a number of major diseases, including coronary artery disease; cancer of the colon, breast, and prostate; stroke; hypertension; type 2 diabetes mellitus; obesity; and osteoporosis.
- Obesity is defined as a body mass index (BMI)—calculated by dividing weight in kilograms by the square of height in meters—of greater than 30. Patients with a BMI between 25 and 30 are overweight.
- Over half of American adults are overweight or obese. A combination of a balanced diet and regular physical activity is the best way to maintain healthy weight.
- There are five major food groups: grains, vegetables, fruit, milk, and meat and beans.
- A variety of grains (bread, cereal, rice, and pasta), especially whole grains—as well as fruits and vegetables—form the basis of a healthy diet.
- Intake of saturated fats (contained in cheese, whole milk, cream, butter, and ice cream) and cholesterol should be limited in order to reduce the risk of hypercholesterolemia and coronary artery disease.
- Total fat intake should not exceed 30 percent of daily calories.
- Intake of foods containing added sugars (eg, soft drinks, cakes, cookies, ice cream, and candy) should be limited in order to limit weight gain and tooth decay.
- Patients should be encouraged to eat less salt in order to lower their risk of developing hypertension.
- The recommended daily intake of calcium for adolescents and adults is 1300 and 1000 mg, respectively.

The majority of adolescent and adult females do not meet these requirements.
- Alcohol should be consumed in moderation (defined as no more than one drink per day for women and no more than two drinks per day for men).

PHYSICAL ACTIVITY

- Adults of any age who participate in even moderate levels of regular physical activity have lower death rates than sedentary adults.
- Regular exercise reduces the risk of coronary artery disease, hypertension, diabetes mellitus, obesity, osteoporosis, colon cancer, and depression.
- The *Healthy People 2010* guidelines published by the Centers for Disease Control and Prevention recommend that adults participate in 30 min of moderate exercise at least 5 days a week or 20 min of vigorous exercise at least three times a week. Moderate activities include those that can be maintained comfortably for at least 60 min (eg, walking); vigorous activities are those that will result in fatigue after 20 min (eg, jogging).
- Only 25 percent of Americans exercise as recommended by *Healthy People 2010*. Barriers to regular physical activity include time constraints, lack of exercise facilities, and lack of a safe environment in which to exercise.

TOBACCO USE

- Cigarette smoking is the most important modifiable cause of disease and death in the United States. It is estimated that cigarette smoking accounts for more than 5 million years of potential life lost annually.

- Smoking is a major risk factor for coronary artery disease, stroke, lung cancer, and chronic obstructive pulmonary disease.
- Approximately 25 percent of American adults smoke cigarettes.
- Exposure to secondhand smoke can cause lung cancer, lower respiratory tract infections, asthma exacerbations, and heart disease in nonsmokers.
- Population-based efforts aimed at reducing cigarette smoking, including increased taxes on cigarettes and antismoking campaigns, have been effective in reducing smoking among adults and adolescents.
- A brief, direct statement informing a patient of the importance of not smoking increases smoking cessation rates by 30 percent.
- Individual or group counseling, telephone help lines, nicotine replacement, and buproprion Hcl (Wellbutrin)—slow-release, 150 mg orally twice daily for 7 to 12 weeks—are also effective smoking cessation interventions.
- Patients who wish to stop smoking should be encouraged to set a "quit date." The first 2 weeks after a patient stops smoking is important, since this is the time when relapse is common.
- Patients who fail in their initial attempts to quit smoking should be told that most patients who do quit smoking are not successful on their first attempt.

PREVENTION OF SEXUALLY TRANSMITTED DISEASES

- Abstention from sexual intercourse is the only method of complete protection from sexually transmitted diseases (STDs).
- People who do not abstain or who are not in a mutually monogamous relationship should be encouraged to use latex condoms consistently and correctly to reduce the risk of STDs (including HIV infection).

INJURY PREVENTION

- Approximately 400 persons in the United States die daily of injuries resulting from motor vehicle accidents, firearms, poisoning, suffocation, falls, fire, and drowning. Most of these deaths result from motor vehicle accidents. Slightly less than half of motor vehicle deaths are alcohol-related.
- Seat belts are the most effective method of preventing injury in motor vehicle accidents.
- Children of age 4 and below always should ride in child safety seats.

- Bicyclists and motorcyclists should be encouraged to wear helmets to reduce the risk of head injury.
- Firearms in homes should be stored in locked containers to reduce the risk of accidental shooting.
- Every home should have a functioning smoke alarm to reduce the risk of death from fire.
- Residential pools should have safety barriers to reduce the risk of drowning.

PREVENTION OF DENTAL DISEASE

- Patients should be encouraged to visit a dental care provider regularly, brush daily with a fluoride-containing toothpaste, and floss daily to reduce the risk of dental caries and periodontal disease.

BIBLIOGRAPHY

Centers for Disease Control and Prevention. *Healthy People 2010.* Available at http://www.healthypeople.gov. Accessed March 2003.

Departments of Health and Human Services and Agriculture. *Nutrition and Your Health: Dietary Guidelines for Americans.* Available at http://health.gov/dietaryguidelines. Accessed March 2003.

U.S. Preventive Services Task Force. *Guide to Clinical Preventive Services,* 2nd ed. Baltimore: Williams & Wilkins, 1996:597.

31 BREAST CANCER SCREENING

John D. Davis

EPIDEMIOLOGY

- Breast cancer is the most common malignancy diagnosed in women in the United States and is the second leading cause of cancer-related deaths in the United States (trailing only lung cancer).
- The lifetime risk of a woman developing breast cancer is one in eight.
- The most significant risk factors for the development of breast cancer are family history of breast cancer in a first-degree relative, previous breast biopsy showing atypical hyperplasia, and first childbirth after age 30.
- Mammography, clinical breast examination (CBE) and breast self-examination (BSE) are the primary methods of screening for breast cancer.

MAMMOGRAPHY

- Women who have mammograms performed regularly reduce their risk of dying from breast cancer by approximately 30 percent.
- While there is little evidence showing that annual mammography reduces breast cancer mortality more effectively than biannual screening, most obstetrician/gynecologists recommend annual mammography beginning at age 40 for average-risk women.
- Women at high risk for breast cancer should begin having mammograms before age 40. Women with an affected first-degree relative should undergo mammography screening beginning at age 35 or when they are 10 years younger than the affected relative was when she was diagnosed with breast cancer.
- There is no specific age when women should stop having mammograms. While most studies of mammography have included few women over the age of 70, these women should continue regular mammographic screening if they are otherwise healthy and have a reasonable life expectancy.
- The chance of developing radiation-induced breast cancer from periodic mammograms is extremely low.
- A mammogram costs approximately $100.

CLINICAL BREAST EXAMINATION

- There are no studies of the effectiveness of CBE alone in reducing mortality from breast cancer.
- Studies comparing mammography alone to mammography with CBE show no significant difference in the reduction of breast cancer mortality.
- Despite these facts, the American College of Obstetricians and Gynecologists (ACOG) recommends that all women over age 18 have an annual CBE.

BREAST SELF-EXAMINATION

- While recent studies have questioned the value of BSE, the ACOG recommends this practice for all women over the age of 18.
- BSE should be performed the week after a woman's menstrual period, the time of her cycle at which hormonal stimulation of the breast tissue will be at a minimum.
- The ideal BSE includes inspection of the breasts for retraction and other skin changes, palpation of the breasts for abnormal masses, and gentle palpation of the nipple and areola to elicit abnormal discharge.
- Patients with abnormalities on BSE should be encouraged to contact their health care provider immediately to arrange for further evaluation.

BIBLIOGRAPHY

American College of Obstetricians and Gynecologists. ACOG Committee Opinion No. 247. Washington, DC: ACOG, December 2000.

U.S. Preventive Services Task Force. *Guide to Clinical Preventive Services*, 3rd ed. U.S. Preventive Services Task Force. Bethesda, MD: 2002–2003.

32 CERVICAL CYTOLOGY

John D. Davis

INTRODUCTION

- Approximately 13,000 new cases of cervical cancer occur annually in the United States; approximately 4100 women die each year from the disease.
- The incidence of invasive cervical cancer in the United States has decreased dramatically over the last half century due primarily to the Papanicolaou ("Pap") test.
- The goal of cytologic screening of the cervix is to identify disease in its early, preinvasive stage, when treatment is safe and nearly 100 percent effective.

EPIDEMIOLOGY

- Well-established risk factors for the development of cervical cancer and cervical intraepithelial neoplasia (CIN) include human papillomavirus (HPV), early onset of sexual activity, multiple sexual partners, HIV infection, and smoking.
- HPV is the cause of virtually all cases of cervical cancer and CIN.
- HPV is a DNA virus. More than 80 types of HPV have been identified, and approximately 25 of these types infect the human genital tract.
- HPV types 6 and 11 are frequently associated with low-grade CIN lesions.
- High-risk HPV types include 16, 18, 31, 33, 35, 39, 45, 51, 52, 56, 58, 59, and 68.
- HPV 18 is commonly associated with adenocarcinoma of the cervix.
- The prevalence of HPV depends on the patient population studied and the method of viral testing used. The majority of patients in high-risk populations will demonstrate HPV infection when tested with sensitive methods.

- While nearly 100 percent of women with cervical cancer or CIN are infected with HPV, less than 5 percent of those infected with HPV develop CIN.

SCREENING

- The Pap test is the primary method of screening for premalignant disease of the cervix.
- The sensitivity of the Pap test in diagnosing premalignant conditions of the cervix is approximately 80 percent.
- Recommendations for the frequency of Pap screening are changing. Until recently, the American Cancer Society, American College of Obstetrics and Gynecology, and National Cancer Institute all recommended that women begin cervical screening at age 18 or at the onset of sexual activity; after three consecutive normal, satisfactory Pap tests, screening may be spaced out at the discretion of the physician.
- In August 2003, the American College of Obstetricians and Gynecologists made the following changes to their recommendations for Pap screening:
  - All women should begin cervical screening 3 years after the onset of sexual activity but no later than age 21.
  - Women under the age of 30 should have Pap tests performed annually.
  - Low-risk women 30 years of age and older who have had three normal Pap tests in a row may undergo screening every 2 to 3 years. Alternatively, these women may have a Pap test and a test for high-risk HPV performed no more frequently than every 3 years.
  - High-risk women (immunocompromised, HIV-positive, history of cervical cancer, history of exposure to diethystilbestrol, or DES) of age 30 and above should undergo annual screening.
  - Screening is not required for patients who have undergone hysterectomy (with removal of the cervix) for indications other than cervical cancer or precancer.
- Conventional Pap testing involves the collection of cells from the ecto- and endocervix and placement of these cells onto a glass slide, where they are fixed, stained, and reviewed. With newer liquid-based cytology, cells from the cervix are collected and placed in a liquid preservative for transport to the laboratory; in the lab the specimen is certrifuged, debris is removed, and a slide containing a single layer of cells is prepared, stained, and reviewed.
- Advantages of liquid-based cytology over conventional Pap testing include the following: most of the specimen obtained from the patient is retained for analysis (with conventional Pap testing much of the specimen can be discarded with the spatula); slides are easier to read because they show less mucus, blood, inflammatory cells, and cell clumping; the number of suboptimal slides is reduced; and residual fluid can be tested for HPV if indicated.
- The Bethesda System is a method of reporting Pap test results using uniform terminology designed to standardize reports, improve communication between cytopathologists and clinicians, and increase correlation between cytologic and histopathologic findings.
- Epithelial cell abnormalities included in the Bethesda System are listed in Table 32-1.

MANAGEMENT OF THE ABNORMAL PAP TEST

- Patients with HSIL and ASC-H Pap tests should undergo immediate colposcopy (examination of the cervix under magnification). While the management of patients with LSIL Pap smears is somewhat more controversial, the majority of patients with LSIL Pap tests should also undergo colposcopy.
- Acceptable management strategies for patients with ASC-US Pap smears include immediate colposcopy, repeat Pap smear in 4 to 6 months, and testing for high-risk HPV types colposcopy for all patients who are positive for high-risk HPV.
- Patients who have liquid-based cytology screening that demonstrates ASC-US can have residual fluid checked for high-risk HPV, eliminating the need to return to clinic to obtain a seperate specimen. This is known as "reflex" HPV testing and has been shown to be a safe, cost-effective way to triage patients with ASC-US Pap smears.
- Patients with atypical glandular cells on their Pap smear should undergo colposcopy, and, if they are not pregnant, endocervical curettage. Patients at risk for endometrial hyperplasia or cancer (for example,

TABLE 32-1   Epithelial Cell Abnormalities

Squamous cell

   Atypical squamous cells
      of undetermined significance (ASC-US)
      cannot exclude high-grade squamous intraepithelial lesion (ASC-H)
   Low-grade squamous intraepithelial lesions (LSIL)
   High-grade squamous intraepithelial lesions (HSIL)
   Squamous cell carcinoma

Glandular cell

   Atypical glandular cells (endocervical, endometrial, or glandular) not otherwise specified
   Atypical glandular cells (endocervical or glandular) favor neoplasia
   Adenocarcinoma

women who are above age 35, who are overweight, or who have experienced abnormal bleeding) should also have endometrial sampling performed.

BIBLIOGRAPHY

Association of Professors of Gynecology and Obstetrics. *Advances in the Screening, Diagnosis, and Treatment of Cervical Disease.* APGO Education Series. Crofton, MD: APGO, September 2002.

Wright TC Jr et al. 2001 consensus guidelines for the management of women with cervical cytological abnormalities. *J Lower Gen Tract Dis* 2002:6:127–143.

33 SCREENING FOR COLORECTAL CANCER

John D. Davis

OVERVIEW

- Colorectal cancer, commonly referred to as colon cancer, is the third most common cancer diagnosed in women and also the third leading cause of cancer-related death in women.
- In 2003, 74,700 women were expected to be diagnosed with colon cancer and 28,800 were expected to die from the disease.
- While nearly 90 percent of colon cancer cases and deaths can be prevented by screening, the majority of patients do not comply with screening guidelines.
- Risk factors for colon cancer are listed in Table 33-1.
- Fecal occult blood testing (FOBT), sigmoidoscopy, colonoscopy, and double-contrast barium enema (DCBE) are all employed as screening tests for colon cancer.

TABLE 33-1 Risk Factors for Colorectal Cancer

Age greater than 50 years
African-American race
Personal or family history of colon cancer or polyps
History of inflammatory bowel disease
Inherited conditions including familial adenomatous polyposis (FAP), hereditary nonpolyposis colorectal cancer (HNPCC), Gardner's syndrome, and Ashkenazi Jewish heritage
Tobacco use
Physical inactivity
High-fat diet

FECAL OCCULT BLOOD TESTING

- FOBT should be performed by patients at home on guaiac-based test cards on three consecutive stool samples.
- Guaiac testing of a single stool specimen obtained during a clinic examination is not an adequate method of screening for colon cancer.
- When performed regularly, FOBT can reduce mortality from colon cancer by 15 to 33 percent.
- According to the American Cancer Society (ACS) guidelines, yearly FOBT combined with sigmoidoscopy every 5 years is preferable to FOBT alone.

SIGMOIDOSCOPY

- Periodic sigmoidoscopic examination can reduce colon cancer mortality by approximately 60 percent.
- Benefits of sigmoidoscopy (compared to colonoscopy) include lower cost (a sigmoidoscopy costs approximately $500), lower risk of bowel perforation or hemorrhage, and more widespread availability (since sigmoidoscopies may be performed by family practitioners and general internists as well as more highly trained gastroenterologists).
- According to the ACS, sigmoidoscopy every 5 years combined with annual FOBT is preferable to periodic sigmoidoscopy alone.

COLONOSCOPY

- Colonoscopy is more sensitive and specific than any other method of detecting colon cancer.
- Drawbacks to colonoscopy include cost (approximately $1500 to $2000 per procedure), greater risk of bowel perforation or bleeding, requirement of conscious sedation (with associated risks), and potentially limited availability owing to the need for more highly trained personnel to perform the procedure.
- When employed as a screening method, colonoscopy should be done every 10 years for patients at average risk.
- Patients who undergo periodic colonoscopy do not require annual FOBT.

DOUBLE-CONTRAST BARIUM ENEMA

- DCBE is an alternative method of examining the entire colon.

TABLE 33-2   American Cancer Society Guidelines for Colorectal Cancer Screening for Individuals at Average Risk

Beginning at age 50, both men and women should follow one of these five screening options:
- Yearly fecal occult blood test (FOBT) plus flexible sigmoidoscopy every 5 years
- Flexible sigmoidoscopy every 5 years[a]
- Yearly fecal occult blood test (FOBT)
- Colonoscopy every 10 years
- Double-contrast barium enema every 5 years

[a]The combination of FOBT and flexible sigmoidoscopy is preferred over either test alone.

- Compared to colonoscopy, DCBE is less expensive (approximately $500 per test) and more readily available; however, DCBE lacks the sensitivity and specificity of colonoscopy, and abnormalities on DCBE or incomplete barium enemas must be followed up with colonoscopy.

RECOMMENDATIONS FOR SCREENING

- All average-risk patients should begin colon cancer screening at age 50.
- ACS guidelines for screening average-risk individuals are listed in Table 33-2.
- Patients at higher risk for developing colon cancer should begin screening before age 50 and should have more frequent screening.

BIBLIOGRAPHY

American Cancer Society. www.cancer.org.
U.S. Preventive Services Task Force. *Screening for Colorectal Cancer: Recommendations and Rationale.* [Originally in *Ann Intern Med* 2002;137:129–131.] Rockville, MD: Agency for Healthcare Research and Quality, July 2002. http://www.ahrq.gov/clnic/3rduspstf/colorectal/colorr.htm.

34 IMMUNIZATIONS

Patrick Duff

INTRODUCTION

- This chapter will reviews the eight immunizations that are of particular importance in adult women:
  - Hepatitis A
  - Hepatitis B
  - Influenza
  - Measles
  - Pneumococcal
  - Rubella
  - Tetanus/diphtheria
  - Varicella

HEPATITIS A VACCINE

- The vaccine is an inactivated agent.
- It is available in two monovalent formulations.
  - Havrix (GlaxoSmithKline)
  - Vaqta (Merck)
- It also is available in a bivalent formulation with the hepatitis B vaccine—Twinrix (GlaxoSmithKline).
- The monovalent vaccine should be administered intramuscularly in two doses 6 months apart.
- The bivalent vaccine should be administered intramuscularly in three doses at 0, 1, and 6 months.
- Candidates for the hepatitis A vaccine include the following:
  - International travelers planning a trip to an area where hepatitis A is endemic
  - Military personnel scheduled for deployment to an area where hepatitis A is endemic
  - Native Americans and Alaskan Eskimos
  - Residents of other areas in the United States where hepatitis A is endemic
  - Patients with chronic liver disease
  - Users of illicit drugs
  - Persons who have clotting factor disorders
  - Residents and staff workers in chronic care facilities
  - HIV-infected patients
  - Persons exposed to someone with hepatitis A
    - In this clinical situation, the vaccine should be administered concurrently with immune globulin.
- The vaccine may be administered safely in pregnancy.
- The most common adverse reaction to the vaccine is soreness, erythema, and induration at the injection site. Serious reactions are extremely rare.
- The vaccine should not be administered to anyone who is allergic to any of the vaccine components:
  - Aluminum hydroxide
  - Phenoxyethanol
  - Polysorbate
  - Sodium chloride
  - Phosphate buffers

HEPATITIS B VACCINE

- The vaccine contains purified hepatitis B surface antigen prepared by recombinant technology.

- It is available in two monovalent forms:
  - Engerix-B (GlaxoSmithKline)
  - Recombivax HB (Merck)
- It also is available in a bivalent form in combination with hepatitis A vaccine—Twinrix (GlaxoSmithKline).
- The vaccine should be administered intramuscularly in three doses at 0, 1, and 6 months. The vaccine is poorly absorbed from the gluteal muscle and therefore should not be injected in this location.
- The Centers for Disease Control and Prevention now recommends universal vaccination for hepatitis B. Women of reproductive age, in particular, should be targeted for this vaccine.
- The vaccine may be administered safely in pregnancy.
- The most common adverse effect of the vaccine is soreness, erythema, and induration at the injection site.
- The vaccine should not be administered to anyone who has a hypersensitivity to the vaccine components:
  - Aluminum hydroxide
  - Thimerosal
  - Sodium chloride
  - Phosphate buffers

INFLUENZA VACCINE

- The vaccine is an inactivated preparation of influenza A and influenza B viral antigens.
- The composition of the vaccine changes annually, in accordance with the viral strains that have been most prevalent in the preceding year.
- Two formulations of the vaccine are available.
  - FluShield (Wyeth-Ayerst)
  - Fluzone (Aventis Pasteur)
- Each formulation is available in a split-virus and whole-virus preparation.
- Adults should receive a single intramuscular dose of the split-virus vaccine.
- The optimal time for annual vaccination is late October through January.
- Appropriate candidates for the vaccine include the following:
  - Health care workers
  - School teachers and day care workers
  - Residents and staff of a chronic care facility
  - Any person with a chronic medical illness
  - Pregnant women
  - Women over the age of 65 years
- In addition, anyone who specifically requests the vaccine should receive the immunization.
- The most frequent adverse reaction is soreness, erythema, and induration at the injection site. A small percentage of patients develop fever, malaise, and myalgias.

- The principal contraindication to the vaccine is an allergy to eggs or egg products or thimerosal.

MEASLES VACCINE

- The measles vaccine (Attenuvax, Merck) is a live-virus vaccine.
- It is usually administered as part of the routine childhood immunizations.
- A second subcutaneous dose of the vaccine is recommended for young men and women and is usually a prerequisite for admission to college.
- The vaccine is available in monovalent, bivalent (measles-rubella), and trivalent forms (measles-mumps-rubella, or MMR).
- Serious side effects of the vaccine are unusual. The most ominous delayed complication of the vaccine is subacute sclerosing panencephalitis (SSPE).
- Contraindications to the vaccine include the following:
  - Pregnancy
  - History of allergic reaction to neomycin
  - Febrile illness
  - Immunodeficiency disorder

PNEUMOCOCCAL VACCINE

- The pneumococcal vaccine (Pneumovax-23, Merck) consists of a mixture of purified capsular polysaccharides from the 23 most prevalent and invasive types of *Streptococcus pneumoniae*.
- The vaccine can be administered intramuscularly or subcutaneously.
- The initial dose should be followed by a booster dose 5 years later.
- Candidates for the pneumococcal vaccine include the following:
  - Immunocompetent persons greater than 65 years of age
  - Immunocompromised persons greater than 2 years of age
  - Persons with chronic medical illnesses, particularly cardiopulmonary disorders, diabetes, renal disease, and sickle cell disease
  - Persons who have had a splenectomy
- The vaccine may be administered safely in pregnancy.
- The most common adverse reactions to the vaccine are soreness, erythema, induration at the injection site, and low-grade fever.
- The vaccine should not be administered to persons who are allergic to any of the vaccine components:
  - Sodium chloride
  - Phenol

RUBELLA VACCINE

- The rubella vaccine (Meruvax II, Merck) is a live-virus vaccine that is administered subcutaneously.
- It usually is administered as part of the routine childhood immunizations in combination with the measles and mumps vaccine (MMR).
- In a small percentage of patients, immunity wanes with age. Therefore all pregnant women should be screened for immunity to rubella. Patients who are susceptible, either because of lack of primary vaccination or waning immunity, should be vaccinated immediately postpartum to ensure immunity in subsequent pregnancies.
- The most frequent adverse reactions to the vaccine are as follows:
  - Fever
  - Headache
  - Malaise
  - Irritability
  - Arthralgias
  - Myalgias
  - Soreness, erythema, and induration at the injection site
- Contraindications to the vaccine include the following:
  - Pregnancy
  - Immunodeficiency disorder
  - Febrile illness
  - Allergy to albumin, neomycin, sorbitol, and gelatin

TETANUS/DIPHTHERIA (T/d) VACCINE

- This vaccine consists of a sterilized combination of tetanus and diphtheria toxoid.
- Tetanus and diphtheria vaccination (diphtheria, pertussis, and tetanus, or DPT) is part of the routine childhood immunization series.
- Booster doses are recommended every 10 years and at the time of an acute penetrating injury.
- The vaccine may be administered safely in pregnancy.
- The most common adverse reaction to the vaccine is soreness, erythema, and induration at the site of injection.
- Contraindications to the tetanus/diphtheria vaccine include the following:
  - Allergy to thimerosal
  - Moderate to severe febrile illness

VARICELLA VACCINE

- The varicella vaccine (Varivax, Merck) is a live-virus immunization.

- The vaccine now is included as part of the routine childhood immunization series.
- Women of reproductive age who are susceptible to varicella should be vaccinated prior to pregnancy or in the immediate postpartum period.
- The vaccine should be administered subcutaneously in two doses 4 to 8 weeks apart.
- The most common adverse reactions are as follows:
  - Fever
  - Soreness, erythema, induration at the injection site
  - Varicella-like rash
- Contraindications to the varicella vaccine include the following:
  - Pregnancy
  - Immunodeficiency disorder or immunosuppressive therapy
  - Active, untreated tuberculosis
  - Febrile illness
  - History of allergic reaction to neomycin

BIBLIOGRAPHY

American College of Obstetricians and Gynecologists. Immunization during pregnancy. *Obstet Gynecol* 2003;101: 207–212.

Broome CV, Breiman RF. Pneumococcal vaccine—Past, present, future. *N Engl J Med* 1991;325:1506–1507.

Duff B, Duff P. Hepatitis A vaccine: ready for prime time. *Obstet Gynecol* 1998;91:468–471.

Duff P. Varicella vaccine. *Infect Dis Obstet Gynecol* 1996;4:63–65.

35 CONTRACEPTION

Patrick Duff

INTRODUCTION

- A variety of reversible methods of contraception are available today to help women make thoughtful choices about the timing of pregnancy.
- In addition, several methods of permanent sterilization are available for women who have completed their childbearing.
- Several factors should be considered by the patient and her physician in planning a method of contraception:
  - Patient motivation
  - Degree of security desired

- Ease of use
- Cost
- Presence of complicating medical conditions:
    - Prior history of thromboembolism—a contraindication to use of combination oral contraceptives
    - Prior history of pelvic inflammatory disease (PID)—a contraindication to use of the IUD

BARRIER METHODS OF CONTRACEPTION

MALE CONDOM

- The male condom fits over the erect penis and prevents the ejaculate from entering the vagina.
- Male condoms are made of latex, polyurethrane, silicone, or lamb's intestine.
- The latex condom is the most resistant to breakage.
- Condoms are highly effective in preventing transmission of sexually transmitted diseases (STDs) such as *Chlamydia,* gonorrhea, syphilis, and HIV infection.
- Failure rates of condoms, due to slippage or breakage, range from a low of 3 percent to a high of 14 percent.

FEMALE CONDOM

- The female condom is made of polyurethrane and is prelubricated with silicone.
- It may be used by itself, without a spermicide.
- It is effective in preventing the transmission of STDs.
- The failure rate of the female condom ranges from 5 to 21 percent, similar to the failure rates associated with the diaphragm or cervical cap.
- The female condom should be inserted no longer than 8 h before coitus. It should be left in place for 6 h thereafter.

DIAPHRAGM

- The diaphragm is made of latex. It fits in the upper vagina and covers the cervix, preventing penetration of sperm into the endocervical canal.
- For maximum effectiveness, it should be used in conjunction with a spermicidal cream or jelly.
- The diaphragm is effective in reducing the risk of transmission of STDs.
- The device should be inserted no longer than 6 h prior to coitus. It should be left in place for 6 h thereafter.
- If a second act of intercourse is planned while the diaphragm is in place, an additional applicatorful of spermicide should be inserted into the upper vagina.

- The failure rate of the diaphragm ranges from 6 to 20 percent.
- The most common adverse effect of the diaphragm is an increased risk of urinary tract infection (UTI).

CERVICAL CAP

- The cervical cap is made of either latex or nonallergenic silicone rubber.
- It is similar in effectiveness to the diaphragm but is harder to fit.
- Its effectiveness is increased when it is used with a spermicide.
- The cap should be inserted no longer than 6 h prior to coitus. It should be left in place for 8 h thereafter.
- The maximum duration of use of the cap is 48 h.

CONTRACEPTIVE SPONGE

- The contraceptive sponge is made of polyurethrane impregnated with a spermicide.
- It absorbs semen and blocks entrance of sperm to the cervical canal.
- The sponge should be inserted no longer than 24 h before coitus and should be left in place for 6 hours thereafter.
- The effectiveness of the sponge is similar to that of the diaphragm or cervical cap.
- The principal adverse effects of the sponge are an allergic reaction and local irritation.

SPERMICIDES

- Several chemicals are used as spermicides. The most common are these:
    - Nonoxynol-9
    - Octoxynol-9
    - Benzalkonium chloride
    - Menfegol
- A spermicide may be prepared as a jelly, cream, foam, tablet, or suppository.
- Spermicides should be inserted just prior to coitus.
- Failure rates range from 6 to 25 percent.
- The most common adverse effect is local irritation.

INTRAUTERINE CONTRACEPTIVE DEVICE (IUD OR IUCD)

- The IUD exerts its effect by creating an intrauterine and intracervical environment that is spermicidal.

- The two IUDs available in the United States are the copper-containing device (TCu-380A) and the levonorgestrel-containing device.
- The copper device can remain in place for 10 years.
- The levonorgestrel-containing device must be replaced in 5 years.
- The failure rate of the IUD is 1 to 3 percent.
- Adverse effects of the IUD include the following:
  ○ Menometrorrhagia
  ○ Intrauterine infection
  ○ Dysmenorrhea
  ○ Expulsion
  ○ Increased risk of ectopic pregnancy if pregnancy occurs
- The IUD should be used primarily in multiparous women who have a stable monogamous relationship and who have no history of PID, uterine anomaly, menometrorrhagia, or severe dysmenorrhea.
- If pregnancy occurs with an IUD in place, the device should be removed if possible. If the IUD cannot be removed, the patient is at increased risk for spontaneous abortion, septic abortion, and preterm delivery.

STEROID CONTRACEPTION

DEPO-MEDROXYPROGESTERONE ACETATE (DEPO-PROVERA)

- Depo-Provera thickens the cervical mucus, alters the endometrium, and prevents ovulation.
- The drug is administered intramuscularly in a dose of 150 mg every 3 months.
- The failure rate is ≤ 1 percent.
- Absolute contraindications to Depo-Provera include the following:
  ○ Pregnancy
  ○ Unexplained genital bleeding
  ○ Severe coagulation disorders
  ○ Hepatic adenoma
- Relative contraindications include:
  ○ Any liver disease
  ○ Severe cardiovascular disease
  ○ Difficulty with intramuscular injections
  ○ Severe depression
  ○ Desire for rapid return to fertility after discontinuation of contraceptive

LEVONORGESTREL IMPLANT (Norplant)

- The Norplant system consists of six silastic capsules that are implanted subcutaneously in the medial aspect of the upper arm.

- Each capsule contains 36 mg of crystalline levonorgestrel.
- The capsules provide effective contraception for 5 years.
- Norplant exerts its effect by inhibiting ovulation and altering the cervical mucus and endometrium.
- The failure rate is ≤ 1 percent.
- Absolute contraindications to use of Norplant include the following:
  ○ Active thrombophlebitis
  ○ Undiagnosed genital tract bleeding
  ○ Acute liver disease
  ○ Benign or malignant liver tumor
  ○ Breast cancer
- Relative contraindications include the following:
  ○ Heavy cigarette smoking (greater than one pack/day)
  ○ History of ectopic pregnancy
  ○ Severe hyperlipidemia
  ○ Severe hypertension
  ○ Cardiovascular disease
  ○ Gallbladder disease

PROGESTIN-ONLY PILL ("Minipill")

- The minipill contains a small dose of a progestational agent. Several different formulations are available.
- It must be taken daily in a continuous manner. It should be taken at the same time each day.
- The minipill exerts its contraceptive effect by altering the cervical mucus and endometrium.
- The failure rate ranges from 1 to 10 percent.
- The most common adverse effect is irregular bleeding.
- The minipill containing levonorgestrel also may cause or exacerbate acne.

COMBINATION ORAL CONTRACEPTIVES

- Combination pills contain an estrogen and a progestin.
- Essentially all of the combination pills currently prescribed use low doses of ethinyl estradiol (≤ 35 μg) as the estrogen.
- Several different progestational agents are used in modern combination pills. Some are more androgenic (eg, levonorgestrel) than others (eg, desogestrel, gestodene, norgestimate).
- The combination pills exert their contraceptive effect primarily by inhibiting ovulation.
- The failure rate is ≤ 1 percent.
- Common minor side effects include the following:
  ○ Breakthrough bleeding
  ○ Emotional lability

○ Breast tenderness
○ Melasma (darkening of certain areas of skin, particularly in the face and areola)
- Serious side effects associated with use of combination oral contraceptives include a *slight* increase in the risk of:
  ○ Superficial and deep vein thrombophlebitis and pulmonary embolism.
  ○ Cerebrovascular accident.
  ○ Myocardial infarction—the excess risk is concentrated almost entirely in women who are > 35 years and who smoke.
  ○ Liver adenoma.
  ○ Cholecystitis.
  ○ Pancreatitis.
- *Absolute* contraindications to use of the combination pills include the following:
  ○ Pregnancy
  ○ Undiagnosed genital tract bleeding
  ○ Heavy smoking and age > 35 years
  ○ Ischemic heart disease
  ○ History of thrombophlebitis or a severe hereditary thrombophilia
  ○ Active liver disease
  ○ Estrogen-dependent tumor
  ○ History of psychotic depression
- *Relative* contraindications to use of the combination pills include the following:
  ○ Hypertension
  ○ Diabetes
  ○ Migraine headaches
  ○ Gallbladder disease
  ○ Prior history of liver disease
  ○ Heavy smoking, age < 35 years

CONTRACEPTIVE PATCH (ORTHO-EVRA)

- The contraceptive patch contains norelgestromin (6 mg) and ethinyl estradiol (0.75 mg).
- The patch delivers a daily dose of norelgestromin (150 μg) and ethinyl estradiol (20 μg).
- The patch is changed weekly for 3 weeks. During the fourth week, the patch is not worn and menses typically occur.
- The patch is similar in effectiveness to the combination oral contraceptive.
- Common side effects of the patch include the following:
  ○ Local irritation
  ○ Nausea and vomiting
  ○ Breast tenderness
  ○ Headache
  ○ Emotional lability

- The absolute and relative contraindications are similar to those of the combination oral contraceptives.

EMERGENCY POSTCOITAL CONTRACEPTION

- Emergency postcoital contraception should be administered within 72 h of a "contraceptive failure."
- The preferred treatment regimen at present is levonorgestrel (0.75 mg) for two doses, 12 h apart. This progestin-only regimen is less likely to cause nausea and vomiting than the regimens that also contain estrogen.
- This formulation is marketed under the trade name of Plan B.
- When administered as an emergency contraceptive, levonorgestrel delays ovulation and alters the endometrium.
- Postcoital contraception is approximately 75 percent effective in preventing pregnancy.

STERILIZATION

- Worldwide, sterilization now is the most common method of contraception in both men and women.
- Female sterilization may be accomplished by either minilaparotomy or laparoscopy. The latter is most commonly used.
- When laparoscopy is performed, the tubes may be occluded by application of a plastic ring or clip or by coagulation.
- Complications associated with surgical sterilization include the following:
  ○ Wound infection
  ○ Pelvic infection
  ○ Vascular injury with resultant hemorrhage
- The long-term failure rate of sterilization procedures is approximately 1 to 2 percent.

BIBLIOGRAPHY

Speroff L, Glass RH, Kase NG. *Clinical Gynecologic Endocrinology and Infertility,* 6th ed. Baltimore: Lippincott Williams & Wilkins, 1999.

Zieman M. Transdermal contraception: Update on clinical management. *OBG* Mgt December 2002; 66–77.

36 NORMAL MENSTRUAL PHYSIOLOGY

Alice Rhoton-Vlasak

OVERVIEW

- A normal menstrual cycle represents an interaction between the hypothalamus, pituitary gland, ovaries, and endometrium.
- The normal menstrual cycle lasts approximately 28 days (normal range of 24 to 35 days), with an average of 14 days in the follicular and 14 days in the luteal phase.
- The menstrual cycle is under control of the hypothalamic/pituitary axis and can be viewed in terms of the endometrial and ovarian cycles.
- The endometrial cycle is divided into two phases:
  ∘ Proliferative
  ∘ Secretory
- The ovarian cycle is divided into three phases:
  ∘ Follicular
  ∘ Ovulatory
  ∘ Luteal
- The precise coordination between the hypothalamic/pituitary axis, ovary, and endometrium—which occurs during each menstrual cycle—allows for the normal flow, lasting from 4 to 7 days, with an average blood loss of 35 mL (Fig. 36-1).

HYPOTHALAMIC/PITUITARY AXIS (HORMONAL REGULATION OF THE NORMAL MENSTRUAL CYCLE)

- The key portions of the brain involved in regulation of the normal menstrual cycle are the hypothalamus and pituitary gland, which are connected by a network of vessels called the hypothalamic-hypophyseal portal system. The hypothalamus secretes gonadotropin-releasing hormone (GnRH), which moves down the portal system to control the secretion of gonadotropins from the anterior pituitary. The gonadotropins are follicle-stimulating hormone (FSH) and luteinizing hormone (LH).
- GnRH is a decapeptide synthesized primarily in the arcuate nucleus. It is secreted in a pulsatile fashion throughout the menstrual cycle.
- The anterior pituitary contains six different cell types that produce six protein hormones: FSH, LH, thyroid-stimulation hormone (TSH), prolactin, growth hormone (GH), and adrenocorticotrophic hormone (ACTH).
- At the start of each menstrual cycle, the pituitary secretes larger amounts of FSH, which, in concert with LH, promotes the maturation of several ovarian follicles.
- The secretion of LH and FSH promotes the production of estradiol from the ovary. Blood levels of estradiol rise and provide negative feedback on the hypothalamic-pituitary secretion of FSH. As estradiol levels rise later in the follicular phase, there is a positive feedback on the release of LH, resulting in an LH surge and ovulation. Ovulation occurs 36 to 44 h after the onset of the midcycle LH surge.
- During the luteal phase, both LH and FSH are significantly suppressed through the negative feedback effect of circulating estradiol and progesterone.
- Should pregnancy fail to occur, inhibition of LH and FSH persists until progesterone and estradiol levels decline near the end of the luteal phase as a result of corpus luteum regression. The net effect is a rise in serum FSH, which initiates follicular growth for the next cycle.

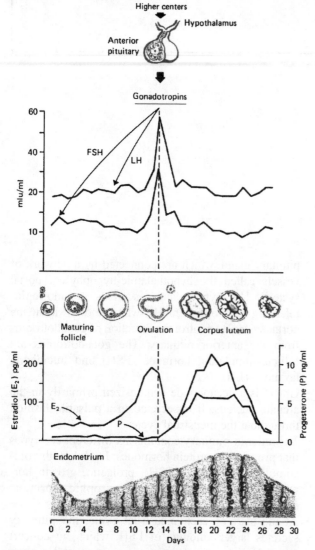

FIG. 36-1 Outlines the hypothalamic, pituitary, endometrial, and ovarian events in the normal menstrual cycle. (From Scott JR, Disaia PJ, Spellacy WN, Hammon DB, eds. *Danforth's Obstetrics and Gynecology*, 5th ed. Philadelphia: Lippincott, 1986:121. With permission.)

OVARIAN PHYSIOLOGY

- Primordial follicles undergo sequential development, differentiation, and maturation until a mature graafian follicle is produced. The follicle then ruptures, releasing the ovum. Subsequently, the follicle undergoes luteinization, resulting in formation of the corpus luteum.

- The three main hormones produced by the ovary during the ovarian cycle are estrogens, progestins, and androgens. Estradiol, the main ovarian estrogen, remains at low levels during early follicular development but begins to rise about 1 week before

ovulation, with maximum levels 1 day before the LH peak. After this peak and before ovulation, there is a marked precipitous fall. During the luteal phase, estradiol levels rise again, with a secondary peak 5 to 7 days after ovulation. They return to baseline shortly before menstruation. Estrone is another ovarian estrogen; it is secreted in lower levels than estradiol.

- The ovary also produces progesterone, which is secreted at low levels during the follicular phase and at higher levels just before ovulation. Levels of progesterone secretion by the corpus luteum reach a peak 8 to 9 days after ovulation and return to baseline shortly before menstruation. When pregnancy occurs, progesterone levels remain elevated.

- The third class of hormones derived from the ovary are androgens. Both the ovary and adrenal glands secrete small amounts of testosterone, but most of the testosterone is derived from the metabolism of androstenedione, which is secreted by both the ovary and the adrenal gland.

- In order for the ovary to produce estrogens, androgens, and progestins, it must undergo growth and development during the follicular, ovulatory, and luteal phases. The cyclic development of the ovarian follicles and the sequential production of hormones create the normal cyclicity of the menstrual cycle.

THE FOLLICULAR PHASE OF THE OVARIAN CYCLE

- At birth, each ovary contains about 400,000 primordial egg cells. The oocyte is initially called a primordial follicle. As the follicular and stromal cells develop in utero, a primary follicle develops. As this follicle forms, two cell layers envelope the developing ovum: the granulosa cells in the inner layer, surrounded by the outer theca interna and theca externa.

- During each cycle, a cohort of follicles is recruited for development. Only one follicle usually continues differentiation and matures into a follicle that ovulates. The remaining follicles undergo atresia. Mature preovulatory follicles reach mean diameters of approximately 18 to 25 mm.

- Follicular maturation is dependent on the local production of receptors for FSH and LH. FSH enhances the induction of LH receptors on the granulosa cells of the follicle that is destined to ovulate. FSH also initiates estradiol production in granulosa cells.

- As the egg matures, the mature or graafian follicle is moved toward the follicular surface, where proteolytic enzymes cause degeneration of the cells on the surface, allowing rupture. The oocyte and corona radiata are expelled into the peritoneal cavity and ovulation takes place. The structural changes that culminate in ovulation are initiated by the preovulatory LH surge.

• Shortly before ovulation, the chromatin in the oocyte is resolved into distinct chromosomes. Meiotic division then takes place, with unequal distribution of the cytoplasm to form a secondary oocyte and the first polar body. Each element contains 23 chromosomes, each in the form of two monads. No further development takes place until after ovulation and fertilization have occurred. A second meiotic division is completed just prior to fertilization to reduce the chromosomal component of the egg pronucleus to 23 single chromosomes (22 plus X or Y). This chromosome number is restored to the usual diploid number at the time of union with the sperm.

LUTEAL PHASE OF THE OVARIAN CYCLE

• After ovulation, the granulosa cells, under the influence of LH, undergo luteinization. The corpus luteum reaches maturity about 8 days after ovulation. The corpus luteum produces copious amounts of progesterone and some estradiol. The normal functional life span of the corpus luteum is about 14 days. If a pregnancy ensues, the corpus luteum will continue to secrete hormones for several more weeks; otherwise, it regresses and is gradually replaced by an avascular scar called the corpus albicans. The events of the ovarian cycle are outlined in Fig. 36-1.

THE ENDOMETRIAL CYCLE

• During the menstrual cycle, sequential changes also occur in the endometrium. The endometrial cycle is divided into two phases. The endometrium is responsive to ovarian hormones, and the cycles correspond directly to the ovarian phases. The endometrium is functionally divided into two zones, consisting of the outer portion, or functionalis, which undergoes cyclic changes during the menstrual cycle, and the inner portion, or basalis, which remains relatively unchanged during each menstrual cycle. The basalis layer provides stem cells for the renewal of the functionalis layer after each episode of menstruation.

• Day 1 of the menstrual cycle is the first day of menstruation. During the menstrual phase, which usually lasts 4 to 7 days, there is disruption and disintegration of the endometrial glands and stroma, leukocyte infiltration, and red blood cell extravasation. Menstruation allows the endometrial wall to be regenerated with each monthly cycle, ensuring a new lining for each possible conceptus.

• The proliferative phase is characterized by endometrial growth secondary to estrogenic stimulation. The large increase in estrogen secretion causes marked cellular proliferation of the epithelial lining, the endometrial glands, and the connective tissue of the stroma. Histologic changes that correlate with the proliferative phase of the endometrium include maximal endometrial growth with elongation of the spiral arteries and straight, narrow-lumened endometrial glands.

• The secretory phase comprises the last 2 weeks, or days 14 to 28, postovulation. After ovulation, progesterone is secreted by the corpus luteum, stimulating the endometrial glandular cells to secrete glycogen and other substances. The glands become torturous, and the lumens become dilated and filled with secretions. Histologically, the spiral arteries continue to extend into the superficial layer of the endometrium and become more convoluted.

• Due to the sequential changes in endometrial histology during the secretory phase, precise dating of the secretory endometrium is possible. Endometrial dating is useful in evaluating patients with infertility or recurrent pregnancy losses because it allows assessment of the adequacy of ovarian progesterone for endometrial development.

• If pregnancy does not occur and the corpus luteum begins to regress, there is a decline in the secretion of progesterone and estradiol. Marked constriction of the spiral arterioles takes place, causing ischemia of the endometrium, followed by leukocyte infiltration and red blood cell extravasation, leading to menstruation a day later.

BIBLIOGRAPHY

Scott JR, Disaia PJ, Spellacy WN, Hammon DB. eds. *Danforth's Obstetrics and Gynecology*, 5th ed. Philadelphia: Lippincott, 1986:121–133.

Yen SC, Jaffe RB, Barbieri RL. eds. *Reproductive Endocrinology: Physiology, Pathophysiology, and Clinical Management*, 4th ed. Philadelphia: Saunders, 1999: 191–256.

37 ABNORMAL UTERINE BLEEDING

Alice Rhoton-Vlasak

EPIDEMIOLOGY

- **Abnormal uterine bleeding** (AUB) is a common indication for gynecologic evaluation.
- AUB may affect women throughout life, from adolescence to menopause.
- Dysfunctional uterine bleeding (DUB) (see Chap. 54) is defined as AUB unrelated to anatomic lesions of the uterus. It is largely caused by aberrations in the hypothalamic-pituitary-ovarian axis. Most DUB occurs around menarche or in the perimenopausal years.
- Of the half-million hysterectomies performed every year in the United States, 50 percent or more are for treatment of AUB.

DEFINITION

- A normal menstrual cycle occurs every 24 to 25 days, with flow of 4 ± 2 days and a mean blood loss of 35 to 40 mL.
- Bleeding more often than every 24 days, or > 7 days of flow, or >80 mL of blood loss is considered abnormal and requires evaluation.
- AUB can be attributed to organic, anatomic, or systemic pathology.
- Table 37-1 outlines various patterns of AUB.

ETIOLOGY

- The causes vary over a woman's lifetime.
- Organic causes, especially neoplasms, increase with advancing age. Table 37-2 lists potential causes of AUB.
- Systemic diseases—including congenital or acquired coagulopathies such as von Willebrand's disease, thrombocytopenia, platelet dysfunction, and/or prothrombin deficiency—may cause AUB.

TABLE 37-1   Patterns of Abnormal Uterine Bleeding

Menorrhagia	Heavy bleeding at regular intervals (>8 days, >80 mL)
Metrorrhagia	Irregular, frequent bleeding
Menometrorrhagia	Prolonged, excessive bleeding at irregular intervals
Amenorrhea	Absence of bleeding for >6 months
Oligomenorrhea	Cycle length >35 days
Polymenorrhea	Cycle length <21 days
Intermenstrual bleeding	Bleeding between normal cycles

TABLE 37-2   Principal Causes of Abnormal Uterine Bleeding

Organic causes
   Uterine leiomyomas
   Endometrial and cervical polyps
   Adenomyosis
   Endometritis/cervicitis
   Endometrial hyperplasia
   Endometrial/cervical carcinoma
Complications of pregnancy
   Abortion
   Ectopic pregnancy
   Gestational trophoblastic disease
Systemic diseases
   Liver disease
   Renal disease
   Hypothyroidism
   Coagulation disorders
Iatrogenic causes
   Hormonal therapy
   Contraceptive devices/hormones
   Heparin/warfarin
   Aspirin
Anovulation (dysfunctional uterine bleeding)

- Although cancer is not the most common cause of AUB, it is the most important. Endometrial exposure to prolonged unopposed estrogen from anovulation may result in the development of endometrial hyperplasia or carcinoma. Figure 37-1 shows a histologic specimen indicating endometrial adenocarcinoma.
- Risk factors for endometrial hyperplasia include body weight >90 kg, age >45 years, infertility, family history of colonic cancer, and nulliparity .
- Iatrogenic causes include the use of oral, transdermal, or injectable contraceptives or hormone replacement.
- DUB is diagnosed when other causes have been excluded. DUB occurs most commonly at the extremes of reproductive age (20 percent of cases in adolescence and 40 percent in patients over age 40).

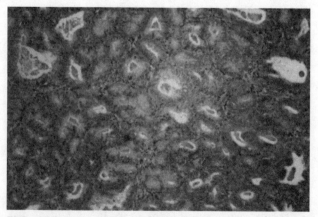

FIG. 37-1 Endometrial biopsy specimen with back-to-back glands, as seen in endometrial adenocarcinoma.

DIAGNOSTIC EVALUATION

- The evaluation should include a history, physical examination, selected laboratory tests, and, in some patients, imaging of the uterine cavity.
- The clinician must distinguish asymptomatic lesions from those causing bleeding.
- The history should include details of bleeding onset, frequency, duration, associated pain, sexual history, use of medications, and possible symptoms of pregnancy.
- The clinician should inquire about easy bruising, family history of bleeding disorders, weight gain or loss, galactorrhea, cold intolerance, and fatigue.
- A detailed physical examination should be performed to assess for conditions such as genital tract infection or mucosal atrophy, cervical polyps, trauma, prolapsed myomas, or cancer.
- An enlarged uterus suggests pregnancy, adenomyosis, or uterine leiomyoma.
- Laboratory evaluation should include the following:
  - Complete blood count
  - Platelet count
  - Urinary/serum B-hCG
  - Cervical cytology
  - Coagulation profile
  - TSH
  - Prolactin
- Several diagnostic procedures may be used to rule out endometrial cancer and identify anatomic causes of AUB (Table 37-3).
- Endometrial biopsy should be performed on patients who fail initial therapy, are at high risk for hyperplasia or cancer, or are >35 years old (Fig. 37-2).
- Pelvic ultrasound imaging identifies endometrial and myometrial abnormalities and evaluates the adnexa. Figure 37-3 demonstrates a saline infusion ultrasound (SIS) image of an intrauterine lesion identified as a benign polyp at hysteroscopy.
- Transvaginal ultrasound also allows measurement of the endometrial thickness. A thickness >10 mm in premenopausal women and 4 mm in postmenopausal women may indicate endometrial pathology requiring further evaluation—ie, with biopsy.

TABLE 37-3 Diagnostic Procedures for Abnormal Uterine Bleeding

Office endometrial biopsy
   Pipelle (flexible curette)
   Novak/Randall (rigid curette)
Dilation and curettage (D&C)
Transvaginal/pelvic ultrasound
Saline infusion ultrasound (SIS)
Hysteroscopy

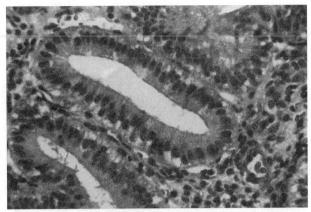

FIG. 37-2 Normal early secretory endometrial glands from a pipelle endometrial biopsy.

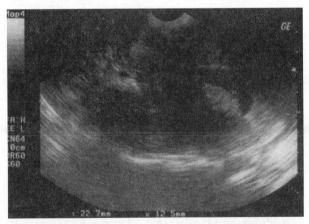

FIG. 37-3 Result of an ultrasound examination following saline infusion in a 35-year-old woman with abnormal uterine bleeding. It demonstrates an intrauterine filling defect likely representing a polyp.

- SIS or hysteroscopy may be used to evaluate the endometrial cavity for polyps, fibroids, or other abnormalities.
- Hysteroscopy may be performed in an office or operating room setting. Resection attachments provide an immediate opportunity to biopsy or remove lesions. Figure 37-4 shows a hysteroscopic view of the polyp seen in Fig. 37-3.
- In most situations, hysteroscopy has replaced the blind dilation and curettage (D&C).

TREATMENT

MEDICAL

- Medical rather than surgical therapy is the preferred management, especially where there is no pelvic pathology. Medications are used to control bleeding

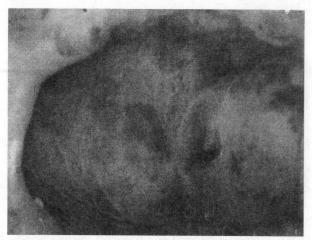

FIG. 37-4 Hysteroscopic view of a benign polyp seen in the patient in Fig. 37-3.

and prevent the development of endometrial hyperplasia or cancer.
- Specific therapy should be used to treat patients with medical conditions such as coagulation disorders, hypothyroidism, liver or renal disease.
- Table 37-4 outlines medical treatments for AUB.

SURGICAL

- Surgical intervention is indicated if bleeding persists despite medical therapy or if diagnostic testing reveals a condition not amenable to medical treatment, such as cancer, or other anatomic abnormalities. Table 37-5 summarizes surgical treatment options for AUB.

TABLE 37-4   Medical Treatment for Abnormal Uterine Bleeding

Iron—325 mg of ferrous sulfate orally two to three
   times daily
Prostaglandin synthetase inhibitors
Daily or cyclic progestins
   Medroxyprogesterone acetate (MPA) 10–20 mg daily or for 10–15
   days per month
High-dose estrogen[a]
   25 mg IV conjugated estrogen every 4–6 h
   2.5 mg oral conjugated estrogen daily for 25 days, then
   MPA 10 mg orally for 7–10 days
Combination oral contraceptives[b]
   Low dose pill orally 2–4 times daily for one week,
   followed by 1 pill/day.*
   Daily oral contraceptive
Gonadotropin releasing hormone agonists/antagonists

[a]For heavy, acute, bleeding.
[b]Oral contraceptives are contraindicated in women over 35 years of age who smoke cigarettes, have undiagnosed abnormal uterine bleeding, active liver disease, or history of thromboembolism and in women who might be pregnant.

TABLE 37-5   Surgical Management Options for Patients with Abnormal Uterine Bleeding

Dilation and curettage[a]
Operative hysteroscopy
Hysteroscopic endometrial ablation
   Electrosurgical techniques
   Hydrothermablator
Non-hysteroscopic endometrial ablation
   Balloon ablation
   Cryoablation
   Bipolar or unipolar electrodes
   Laser
   Microwave
Hysterectomy
   Abdominal
   Vaginal
   Laparoscopically assisted (LAVH)
Myomectomy[b]

[a]Indicated only for patients who fail medical therapy or those undergoing hysteroscopy.
[b]Indicated for symptomatic uterine fibroids when preservation of the uterus and fertility is desired.

- Hysterectomy (either abdominal or vaginal) is the most common surgery for AUB. Figure 37-5 shows a hysterectomy specimen demonstrating multiple uterine fibroids.
- Hysterectomy is no longer considered the only definitive cure for patients with benign AUB because of the availability of hysteroscopic and nonhysteroscopic endometrial ablation techniques. Hysterectomy should be reserved for patients who have endometrial cancer or who fail to respond to conservative surgical procedures.
- Hysteroscopy largely has replaced blind D&C. The advantages of hysteroscopy include the following:
  - Ability to diagnose and resect polyps or fibroids, and ablate endometrium in one surgical procedure.
  - Relatively inexpensive.

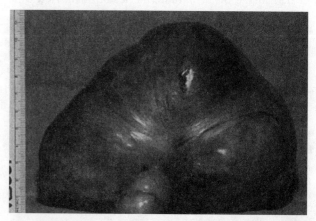

FIG. 37-5 A hysterectomy specimen with multiple uterine fibroids, which caused abnormal uterine bleeding. (Photograph courtesy of John Davis, MD.)

- Contraindications to hysteroscopy include:
  - Presence of infection
  - Endometrial hyperplasia or cancer
  - Intrauterine lesion >5 cm
- Endometrial ablation (destruction) at the time of hysteroscopy results in amenorrhea in 50 to 75 percent of patients and improvement of bleeding in others. Ablation techniques are used in patients who have personal or medical contraindications to hysterectomy.

BIBLIOGRAPHY

Farquhar CM, Lethaby A, Sowter M, et al. An evaluation of risk factors for endometrial hyperplasia in premenopausal women with abnormal menstrual bleeding. *Am J Obstet Gynecol* 1999;181:525–529.

Ferenczy A. Pathophysiology of endometrial bleeding. *Maturitas* 2003;45(1):1–14.

Munro MG. Abnormal uterine bleeding in the reproductive years. Part I: Pathogenesis and clinical investigation. *J Am Assoc Gynecol Laparosc* 1999; 6:391–418.

Munro MG. Abnormal uterine bleeding in the reproductive years. Part II: Medical management. *J Am Assoc Gynecol Laparosc* 2000;1:17–34.

Munro MG. Abnormal uterine bleeding: Surgical management: Part III. *J Am Assoc Gynecol Laparosc* 1999;7(4):18–47.

Seltzer VL, Benjamin F, Deutsch S. Perimenopausal bleeding patterns and pathologic findings. *J Am Med Women's Assoc* 1990;45:132–134.

38 VAGINAL INFECTIONS

Patrick Duff

Vaginal infections are among the most common reasons for urgent office visits. They may be divided into three types: bacterial vaginosis, candidiasis, and trichomoniasis. While most vaginal infections are easily treated, some may be associated with more serious complications, such as premature delivery, maternal and neonatal infection, pelvic inflammatory disease, and severe systemic infection.

BACTERIAL VAGINOSIS

EPIDEMIOLOGY

- **Bacterial vaginosis** (BV) is a polymicrobial infection caused by a disruption in the normal vaginal flora. It is responsible for approximately 45 percent of vaginal infections.
- The principal pathogens are *Gardnerella vaginalis*, *Mobiluncus species*, anaerobes, and mycoplasmas.
- In pregnant women, BV has been associated with preterm delivery, **preterm premature rupture of the membranes** (PPROM), and maternal and neonatal infection.
- In nonpregnant women, BV is an important risk factor for pelvic inflammatory disease.

CLINICAL MANIFESTATIONS

- Some patients with BV are relatively asymptomatic.
- Symptomatic patients typically note a profuse, thin, gray-colored vaginal discharge. The discharge has the odor of spoiled fish, and the odor is often accentuated after intercourse. Pruritus is not a characteristic symptom, and the vaginal mucosa is not inflamed.

DIAGNOSIS

- In affected patients, the vaginal pH is greater than or equal to 4.5.
- When vaginal secretions are mixed with a drop of 10% potassium hydroxide, a characteristic amine odor (spoiled fish) is liberated ("whiff test").
- Saline microscopy typically shows decreased or absent lactobacilli, many cocci and small bacilli, and clue cells.
- Gram's stain of vaginal secretions is the usual method for identifying BV in research studies (Fig. 38-1), but saline microscopy, pH assessment, and the amine test are the most useful diagnostic studies in clinical practice.

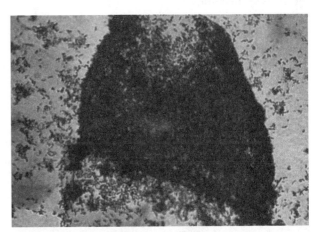

FIG. 38-1 Gram's stain shows an epithelium that is virtually covered with small cocci and bacilli. These same bacteria are present in the background, and lactobacilli are absent.

- Culture for bacteria or mycoplasmas is virtually never indicated in patients with suspected BV.

TREATMENT

- The most cost-effective treatment for BV in both pregnant and nonpregnant women is oral metronidazole.
- Pregnant women should be treated with metronidazole, 250 mg three times daily for 7 days. An alternative regimen is clindamycin, 300 mg orally twice daily for 7 days. Clindamycin is considerably more expensive than metronidazole and is more likely to cause diarrhea.
- Nonpregnant women should be treated with metronidazole, 500 mg twice daily for 7 days. Alternative regimens are oral clindamycin (300 mg twice daily for 7 days), metronidazole gel 0.75% (one applicatorful intravaginally daily for 5 days), or clindamycin cream 2% (one applicatorful intravaginally daily for 7 days).
- Treatment of the sexual partner is not recommended as a matter of routine. However, treatment of the partner should be considered in patients with persistent or recurrent infections.

CANDIDIASIS

EPIDEMIOLOGY

- Vaginal candidiasis accounts for approximately 35% of vaginal infections.
- Vaginal candidiasis is caused by fungal organisms that are part of the normal vaginal flora. It is **not** a sexually transmitted disease.
- The most common fungal organism is *Candida albicans*. *Candida tropicalis* and *Candida glabrata* are also important pathogens, particularly in women with recurrent infections.
- Several factors may predispose a patient to vaginal candidiasis:
  ◦ Recent broad-spectrum antibiotic therapy
  ◦ Diabetes
  ◦ Pregnancy
  ◦ Immunosuppressive disorder (eg HIV infection)
  ◦ Use of oral contraceptives
  ◦ Use of oral corticosteroids

CLINICAL MANIFESTATIONS

- Symptomatic patients typically have intensive vulvar and vaginal pruritus in association with a white, curd-like ("cottage cheese") vaginal discharge that may be adherent to the vaginal mucosa. When the discharge is removed, pinpoint hemorrhages may be evident.

- The vaginal mucosa and skin of the vulva are usually inflamed. Erythematous papules ("satellite lesions") may be present in the groin.

DIAGNOSIS

- Patients with candidiasis invariably have a normal vaginal pH, <4.2.
- The diagnosis is most quickly confirmed by observing hyphae and budding yeast in a 10% potassium hydroxide preparation (Fig. 38-2). Culture of fungal organisms is also possible but more time-consuming. Culture is of greatest value in identifying unusual organisms such as *C. tropicalis* and *C. glabrata* in patients with recurrent infections.

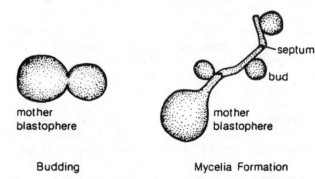

REPRODUCTION OF YEAST

mother blastophere

Budding

septum

bud

mother blastophere

Mycelia Formation

FIG. 38-2 Schematic drawing of mycelia with budding yeast.

TREATMENT

- Many different topical treatments are acceptable for treatment of uncomplicated vulvovaginal candidiasis, (Table 38-1).
- Patients also can be treated with oral fluconazole, 150 mg in a single dose.

RECURRENT VULVOVAGINAL CANDIDIASIS

- Recurrent vulvovaginal candidiasis is defined as four or more symptomatic episodes in a year. Most affected patients have no obvious predisposing risk factor for recurrent infection.
- When patients with recurrent vulvovaginal candidiasis have a symptomatic infection, they should be treated with topical medication for a minimum of 7 to 14 days. If they are treated orally with fluconazole, they should receive an initial dose of 150 mg,

Table 38-1 Treatment Regimens for Uncomplicated Vulvovaginal Candidiasis

DRUG	DOSE AND DURATION OF TREATMENT
Butoconazole 2% cream[a]	5 g intravaginally × 3 days
Butoconazole 2% cream, sustained release	5 g intravaginally × 1 dose
Clotrimazole 1% cream[a]	5 g intravaginally × 7-14 days
Clotrimazole	100 mg vaginal tablet × 7 days
Clotrimazole	Two 100 mg vaginal tablets × 3 days
Clotrimazole	500 mg vaginal tablet × 1 dose
Miconazole 2% cream[a]	5 g intravaginally × 7 days
Miconazole[a]	100 mg vaginal suppository × 7 days
Miconazole[a]	200 mg vaginal suppository × 3 days
Tioconazole 6.5% ointment[a]	5 g intravaginally × 1 dose
Terconazole 0.4% cream	5 g intravaginally × 7 days
Terconazole 0.8% cream	5 g intravaginally × 3 days
Terconazole	80 mg vaginal suppository x 3 days

[a]Available over the counter.

followed in 3 days by a second dose. They should then be placed on one of the maintenance (prophylactic) regimens listed in Table 38-2 for 6 months.

TRICHOMONIASIS

EPIDEMIOLOGY

- Trichomoniasis is a vaginal infection caused by the protozoan *Trichomonas vaginalis*. It accounts for approximately 20 percent of vaginal infections.
- Trichomoniasis is a highly contagious sexually transmitted disease and therefore is more common in women who are young and unmarried and who have multiple sexual partners.

CLINICAL MANIFESTATIONS

- Many patients with trichomoniasis are asymptomatic.
- Symptomatic patients typically have a yellow-green, frothy vaginal discharge in association with dysuria and dyspareunia. The vaginal mucosa usually is erythematous, and the cervix may have multiple punctate hemorrhages ("strawberry cervix").

Table 38-2 Maintenance (Prophylactic) Regimens for Recurrent Vulvovaginal Candidiasis

DRUG	DOSE[a]
Clotrimazole	500 mg vaginal suppository once weekly
Ketoconazole	100 mg orally daily
Fluconazole	100-150 mg orally once weekly
Itraconazole	100 mg once daily
	OR
	400 mg monthly

[a]All medications should be continued for 6 months.

DIAGNOSIS

- Patients with trichomoniasis have an elevated vaginal pH, greater than or equal to 4.5.
- The diagnosis is most quickly confirmed by observing motile trichomonads in a wet mount or saline microscopy preparation (Fig. 38-3).

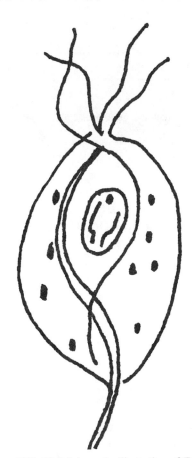

FIG. 38-3 Schematic illustration of *Trichomonas vaginalis*.

- Saline microscopy has a sensitivity of 60 to 70 percent. Therefore, in problematic cases, culture may be necessary to confirm the diagnosis.

TREATMENT

- The treatment of choice for trichomoniasis in both nonpregnant and pregnant women is metronidazole, 2 g orally in a single dose.
- An alternative regimen is metronidazole, 500 mg orally twice daily for 7 days.
- Topical metronidazole is not recommended for the treatment of trichomoniasis.
- The patient's sexual partner(s) should be referred for treatment.
- The patient should be reevaluated soon after treatment to be certain the infection is eradicated. If the infection persists, the patient should be retreated with metronidazole, 500 mg orally twice daily for 7 days. If treatment failure occurs again, she should receive metronidazole, 2 g orally for 5 days.
- Failure of the woman's sexual partner to receive treatment is the most important cause of persistent infection or reinfection.

BIBLIOGRAPHY

Sexually transmitted diseases treatment guidelines 2002. *MMWR* 2002;51:1-80.

39 SCREENING FOR STDS: CHLAMYDIA, GONORRHEA, AND SYPHILIS

Patrick Duff

CHLAMYDIA

EPIDEMIOLOGY

- Chlamydial infections are caused by *Chlamydia trachomatis,* which is an obligate intracellular bacterium.
- Chlamydia is the most common sexually transmitted bacterial disease in western countries.

- Chlamydial infections are three to five times as common as gonococcal infections. The prevalence of chlamydial infection in an obstetric population is about 3 to 5 percent.
- The infection is transmitted primarily by sexual contact. It can also be transmitted from an infected mother to her baby during childbirth.

CLINICAL MANIFESTATIONS IN ADULT WOMEN

- Urethritis
- Proctitis
- Endocervicitis
- Pelvic inflammatory disease
- Perihepatitis (Fitz-Hugh–Curtis syndrome)
- Conjunctivitis

CLINICAL MANIFESTATIONS IN NEONATES

- Conjunctivitis is the most common manifestation.
- Pneumonitis is a less frequent sequela of perinatal transmission.

DIAGNOSIS

- **All** pregnant women and **all at-risk** nonpregnant women should be screened for chlamydial infection.
- The best screening test is a nucleic acid probe [polymerase chain reaction (PCR) or ligase chain reaction (LCR)]. These tests can be performed on several different fluid samples, including urine; endocervical, urethral, or rectal exudate; and conjunctival fluid.

TREATMENT

- From the perspective of convenience, efficacy, safety, tolerance, and cost, azithromycin powder (1 g orally in a single dose) is an excellent choice for the treatment of chlamydial infection in pregnant and nonpregnant women.
- In nonpregnant women, doxycycline (100 mg orally twice daily for 7 days) also is an appropriate selection. This regimen is less expensive but also less convenient than the single-dose regimen of azithromycin.
- In pregnant women, erythromycin (500 mg orally four times daily for 7 days) is an effective treatment

regimen. However, the multiple daily doses, extended duration of treatment, and gastrointestinal side effects of erythromycin make it less appealing than azithromycin.

GONORRHEA

EPIDEMIOLOGY

- Gonococcal infections are caused by the gram-negative diplococcus *Neisseria gonorrhoeae.*
- Gonorrhea is less common than chlamydial infection. Its prevalence in an obstetric population is about 1 percent.
- The infection is transmitted principally by sexual contact. It can also be transmitted perinatally from an infected mother to her baby.

CLINICAL PRESENTATION IN ADULT WOMEN

- Urethritis
- Proctitis
- Endocervicitis
- Pelvic inflammatory disease
- Pharyngitis
- Disseminated infection
  - Arthritis
  - Dermatitis
  - Perihepatitis
  - Pericarditis
  - Endocarditis
  - Meningitis

CLINICAL PRESENTATION IN NEONATES

- Ophthalmia neonatorum is the principal manifestation of gonococcal infection in the neonate.
- Gonococci have also been isolated from localized scalp abscesses in infants who have had scalp electrodes in place during labor.

DIAGNOSIS

- **All** pregnant women and **all at-risk** nonpregnant women should be screened for gonococcal infection.
- The **least expensive screening test** is culture of secretions from the urethra, endocervix, or rectum on selective agar such as Thayer-Martin medium.

- The **most convenient and rapid screening test** is a nucleic acid probe (PCR or LCR). These tests can easily be performed on urine or urethral, endocervical, or rectal secretions.

TREATMENT

- The recommended treatment for uncomplicated, localized gonococcal infection is ceftriaxone (125 mg IM in a single dose).
- If a pregnant woman is allergic to beta-lactam antibiotics, the treatment of choice for gonorrhea is spectinomycin, 2 g IM in a single dose.
- In nonpregnant women who are allergic to beta-lactam antibiotics, the quinolone antibiotics—such as ciprofloxacin, ofloxacin, and levofloxacin—may be used to treat gonorrhea. All of these drugs may be administered in single-dose oral regimens.

SYPHILIS

EPIDEMIOLOGY

- The microorganism that causes syphilis is the spirochete *Treponema pallidum.*
- The incidence of syphilis has increased in recent years, coincident with the rise in frequency of HIV infection.
- The organism is transmitted primarily by sexual contact. However, it can also be transmitted transplacentally and may cause serious infection, even death in utero, in the developing fetus.

CLASSIFICATION OF INFECTION

- **Primary**—characteristic lesion is the chancre.
- **Secondary**—characteristic lesions are the erythematous maculopapular lesions on the palms and soles and wart-like growths on the genitalia (condylomata lata).
- **Latent**—no physical findings or symptoms are present.
  - **Early latent**—duration of infection is less than 1 year
  - **Late latent**—duration of infection is indeterminate or greater than 1 year.
- **Tertiary syphilis**
  - The characteristic lesion of tertiary syphilis is the destructive **gumma.**
  - Cardiovascular disease (**aortitis**) also may be present at this stage of the disease.
- **Neurosyphilis**
  - The typical clinical manifestations are **generalized paresis** and **tabes dorsalis.**

PERINATAL TRANSMISSION

• In the absence of treatment, perinatal transmission can occur at all stages of pregnancy.
• The risk of transmission depends on the stage of maternal disease (Table 39-1).

TABLE 39-1   Risk of Congenital Syphilis

STAGE OF MATERNAL DISEASE	APPROXIMATE RISK OF CONGENITAL SYPHILIS
Primary	50%
Secondary	50%
Early latent	40%
Late latent or tertiary	10%

DIAGNOSIS

• Patients with characteristic physical findings may be correctly diagnosed by clinical examination.
• However, the mainstay of diagnostic tests in asymptomatic patients is serology.
• **All** pregnant women and **all at-risk** nonpregnant women should be screened for syphilis.
• The initial screening test is a non-treponemal assay such as the **Venereal Disease Research Laboratory** (VDRL) test or **rapid plasma reagin** (RPR) test.

• Because nontreponemal tests may produce false-positive results, a positive test must always be confirmed by a specific treponemal test such as the **fluorescent treponemal antibody** (FTA) assay or **microhemagglutination** (MHA) test.
  ○ The specific treponemal test will usually remain positive for the lifetime of the patient even though effective treatment is administered. The nontreponemal test typically becomes negative or declines to a low antibody titer.
  ○ Recurrent infection is confirmed by reappearance of a positive VDRL or RPR or a fourfold increase in the quantitative titer of one of these tests.

TREATMENT

• The drug of choice for treatment of syphilis in both pregnant and nonpregnant women is penicillin.
• Treatment regimens are summarized in Table 39-2.

BIBLIOGRAPHY

Centers for Disease Control and Prevention. Sexually transmitted diseases treatment guidelines 2002. *MMWR* 2002;51(No. RR-6):1–80.

TABLE 39-2   Treatment of Syphilis

STAGE OF DISEASE	PRIMARY TREATMENT	ALTERNATIVE TREATMENT (FOR PENICILLIN-ALLERGIC PATIENTS[a])
Primary	Benzathine penicillin G—2.4 million U IM	Doxycycline—100 mg orally twice daily × 14 days OR Tetracycline—500 mg orally four times daily × 14 days
Secondary and early latent	Benzathine penicillin G—2.4 million U IM	Same as above
Late latent or undetermined duration	Benzathine penicillin G—2.4 million U IM weekly × 3 doses	Doxycycline—100 mg orally twice daily × 28 days OR Tetracycline—500 mg orally four times daily × 28 days
Tertiary	Benzathine penicillin— 2.4 million units IM weekly × 3 doses	Same as above
Neurosyphilis	Aqueous crystalline penicillin G—24 million U, administered as 4 million U IV every 4 h or by continuous infusion for 10–14 days OR Procaine penicillin 2.4 million U IM once daily plus probenecid, 500 mg orally four times a day, both for 10–14 days	Ceftriaxone—2 g IM or IV × 10–14 days

[a]Pregnant patients who are allergic to penicillin should be desensitized and then treated with the appropriate dose of penicillin.

40 PELVIC INFLAMMATORY DISEASE

Patrick Duff

EPIDEMIOLOGY

- Pelvic inflammatory disease (PID) is a serious infection of the upper genital tract (endometritis, salpingitis, oophoritis) and the pelvic peritoneum.
- Approximately 200,000 to 300,000 women are hospitalized each year for treatment of acute PID. At least two to three times as many are treated as outpatients.
- The principal risk factors for PID are:
  - ○ Young age
  - ○ Multiple sexual partners
  - ○ Unprotected intercourse
  - ○ Preexisting lower genital tract infection—ie, gonococcal or chlamydial endocervicitis
  - ○ Instrumentation of the upper genital tract

MICROBIOLOGY

- PID is a polymicrobial, mixed aerobic-anaerobic infection.
- *Neisseria gonorrhoeae* and *Chlamydia trachomatis* are major causes of PID, particularly the initial acute episode.
- Aerobic gram-negative bacilli (*E. coli, Klebsiella pneumoniae, Proteus* species), anaerobic gram-negative bacilli (*Gardnerella vaginalis, Bacteroides* species, *Prevotella* species), aerobic gram-positive cocci (*Streptococcus agalactiae,* enterococci), and genital mycoplasmas also are important pathogens.

CLINICAL MANIFESTATIONS

- The usual clinical manifestations of acute PID are listed in Table 40-1.

TABLE 40-1   Principal Clinical Manifestations of Pelvic Inflammatory Disease

Fever
Chills
Malaise
Severe lower abdominal pain and tenderness
Pelvic peritoneal irritation
Uterine and adnexal tenderness
Cervical motion tenderness
Mucopurulent cervical exudate
Irregular uterine bleeding

- Patients with recurrent episodes of PID are less likely to have all of the major manifestations listed in the table. They typically have only a low-grade fever and less severe pelvic pain and tenderness.

DIAGNOSIS

- The differential diagnosis of PID includes threatened abortion, ectopic pregnancy, adnexal torsion, ruptured ovarian cyst, appendicitis, and diverticulitis.
- Distinction among these disorders usually is possible by judicious use of the laboratory studies summarized in Table 40-2.

TREATMENT

- Compliant patients with mild PID who have a good support system at home may be treated as outpatients. They should be reevaluated approximately 48 h after the start of therapy. If they are not improving, they should be hospitalized for treatment with parenteral antibiotics. Table 40-3 presents two acceptable outpatient treatment regimens.

TABLE 40-2   Diagnostic Studies of Value in the Evaluation of Patients with Suspected Pelvic Inflammatory Disease

DIAGNOSTIC TEST	OBJECTIVE OF TEST
Quantitative beta-Hcg	Negative test rules out the diagnosis of threatened abortion or ectopic pregnancy.
Complete blood count	Elevated white blood cell count supports diagnosis of infection. Decreased hematocrit may indicate hemoperitoneum from ectopic pregnancy or ruptured ovarian cyst.
Endovaginal ultrasound	Helpful in assessing for an adnexal mass (ectopic pregnancy, tuboovarian abscess, ovarian cyst or torsion) Also helpful in identifying intraperitoneal fluid (pus, blood, cystic fluid)
Endocervical sampling for nucleic acid probes	Most rapid test for identification of gonorrhea and chlamydia
Rapid plasma reagin test (RPR) HIV, hepatitis B serology	Patient should be tested for other STDs
CT scan of the abdomen	Key test for diagnosis of appendicitis. Would also demonstrate free air in abdomen resulting from ruptured diverticulum.
Diagnostic laparoscopy	May be necessary when diagnosis remains uncertain or patient has poor initial response to empiric therapy.

TABLE 40-3   Outpatient Treatment Regimens for Pelvic Inflammatory Disease

REGIMEN A	REGIMEN B
Ofloxacin, 400 mg orally twice daily for 14 days	Ceftriaxone, 250 mg IM in a single dose
OR	PLUS
Levofloxacin, 500 mg orally once daily for 14 days	Doxycycline, 100 mg orally twice daily for 14 days
PLUS	PLUS
Metronidazole, 500 mg orally twice daily for 14 days	Metronidazole, 500 mg orally twice daily for 14 days

- Patients who meet any of the following criteria should be treated as inpatients:
  - Seriously ill
  - Suspected pelvic mass
  - Immunosuppressive disorder
  - Noncompliant
  - Inadequate support system
  - Coexisting pregnancy
  - IUD in place
  - Uncertain diagnosis
- One recommended regimen for inpatient treatment of PID is the combination of cefotetan, 2 g IV every 12 h, plus doxycycline, 100 mg IV or orally every 12 h.
- An alternative and slightly less expensive treatment regimen is the combination of clindamycin, 900 mg IV every 8 h, plus gentamicin, 7.5 mg/kg ideal body weight IV every 24 h.
- Parenteral antibiotics should be continued until the patient has been afebrile and relatively asymptomatic for 24 h. The patient then should receive doxycycline, 100 mg orally twice daily, to complete 14 days of treatment.
- Patients with a tuboovarian abscess may require surgical drainage if the abscess ruptures or they fail to improve with medical therapy.
- The sexual partners of patients with PID should be counseled to have testing for sexually transmitted diseases such as gonorrhea, chlamydia, HIV, syphilis, and hepatitis B.

LONG-TERM SEQUELAE OF PID

- Even when treated properly, PID may cause three important long-term sequelae:
- One possible outcome is subsequent infertility due to tubal obstruction (Figs. 40-1 and 40-2).
- PID is also the most important risk factor for ectopic pregnancy, which occurs approximately once in every 100 pregnancies.
- PID is also the most important cause of chronic pelvic adhesive disease, which, in turn, may lead to chronic pelvic pain.

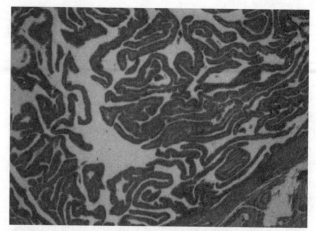

FIG. 40-1 Histologic section of a normal fallopian tube.

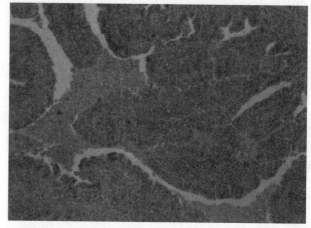

FIG. 40-2 Histologic section of a fallopian tube in a patient with acute PID. Note inflammatory exudate, which completely fills the tube's lumen.

BIBLIOGRAPHY

Sexually transmitted diseases treatment guidelines 2002. *MMWR* 2002;51:1–80.

41   HUMAN IMMUNODEFICIENCY VIRUS INFECTION

Patrick Duff

VIROLOGY

- Human immunodeficiency virus (HIV) infection is caused by an RNA retrovirus.
- The two major strains of HIV are HIV-1 and HIV-2.
- Each strain has several subtypes.

- Structure of the virus:
  - **Lipid bilayer**
  - **Outer envelope protein**—facilitates viral entry into host cell by binding to CD4 receptor.
  - **Transmembrane protein**—facilitates fusion of viral envelope with cell membrane.
  - **Viral capsid.**
  - Principal **enzymes:**
    - **Reverse transcriptase**—transcribes viral RNA into double-stranded DNA.
    - **Integrase**—facilitates integration of viral DNA into host genome.
    - **Protease**—produces individual viral proteins by proteolysis of precursors.

PRINCIPAL MECHANISMS OF TRANSMISSION OF HIV INFECTION

- Sexual contact:
  - Homosexual
  - Bisexual
  - Heterosexual
- Contaminated needles shared by intravenous drug addicts
- Vertical transmission from mother to infant
- Infection as a result of blood transfusion, organ donation, or artificial insemination is extremely rare.

EPIDEMIOLOGY

- On a global scale, approximately half of all individuals infected with HIV are women and half are men.
- In the United States, approximately 30 percent of **all** cases are in women. However, almost half of **new** cases are in women.
- Worldwide, more than 25 million adults and 1.5 million children are infected with HIV.
- In the United States, more than 1 million individuals are infected.
- In U.S. women, the two most common mechanisms of transmission of HIV infection are heterosexual contact with high-risk men and intravenous drug use.
- The principal risk factors for heterosexual transmission of HIV infection are as follows:
  - Multiple partners
  - Receptive anal intercourse
  - Concurrent intravenous drug use or crack cocaine addiction
  - Presence of ulcerated genital tract lesions—syphilis, herpes, chancroid
  - Other STDs
  - Sex during menses

- Traumatic acts of intercourse—eg, during sexual assault
- HIV infection typically progresses through four general stages:
  - **Acute retroviral illness**
    - Occurs 5 to 30 days after exposure
    - Characterized by flu-like symptoms
  - **Latent phase of illness**—median duration now approaches 10 years
  - **Symptomatic illness**
  - **Acquired immunodeficiency syndrome (AIDS)**—once this stage of the illness is reached, life expectancy usually does not exceed 5 years.

CLINICAL MANIFESTATIONS

- HIV infection is a multisystem disease characterized by severe immunodeficiency.
- Nonspecific symptoms and signs include the following:
  - Malaise
  - Fatigue
  - Weight loss
  - Generalized lymphadenopathy
  - Anorexia
  - Nausea and vomiting
  - Diarrhea
  - Wasting syndrome (cachexia)
- Opportunistic infections are the hallmark of HIV infection. The principal opportunistic diseases in women include:
  - *Pneumocystis carinii* pneumonia
  - Esophageal and vaginal candidiasis
  - *Mycobacterium avium intracellulare* (MAC) infection
  - Toxoplasmosis
  - Tuberculosis
  - Cytomegalovirus (CMV) infection
  - Cryptococcal infection
    - Pulmonary infection
    - Meningitis
  - Cryptosporidiosis
- The most common malignancies are as follows:
  - Kaposi's sarcoma—common in men but rare in women
  - Non-Hodgkin's lymphoma

DIAGNOSIS

- Detection of antibody to HIV is the most common diagnostic test.
  - The initial screening test is an enzyme immunoassay (EIA). Rapid tests now are available that can be completed in the office or clinic within 1 h.

◦ If this test is positive, a confirmatory test should be performed.
  ▪ Western blot (WB)
  ▪ Immunofluorescent assay (IFA)
◦ If both the EIA and confirmatory test are positive, the probability of a false-positive result is less than 1:10,000.
• Viral culture—virus may be cultured from plasma, lymphocytes, and monocytes.
• Detection of viral antigen by polymerase chain reaction (PCR).
  ◦ This test is usually used to monitor response to therapy by quantitating viral load rather than for diagnosis of infection. However, it can be used as a diagnostic test in patients who have an indeterminate Western blot or immunofluorescent assay.
• In the United States, the dominant viral strain is HIV-1 and testing is usually directed only at this organism. However, the following patients also should be tested for HIV-2 infection:
  ◦ Sexual contact or needle-sharing partner of a person from a country where HIV-2 is endemic (eg, West Africa, Portugal, France).
  ◦ Person who has received a transfusion or nonsterile injection in a country where HIV-2 is endemic.
  ◦ Children of high-risk women.
  ◦ Patient who has clinical evidence of HIV infection but has negative tests for HIV-1.

TREATMENT

• The drugs currently available for the treatment of HIV-infected patients are listed in Table 41-1.
• The current standard of care is to offer all patients treatment with at least three drugs.
• One of the most popular treatment regimens employs the combination of two nucleoside reverse transcriptase inhibitors (zidovudine plus lamivudine) plus a protease inhibitor (nelfinavir). These three drugs offer an excellent combination of safety, effectiveness, and tolerability. Zidovudine and lamivudine can be administered in a single tablet—Combivir.
• Response to treatment is monitored by quantitation of viral load by PCR. The goal of therapy is to depress the viral load to a nondetectable range (<50 copies/mL).
• If the patient fails to respond appropriately to therapy, there are two possible explanations—poor compliance or resistant organism.
• In this situation, the sensitivity of the virus to the treatment agents should be assessed. If resistance is documented, the entire treatment regimen should be changed.

• In addition to antiviral chemotherapy, patients should receive prophylactic antibiotics to prevent selected opportunistic infections. The indications and agents for prophylaxis are summarized in Table 41-2.
• Patients should also receive certain vaccines to ensure protection against other potentially serious infections.
  ◦ Pneumococcal vaccine—administered initially, followed by a booster dose in 5 years.
  ◦ Influenza vaccine—administered annually during the period of late October through January.
  ◦ Hepatitis A vaccine—administered in a series of two vaccines.
  ◦ Hepatitis B vaccine—administered in a series of three vaccines.

HIV INFECTION IN PREGNANCY: SPECIAL CONSIDERATIONS

• Virtually all cases of HIV infection in children result from perinatal transmission.
• The mechanisms of perinatal transmission include the following:
  ◦ **Intrapartum exposure** to maternal blood and genital tract secretions; this is of the greatest importance.
  ◦ **Transplacental dissemination,** which may occur spontaneously or as the result of invasive procedures such as amniocentesis or chorionic villus sampling.
  ◦ **Breast feeding.**
• Several factors significantly increase the risk of perinatal transmission of HIV infection (Table 41-3).
• In the absence of any obstetric intervention, the risk of perinatal transmission is approximately 20 to 30 percent.
• Antiviral chemotherapy is effective in preventing perinatal transmission. With use of the highly active treatment regimens described previously, the risk of perinatal transmission should be less than 3 percent.
• Women who are receiving multiagent chemotherapy and who have an undetectable viral load are appropriate candidates for vaginal delivery.
  ◦ They should be treated intrapartum with intravenous zidovudine (2 mg/kg loading dose followed by 1 mg/kg/h until delivery).
  ◦ Every effort should be made to avoid rupture of membranes, invasive monitoring (ie, scalp electrode, scalp pH determination), instrumental delivery, and episiotomy.
• Women who have a detectable viral load should be scheduled for cesarean delivery at approximately 38 weeks, **before** rupture of membranes and onset of labor. These

TABLE 41-1 Drugs for Treatment of HIV Infection

AGENT	FDA PREGNANCY CATEGORY	USUAL ADULT DOSE	REMARKS	COST OF 30-DAY TREATMENT[a]
NUCLEOSIDE REVERSE TRANSCRIPTASE INHIBITORS				
Abacavir	C	300 mg bid	Most serious adverse effect is a hypersensitivity reaction (2-5% of patients).	$349.00
Didanosine (DDI, Videx)	B	200 mg bid	Most serious adverse effects are pancreatitis and peripheral neuropathy.	$194.00
Lamivudine (3TC, Epivir)	C	150 mg bid	Adverse effects are similar to those of zidovudine but are less frequent. Drug is eliminated by renal excretion.	$230.00
Stavudine (d4T, Zerit)	C	40 mg bid	Main adverse effect is peripheral sensory neuropathy.	$254.00
Zalcitabine (ddC, HIVID)	C	0.75 mg q 8 h	Most serious adverse effect is peripheral neuropathy. Pancreatitis also can occur. Least potent of the nucleoside analogues.	$207.00
Zidovudine (Retrovir)	C	300 mg bid	Main adverse effect is marrow suppression.	$287.00
NONNUCLEOSIDE REVERSE TRANSCRIPTASE INHIBITORS				
Delavirdine (Rescriptor)	C	400 mg tid	Most common side effect is rash; it is usually less severe than the rash associated with nevirapine. Hepatitis also can occur.	$222.00
Nevirapine (Viramure)	C	200 mg bid	Most common adverse effect is rash. If the rash is extensive, the drug should be permanently discontinued. Hepatitis is a rare side effect.	$248.00
Efavirenz (Sustiva)	C	600 mg qd	Most common adverse effects are rash and CNS changes. The drug is teratogenic and should not be used in pregnancy.	$394.00
PROTEASE INHIBITORS				
Amprenavir	C	1200 mg bid	Most common adverse effects are rash and GI irritation.	$605.00
Indinavir (Crixivan)	C	800 mg q 8 h	Well tolerated. Most serious adverse effect is nephrolithiasis. Most common side effect is GI upset. Less expensive than ritonavir.	$450.00
Lopinavir/ritonavir (Kaletra)	C	3 gelatin capsules (133.3mg/33.3 mg) bid 5 mL solution (80 mg/20mg/mL) bid	Most common adverse effects are diarrhea, nausea, fatigue, headache, asthenia.	$677.00
Nelfinavir (Viracept)	B	1250 mg in a.m. 1000 mg in p.m.	Clinical efficacy data are limited. Most common adverse effects are diarrhea, fatigue, poor concentration.	$557.00
Ritonavir (Norvir)	B	600 mg q 12 h	Most likely drug in this class to cause adverse effects. Can be given in a convenient twice-daily dosing regimen. Major side effect is GI irritation. Should be taken with meals. It has major potential for interactions with other drugs.	$668.00
Saquinavir (Invirase and Fortovase)	B	600 mg tid	Least effective of the protease inhibitors. Should not be used as monotherapy. Drug has low oral bioavailability and must be taken with a high-fat meal.	$572.00

[a]Cost to pharmacist.

TABLE 41-2   Prophylactic Antibiotics for Selected Opportunistic Infections

INFECTION	INDICATION FOR PROPHYLAXIS	ANTIBIOTIC
Pneumocystis *carinii*	Prior infection or CD4 cell count $<200/mm^3$	Trimethoprim/sulfamethoxazole, double strength-one tablet PO daily or three times weekly
Toxoplasmosis	Positive serology and CD4 cell count $<100/mm^3$	Trimethoprim/sulfamethoxazole, double strength-one tablet PO daily
Tuberculosis	Positive PPD >5 mm	Isoniazid, 300 mg PO daily, plus pyridoxine, 50 mg daily
MAC	CD4 cell count $<50/mm^3$	Azithromycin, 1200 mg orally each weekly
Candidiasis	Recurrent symptomatic infection	Fluconazole, 150 mg PO daily
Herpes simplex	Recurrent symptomatic infection	Acyclovir, 400 mg PO twice daily

Key: PPD purified protein derivative (tuberculin); MAC, *mycobacteruim avium* complex.

TABLE 41-3   Risk Factors for Perinatal Transmission of HIV Infection

RISK FACTOR	MECHANISM
Higher viral load in mother	Greater exposure of fetus to infectious virus
$HIV_1>>HIV_2$	HIV_1 is more virulent than HIV_2
History of previous child with AIDS	Higher viral inoculum in mother
Overt AIDS in mother	Higher viral inoculum in mother
Prematurity	Decreased immune defenses in neonate
Decreased T4 cell count	Impaired maternal defenses
Invasive procedure during antepartum period (amniocentesis, CVS, amnioscopy)	Inovulation of virus directly into fetal circulation
Concurrent STD	Impairment of host immunity, disruption of mucosal barriers
First twin	Greater exposure to infected maternal blood and genital tract secretions
Chorioamnionitis	Transmission due to vascular injury within placenta
Increased intrapartum blood exposure	Exposure of neonate to higher viral inoculum
Rupture of membranes >4 h	Exposure of neonate to higher viral inoculum
Illicit drug use during pregnancy	Impaired maternal immune system

Key: CVS, chorionic villus sampling; STD, sexually transmitted disease.

patients should be treated with intravenous zidovudine for at least 3 h prior to delivery.

• Postnatally, the neonates should be evaluated by a specialist in pediatric infectious diseases and treated with chemotherapy.

BIBLIOGRAPHY

U.S. Public Health Service Task Force recommendations for use of antiretroviral drugs in pregnant HIV-1-infected women for maternal health and interventions to reduce perinatal HIV-1 transmission in the United States. *MMWR (Suppl)* 2002; 51(No. RR-18):1–38.

Wahs DH. Management of human immunodeficiency virus infection in pregnancy. *N Engl J Med* 2002;346:1879–1891.

42 VULVAR DYSTROPHIES AND DERMATOSES

John D. Davis

INTRODUCTION

• Vulvar dystrophies and dermatoses, also known as vulvar nonneoplastic epithelial disorders, include lichen sclerosus, squamous cell hyperplasia, lichen simplex chronicus, and lichen planus.

• Vulvar biopsy should be performed liberally in evaluating patients with vulvar lesions in order to establish the correct diagnosis and rule out malignancy.

LICHEN SCLEROSUS

- Lichen sclerosus is a benign disorder of the vulvar epithelium characterized by depigmentation and thinning of the skin, shrinkage and agglutination of the labia, and introital stenosis.
- The condition occurs most frequently in postmenopausal and premenarchal females; the cause is unknown.
- The most common symptom experienced by patients with lichen sclerosus is pruritus.
- Physical examination of affected patients demonstrates thin, pale, paper-like vulvar epithelium that may have fissures, superficial ulcerations, and ecchymotic areas (Fig. 42-1).
- While lichen sclerosus may be suspected clinically, the diagnosis should be confirmed with biopsy. Typical histologic changes include thinning of the epidermis, loss of the rete ridges, and edema and fibrosis of the dermis (Fig. 42-2).
- The mainstay of treatment for lichen sclerosus is high-potency topical steroids, such as 0.05% clobetasol propionate, applied twice daily for 2 to 3 weeks. High-potency steroids can be continued once daily until symptoms resolve; then medium- to low-potency steroids can be prescribed for maintenance therapy.
- While lichen sclerosus is not considered a premalignant condition, 3 to 9 percent of patients with lichen sclerosus can have an associated vulvar carcinoma.

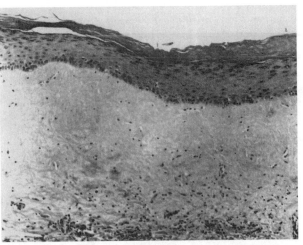

FIG. 42-2 Lichen sclerosus with typical thin epithelium, absent rete ridges, and subepithelial edema. (From Friedrich EG Jr. *Vulvar Disease,* 2d ed. Philadelphia: Saunders, 1983:132. With permission.)

SQUAMOUS CELL HYPERPLASIA

- Squamous cell hyperplasia, previously known as hyperplastic dystrophy, is a benign disorder of the vulvar epithelium characterized by depigmentation and thickening of the skin. The cause of the condition is not known.
- As with lichen sclerosus, most patients present with vulvar pruritus. Examination shows thickened vulvar skin that is white or gray in color (Fig. 42-3).

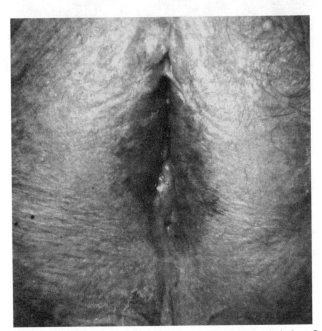

FIG. 42-1 Thin, pale paper-like epithelium characteristic of lichen sclerosus. (From Friedrich EG Jr. *Vulvar Disease,* 2d ed. Philadelphia: Saunders, 1983:135. With permission.)

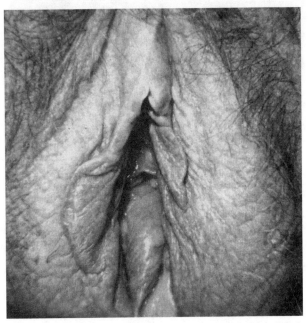

FIG. 42-3 Squamous cell hyperplasia. (From Friedrich EG Jr. *Vulvar Disease,* 2d ed. Philadelphia: Saunders, 1983:139. With permission.)

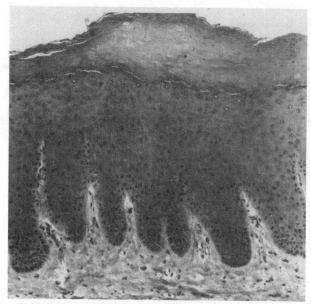

FIG. 42-4 Thickened epithelium and deep, broad rete ridges characteristic of squamous cell hyperplasia. (From Friedrich EG Jr. *Vulvar Disease,* 2d ed. Philadelphia: Saunders, 1983:133. With permission.)

- Histopathologic findings of squamous cell hyperplasia include thickened, acanthotic epithelium. The rete ridges are broad and deep. Dermal inflammation is not present (Fig. 42-4).
- Squamous cell hyperplasia should be treated with medium-strength topical steroids (such as 0.1% betamethasone valerate) twice daily until the lesion resolves.

LICHEN SIMPLEX CHRONICUS

- Lichen simplex chronicus is another benign disorder characterized by thickening of the vulvar skin. Clinically, lichen simplex chronicus may be indistinguishable from squamous cell hyperplasia.
- The chief complaint of patients with lichen simplex chronicus is vulvar pruritus. On examination, the skin has a thickened, leathery appearance (Fig. 42-5).
- Histopathologically, lichen simplex chronicus appears similar to squamous cell hyperplasia. However, unlike squamous cell hyperplasia, biopsy

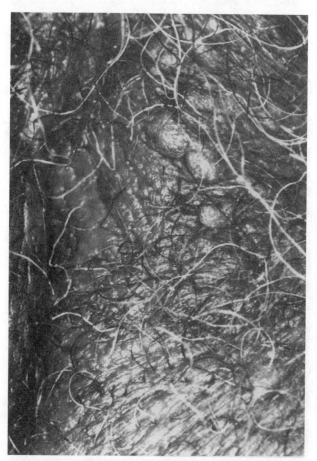

FIG. 42-5 Lichen simplex chronicus. (From Wilkinson EJ, Stone IK. *Atlas of Vulvar Disease.* Baltimore: Williams & Wilkins, 1995:83. With permission.)

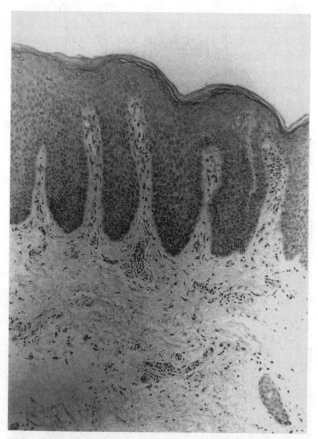

FIG. 42-6 Lichen simplex chronicus. Note the inflammatory cells in the superficial dermis. (From Wilkinson EJ, Stone IK. *Atlas of Vulvar Disease.* Baltimore: Williams & Wilkins, 1995:83. With permission.)

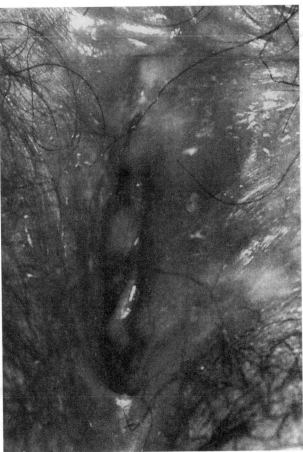

FIG. 42-7 Lichen planus. (From Wilkinson EJ, Stone IK. *Atlas of Vulvar Disease.* Baltimore: Williams & Wilkins, 1995:29. With permission.)

specimens from patients with lichen simplex chronicus show inflammatory cells in the superficial dermis (Fig. 42-6).

- Treatment of lichen simplex chronicus is similar to treatment of squamous cell hyperplasia. In addition, avoidance of irritants and allergens is recommended.

LICHEN PLANUS

- Lichen planus is a chronic inflammatory dermatosis that may involve the vulva, vagina, oral mucosa, and nongenital cutaneous sites; the etiology of the disorder is unknown. Without treatment, vulvovaginal lichen planus can lead to vaginal scarring and complete vaginal stenosis.
- Patients with vulvovaginal lichen planus often present with varying degrees of desquamative vulvovaginitis (Fig. 42-7). Symptoms include dyspareunia, a sensation of vaginal narrowing, and a bloody vaginal discharge.

- There is a strong association between lichen planus and hepatitis C.
- A strong clinical suspicion is required to make the diagnosis, since biopsy may demonstrate only non-specific changes such as loss of epithelium and inflammation.
- Topical steroids (such as medium-potency 0.1% betamethasone valerate, applied twice daily to the vulva, and low-potency hydrocortisone, 25 mg suppositories inserted vaginally once daily), griseo-fulvin, dapsone, isotretinoin, cyclosporine and vaginal dilators have all been suggested as treatments for lichen planus. Topical tacrolimus (0.1% ointment applied twice daily) is effective for some patients.
- As with lichen sclerosus, patients with lichen planus may be at increased risk of developing vulvar carcinoma.

BIBLIOGRAPHY

American College of Obstetricians and Gynecologists. Vulvar nonneoplastic epithelial disorders. *ACOG Educ Bull* no. 241, October 1997.

Foster DC. Vulvar disease. *Obstet Gynecol* 2002;100:145–163.

Wilkinson EJ, Stone IK. *Atlas of Vulvar Disease.* Baltimore: Williams & Wilkins, 1995:27–29.

43 PELVIC SUPPORT DEFECTS

John D. Davis

NORMAL ANATOMIC SUPPORT

- The levator ani muscle—composed of the pubococcygeal, iliococcygeal, and coccygeal muscles—forms the muscular floor of the pelvis (or pelvic diaphragm) and is the main source of support for the pelvic organs (Fig. 43-1).
  - Laterally, the levator ani muscle attaches to the fascia of the obturator internus muscle along the arcus tendineus levator ani, or white line of the pelvis. Anteriorly and posteriorly, the levator ani attaches to the pubic bone and ischial spine of the superior pubic ramus, respectively.
  - The region of the levator ani between the anus and coccyx, formed by the muscular raphe, is called the levator plate.

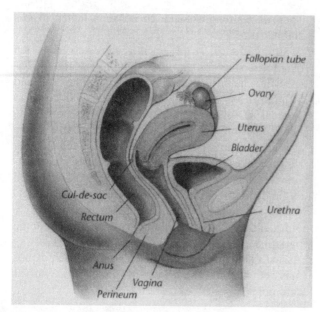

FIG. 43-1 Normal female anatomy. (From the American College of Obstetricians and Gynecologists. *Gynecologic Problems: Pelvic Support Problems.* ACOG Patient Education pamphlet. Washington, DC: ACOG, September 1999. With permission.)

○ The opening in the central portion of the levator ani through which the urethra, vagina, and rectum pass is called the urogenital hiatus. When a woman is in an upright position, the vagina is nearly horizontal and is supported, along with the uterus and rectum, by the levator plate.
- Support for the pelvic organs also is provided by connective tissue attachments and the endopelvic fascia.
  ○ The dense connective tissue at the base of the broad ligament is the cardinal ligament; this structure supports the cervix and upper vagina. The uterosacral ligament also helps to maintain the cervix in its normal anatomic position.
  ○ The endopelvic fascia is a layer of strong connective tissue that surrounds the vagina, attaches to the pubic symphysis and the arcus tendineus, envelopes the cervix, and ultimately attaches to the pelvic side wall.
- Other important sources of pelvic support include the perineal membrane and perineum.
  ○ The perineal membrane is dense connective tissue located at the anterior triangle of the pelvic outlet, which attaches to the inferior pubic rami bilaterally. This membrane supports the urethra, distal vagina, and perineal body.
  ○ The muscles of the perineum—including the bulbocavernosus, ischiocavernosus, and superficial transverse perineal muscles—support the distal vagina and rectum.

ETIOLOGY, PREVALENCE, AND SYMPTOMS

- The most important risk factor for pelvic organ prolapse is a history of a vaginal delivery.
- Vaginal delivery may contribute pelvic support defects by causing trauma to structures of pelvic support and a pudendal neuropathy.
- Other factors associated with uterovaginal prolapse include older age, estrogen deficiency, pregnancy (regardless of route of delivery), obesity, chronic cough, chronic constipation, prior hysterectomy, and congenital connective tissue abnormalities.
- The incidence of pelvic organ prolapse is difficult to determine accurately. Approximately 10 percent of women in the United States will undergo surgery for pelvic relaxation before the age of 80.
- Women with pelvic organ prolapse may comment about tissue protruding from the vagina, pelvic pressure, back discomfort, dyspareunia, urinary incontinence or hesitancy, and bowel dysfunction.

DEFINITIONS AND CLASSIFICATION

- Historically, the terms *cystocele, rectocele,* and *enterocele* have been used to describe presumed prolapse of the bladder, rectum, and small bowel, respectively. Often, intraoperative findings do not correlate with the preoperative diagnosis.
- Currently, the terms *anterior support defect, posterior support defect, and apical support defect* are preferred. Examples of common pelvic support defects are depicted in Fig. 43-2.
- A number of classification systems exist for staging pelvic organ prolapse:
  ○ Pelvic support defects are commonly graded as **first-degree** if they extend into the upper half of the vagina, **second-degree** if they extend into the lower half of the vagina but not beyond the hymenal ring, **third-degree** if they extend partially beyond the hymenal ring, and **fourth-degree** if they are completely prolapsed.
  ○ The Pelvic Organ Prolapse Quantification (POP-Q) System was proposed in 1995 and uses six points of reference on the anterior, superior, and posterior vagina to grade prolapse. This system has been criticized for being difficult to use and for not addressing all potential pelvic support defects.
  ○ The Revised New York Classification System addresses some deficiencies of the POP-Q System and has been proposed as an alternative staging system.

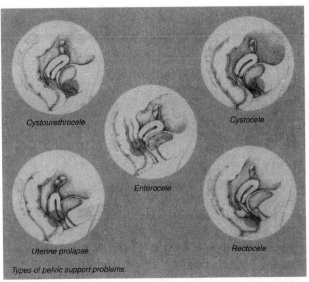

FIG. 43-2 Types of pelvic support problems. (From the American College of Obstetricians and Gynecologists. *Gynecologic Problems: Pelvic Support Problems.* ACOG Patient Education pamphlet. Washington, DC: ACOG, September 1999. With permission.)

EVALUATION

- Patients with pelvic organ prolapse should undergo a detailed pelvic examination to identify all sites of damage. They should be asked to perform a Valsalva maneuver during the examination to determine the full extent of the prolapse.
- The sites that should be examined for support defects include the urethra, urethrovesical junction, central and lateral anterior vaginal wall, cervix or vaginal cuff, posterior cul-de-sac, central and lateral posterior vaginal wall, perineum, and anal sphincter.

TREATMENT

- Nonsurgical therapies for pelvic support defects include lifestyle modification and use of a pessary.
- Lifestyle changes that may prevent damage to the pelvic floor include weight loss, avoidance of heavy lifting, smoking cessation, pelvic floor exercises, and avoidance of constipation.
- Pessaries, devices placed in the vagina to provide support for pelvic organs, are usually made of silicone and come in a variety of shapes and sizes.
- The traditional surgical procedure used to treat defects in the anterior vaginal wall is the anterior colporrhaphy. Repairs of paravaginal defects, done abdominally or vaginally, and site-specific repairs have been introduced relatively recently.

- Common surgical procedures used to suspend the vaginal apex include the abdominal sacrocolpopexy and sacrospinous ligament fixation.
- Defects in the posterior wall are usually treated with either a posterior colporraphy or a site-specific repair.

BIBLIOGRAPHY

American College of Obstetricians and Gynecologists. *Precis, Gynecology: An update in obstetrics and gynecology,* 2nd ed. Washington, DC: ACOG; 2001:42–54.

Koduri S, Sand PK. Recent developments in pelvic organ prolapse. *Curr Opin Obstet Gynecol* 2000;12:399–404.

Rovner ES. Pelvic organ prolapse: A review. *Ostomy/Wound Mgt* 2000;46:24–37.

Shull BL. Pelvic organ prolapse: Anterior, superior, and posterior vaginal segment defects. *Am J Obstet Gynecol* 1999;181:6–11.

44 EVALUATION AND MANAGEMENT OF THE PELVIC MASS

John D. Davis

DIFFERENTIAL DIAGNOSIS

- Pelvic masses may arise from the ovary, uterus, fallopian tube, urinary tract, gastrointestinal tract, musculoskeletal system, nervous system, and vascular-lymphatic system.
- Principal causes of a pelvic mass are listed in Table 44-1.

HISTORY

- Age is an important factor in evaluating a patient with a pelvic mass. An ovarian malignancy should be strongly considered as the cause of a pelvic mass in premenarcheal girls and postmenopausal women, while reproductive-age women are more likely to have nonmalignant conditions such as functional cysts, mature cystic teratomas, endometriomas, or fibroids.
- Ectopic pregnancy should be considered in a patient with a pelvic mass who is late for her menstrual period.
- Women using oral contraceptive pills are less likely to develop functional cysts; therefore other causes of a pelvic mass should be considered more strongly in such patients.

TABLE 44-1   Principal Causes of a Pelvic Mass

Ovary
  Functional cyst
    Follicular cyst
    Corpus luteum cyst
    Theca lutein cyst
  Neoplasm
    Benign
      Serous cystadenoma
      Mucinous cystadenoma
      Mature cystic teratoma (dermoid cyst)
      Fibroma
    Malignant (a detailed classification of ovarian malignancies is
      given in Chap. 64)
  Other
    Endometrioma
    Tuboovarian abscess
Uterus
  Leiomyoma
  Adenomyoma
  Pregnancy
  Congenital uterine anomaly
  Endometrial cancer
  Sarcoma
Fallopian tube
  Ectopic pregnancy
  Hydrosalpinx/pyosalpinx
  Tuboovarian abscess
  Paratubal cyst
  Malignancy
Urinary tract
  Distended bladder
  Pelvic kidney
Gastrointestinal tract
  Impacted stool
  Diverticular abscess
  Appendiceal abscess
  Colorectal cancer
Others
  Presacral teratoma
  Lymphoma

- Patients with a pelvic mass, menorrhagia, and dysmenorrhea may have leiomyomata uteri.
- Nulliparous patients with severe dysmenorrhea and a pelvic mass may have an endometrioma.
- Tuboovarian abscess (TOA) should be considered in a patient having unprotected intercourse or intercourse with multiple sexual partners who presents with pain, fever, and a pelvic mass.
- Adnexal torsion (often with a related dermoid) should be considered in women of reproductive age with acute, severe pain and a pelvic mass.
- Ovarian malignancy should be considered in postmenopausal patients with vague symptoms such as early satiety and increasing abdominal girth.
- Colon cancer should be considered in an older patient with altered bowel pattern, heme-positive stools, and a pelvic mass.

PHYSICAL EXAMINATION

- If a mass is palpable during the pelvic examination, its location, size, consistency, mobility, and tenderness should be determined.
- The pelvic examination should be performed with the patient's bladder empty.
- Solid midline masses contiguous with the uterus are consistent with fibroids.
- Fixed, tender adnexal masses may represent an endometrioma, TOA, or malignancy, while mobile adnexal masses may be due to a functional cyst or a dermoid.
- Patients suspected of having a gastrointestinal source of a pelvic mass should have a digital rectal examination and a stool guaiac test.

PELVIC ULTRASOUND

- Pelvic ultrasound, usually done transvaginally, is the preferred test for identifying and characterizing masses originating from the uterus, tubes, or ovaries. Sonograms of some benign pelvic masses are shown in Figures 44-1 through 44-4.
- Ultrasound findings consistent with a malignant ovarian growth are listed in Table 44-2. A sonogram of an ovarian malignancy is shown in Fig. 44-5.

OTHER DIAGNOSTIC TESTS

- Computed tomography of the pelvis also may be of value in the evaluation of a pelvic mass. Certain conditions that may not be readily evident on

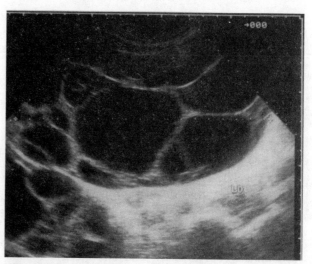

FIG. 44-1 Transvaginal sonogram of a multicystic ovary.

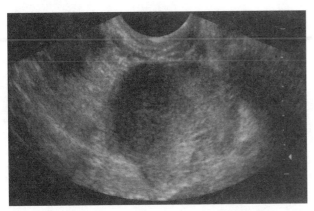

FIG. 44-2 Transvaginal sonogram of an endometrioma.

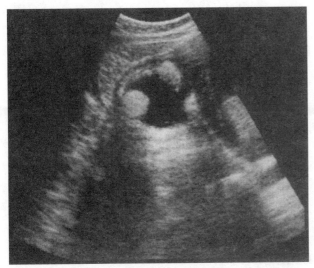

FIG. 44-3 Transvaginal sonogram of a mature cystic teratoma.

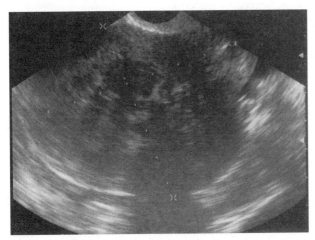

FIG. 44-4 Transvaginal sonogram of a leiomyoma.

TABLE 44-2 Sonographic Characteristics of an Adnexal Mass That May Be Associated with Malignancy

Large size (>10 cm)
Thick septations
Solid components
Papillations or excrescences
Bilateral in location
Associated ascites
Low impedance to flow (when evaluated with Doppler)

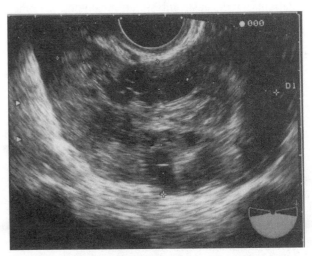

FIG. 44-5 Transvaginal sonogram of an ovarian malignancy.

transvaginal ultrasound (such as hydronephrosis, colon cancer, appendiceal abscess, omental tumor involvement, and lymphadenopathy) may be identified on CT scan.

- Magnetic resonance imaging is often reserved for characterizing congenital anomalies of the reproductive tract.

- Cancer antigen 125 (CA 125) is a glycoprotein found on the surface of epithelial cells of tissue derived from coelomic epithelium. Epithelial cells lining the fallopian tube, endometrium, endocervix, peritoneum, pleura, pericardium, and bronchus all normally produce CA 125.

- Serum CA 125 levels are elevated in 50 to 80 percent of patients with non mucinous epithelial ovarian tumors, and measurements of CA 125 have been suggested as a means of distinguishing between malignant and benign neoplasms of the ovary.

- In women of reproductive age, many benign conditions—including endometriosis, pelvic inflammatory disease, leiomyomata, and pregnancy— can cause elevated levels of CA 125.

- Since CA 125 levels are not elevated in all patients with ovarian cancer and many benign conditions can be associated with elevated values, measurements of

CA 125 cannot reliably distinguish malignant from benign masses.

MANAGEMENT

- Patients with leiomyomata uteri, ectopic pregnancy, pelvic inflammatory disease (PID) with a TOA, or obvious malignancy of the uterus or ovary should be managed as described elsewhere in this book. Patients with gastrointestinal, urologic, or other nongynecologic conditions should be referred appropriately.
- The management of other patients with adnexal masses depends on the age of the patient, whether she is symptomatic or not, and the ultrasound characteristics of the mass.
- Asymptomatic women of reproductive age with small (≤6 cm) cystic adnexal masses noted on pelvic examination likely have functional cysts. These patients may be reexamined in 4 to 6 weeks to see whether the cyst has resolved.
- Asymptomatic women of reproductive age with large (>6 cm) or solid masses or in whom smaller cystic masses fail to resolve over 4 to 6 weeks should have a pelvic ultrasound performed.
- All postmenopausal patients with adnexal masses identified on pelvic examination should undergo a pelvic ultrasound to further characterize the mass.
- Indications for surgical intervention in patients with an adnexal mass include sonographic evidence of malignancy, secondary symptoms such as pain, and persistence of the mass over time.
- When a malignancy is likely, surgical exploration should be performed through a vertical midline incision in order to allow complete surgical staging, as described in Chap. 64.
- Patients less likely to have a malignancy may initially be evaluated by laparoscopy. If intraoperative evaluation, including frozen section of the involved adnexa, rules out malignancy, no further intervention is required. If a malignancy is identified grossly or on frozen section, the patient should undergo immediate laparotomy with staging or should be referred without delay to a gynecologic oncologist for surgical staging.
- Adnexal torsion should be suspected in patients with acute, severe pain and an adnexal mass. Such patients should undergo immediate surgical exploration, and the affected ovary should be evaluated to see if it is viable. If so, the adnexa may be untorsed, the mass removed, and the ovary saved. If the adnexa does not appear viable, it should be removed.

BIBLIOGRAPHY

American College of Obstetricians and Gynecologists. Benign disorders of the ovaries. *Precis, Gynecology: An update in obstetrics and gynecology,* 2nd ed. Washington, DC: ACOG, 2001:86–90.

Stenchever MA. Differential diagnosis of major gynecologic problems by age groups. In: Stenchever MA, Droegemueller W, Herbst AL, Mishell DR Jr, eds. *Comprehensive Gynecology.* St. Louis: Mosby, 2001.

45   CHRONIC PELVIC PAIN

John D. Davis

BACKGROUND

- Chronic pelvic pain is defined as noncyclic pain located in the pelvis that is present for at least 6 months.
- Patients with chronic pelvic pain account for approximately 10 percent of all outpatient gynecologic evaluations.
- Approximately one-third of all laparoscopies performed by gynecologists are for patients experiencing chronic pelvic pain.

ETIOLOGY

- Chronic pelvic pain is a complex disorder in which biologic disorders, psychologic variables, and social factors all interact to influence the degree of pain experienced by patients.
- Organic disease processes that have been implicated as causes of chronic pelvic pain include endometriosis, pelvic adhesive disease, atypical menstrual pain, urinary tract disorders (especially interstitial cystitis), bowel disorders (such as irritable bowel syndrome and inflammatory bowel disease), and trigger points (discrete hypersensitive foci thought to be caused by trauma to local nerves).
- There is a strong correlation between chronic pelvic pain and certain psychiatric disorders. Approximately 50 percent of patients with chronic pelvic pain have depression; up to 50 percent of such patients are past or current victims of physical and/or sexual abuse.

EVALUATION

- The directed history that should be obtained from patients with chronic pelvic pain includes the following:
  - Standard pain history components—ie, location, onset, character, intensity, alleviating and aggravating factors, associated symptoms, and radiation.
  - The relationship of the patient's pain to menses, intercourse, urination, and defecation.
  - Exacerbation of the patient's pain during periods of stress.
  - Specific questioning regarding urinary tract or bowel symptoms.
    - Past history of endometriosis, pelvic inflammatory disease, sexually transmitted diseases, pelvic surgery, or infertility.
    - Previous treatment for pelvic pain, including all past medical and surgical therapy.
- The abdominal and pelvic examination should be directed toward identifying the specific source of the patient's pain.
  - The abdominal wall should be inspected for scars from previous surgical procedures.
  - After asking the patient to identify the area of maximum pain, the examiner should palpate the abdomen for direct and rebound tenderness, voluntary and involuntary guarding, and masses.
  - To evaluate for trigger points, the abdomen should be examined with the patient doing a straight leg raise. Areas of tenderness still present when the patient does this maneuver may indicate a trigger point.
  - The external genitalia, vagina, and cervix should be inspected for lesions and discharge.
  - A bimanual examination should be performed to identify adnexal tenderness and/or masses, uterine tenderness and/or enlargement, cervical motion tenderness, nodularity in the posterior cul-de-sac, (sometimes noted in patients with endometriosis), bladder tenderness, and focal areas of tenderness which may indicate pelvic trigger points.
  - A rectovaginal examination should be performed if indicated on the basis of the patient's history or pelvic examination findings.
- Simple laboratory studies that should be performed on patients with chronic pelvic pain (depending on their history and physical examination findings) include cervical cultures, urinalysis, complete blood count, testing for fecal occult blood, and wet-mount examination of vaginal discharge.
- Ultrasound examination of the pelvis should be reserved primarily for patients suspected of having an adnexal mass.

MANAGEMENT

- In general, patients with chronic pelvic pain should initially be treated with nonsurgical therapy.
- First-line medical therapy often includes treatment with hormonal formulations (such as oral contraceptives) and nonsteroidal anti-inflammatory drugs (given on a scheduled rather than "as needed" basis).
- Treatment with other medications, such as antidepressants and antispasmodics, may be indicated based on the initial evaluation of the patient. Fiber supplements should be considered for patients with bowel symptoms. Empiric antibiotic therapy should not be part of the treatment in patients with chronic pelvic pain.
- A multidisciplinary approach to pain management—including psychologic evaluation and counseling, physical therapy, acupuncture, and local injection of anesthetics and steroids—is also helpful for some patients with chronic pelvic pain.
- Patients with chronic pelvic pain who do not respond to nonsurgical therapy may benefit from diagnostic laparoscopy.
- Laparoscopic evaluation of patients with pelvic pain may (1) identify the cause of pain, (2) allow treatment of any pathology identified (such as ablation of endometriosis or lysis of adhesions), and (3) provide reassurance to the patient if no abnormalities are identified.
- The decision to proceed with hysterectomy in patients with chronic pelvic pain should be made with great caution. While approximately 75 percent of patients who undergo hysterectomy experience pain relief, 25 percent will have persistent pain. Moreover, other patients may have only temporary relief of pain, and some will develop new chronic symptoms (such as migraine headaches or low back pain) if other underlying issues related to the pelvic pain go unaddressed.

BIBLIOGRAPHY

Milburn A, Reiter RC, Rhomberg AT. Multidisciplinary approach to chronic pelvic pain. *Obstet Gynecol Clin North Am* 1993;20(4):643–662.

Parsons LH, Stovall TG. Surgical management of chronic pelvic pain. *Obstet Gynecol Clin North Am* 1993;20(4):765–778.

46   ENDOMETRIOSIS

Alice Rhoton-Vlasak

EPIDEMIOLOGY

- Endometriosis is a benign condition characterized by the presence of endometrial glands and stroma outside the endometrial cavity.
- Endometriosis occurs in approximately 15 percent of women. Pelvic endometriosis is present in 6 to 43 percent of women undergoing sterilization, 12 to 32 percent of women undergoing laparoscopy for pelvic pain, and 21 to 78 percent of women undergoing laparoscopy for infertility.

PATHOGENESIS

- The exact cause is unknown, but there are several theories.
- **Retrograde menstruation theory of Sampson**. Endometrial fragments shed out the fallopian tubes at menstruation implant and grow in the pelvis.
- **Lymphatic/hematogenous spread**. This theory helps explain the presence of endometriosis in such distant organs as the brain, lung, kidney, pericardium, and thigh.
- **Müllerian metaplasia**. This theory proposes that endometriosis results from the metaplastic transformation of peritoneal mesothelium into endometrium.
- **Genetic predisposition to endometriosis**.
- **Alterations in pelvic cellular immunity**.

SITES OF OCCURRENCE

- Endometriosis most commonly occurs in the
  ◦ Ovaries
  ◦ Broad ligament
  ◦ Peritoneal surfaces of the cul-de-sac
  ◦ Rectovaginal septum
- Occasionally it will occur in the bowel, appendix, bladder, and other distant sites.

PATHOLOGY

- Laparoscopy with biopsy is the definitive diagnostic method.
- Endometriotic implants have a variety of appearances, ranging from clear to red superficial macules or nodules to a brown, blue, or black "powder burn."
- Repetitive bleeding within the implants gives them the dark color.

- Lesions may be locally invasive and cause significant adhesion formation.
- Endometriomas are cystic structures that usually involve the ovary. They may range in size from 1 to 10 cm and are usually filled with thick red to black fluid.
- The four major histologic components of endometriosis are as follows:
  ◦ Endometrial glands
  ◦ Endometrial stroma
  ◦ Fibrosis
  ◦ Hemorrhage
  ◦ These components are illustrated in Fig. 46–1.

CLINICAL PRESENTATION

- Symptoms include pelvic pain, dysmenorrhea, dyspareunia, dyschezia (difficult or painful evacuation of feces from the rectum), and infertility.
- Neither the amount of pain nor the presence of infertility correlates well with the amount of disease identified at laparoscopy.
- Findings on physical examination include cul-de-sac or uterosacral nodules/tenderness, fixed tender pelvic mass, and vaginal or cervical lesions.

CLASSIFICATION

- The most frequently used classification system is the American Society for Reproductive Medicine (ASRM) scoring system.
- Endometriosis is staged as minimal (stage I), mild (stage II), moderate (stage III), or severe (stage IV) based on disease location, size of implants, depth of implants, and presence of adhesions. Figure 46–2 outlines the ASRM scoring system.

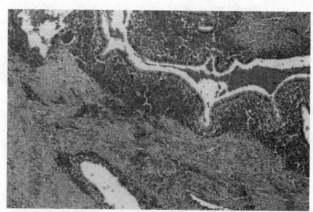

FIG. 46-1 Histologic findings of endometriosis demonstrating endometrial glands and stoma in an ectopic site. (Courtesy of Edward Wilkinson, MD.)

AMERICAN SOCIETY FOR REPRODUCTIVE MEDICINE
REVISED CLASSIFICATION OF ENDOMETRIOSIS

Patient's Name _____ Date_____

Stage I (Minimal) · 1-5
Stage II (Mild) · 6-15
Stage III (Moderate) · 16-40
Stage IV (Severe) · >40
Total_____

Laparoscopy_____ Laparotomy_____ Photography_____
Recommended Treatment_____

Prognosis_____

PERITONEUM	**ENDOMETRIOSIS**	<1cm	1-3cm	>3cm
	Superficial	1	2	4
	Deep	2	4	6
OVARY	R Superficial	1	2	4
	Deep	4	16	20
	L Superficial	1	2	4
	Deep	4	16	20

	POSTERIOR CULDESAC OBLITERATION	Partial	Complete
		4	40

	ADHESIONS	<1/3 Enclosure	1/3-2/3 Enclosure	>2/3 Enclosure
OVARY	R Filmy	1	2	4
	Dense	4	8	16
	L Filmy	1	2	4
	Dense	4	8	16
TUBE	R Filmy	1	2	4
	Dense	4*	8*	16
	L Filmy	1	2	4
	Dense	4*	8*	16

*If the fimbriated end of the fallopian tube is completely enclosed, change the point assignment to 16.

Denote appearance of superficial implant types as red [(R), red, red-pink, flamelike, vesicular blobs, clear vesicles], white [(W), opacifications, peritoneal defects, yellow-brown], or black [(B) black, hemosiderin deposits, blue]. Denote percent of total described as R____%, W____% and B____%. Total should equal 100%.

Additional Endometriosis: _____   Associated Pathology: _____
_____   _____
_____   _____

To Be Used with Normal
Tubes and Ovaries

L .... R

To Be Used with Abnormal
Tubes and/or Ovaries

L .... R

FIG. 46-2 Revised American Society for Reproductive Medicine classification of endometriosis. (From the American Society for Reproductive Medicine. *Fertil Steril* 1997;67:817–821. With permission.)

DIAGNOSIS

- Laparoscopy, with direct visualization of endometriotic implants, is the "gold standard" for diagnosis.

- The diagnosis also can be confirmed by biopsy when endometriotic implants are present in sites such as the cervix, the vagina, or within a surgical scar.

DIFFERENTIAL DIAGNOSIS

- Acute or chronic pelvic inflammatory disease
- Hemorrhagic corpus luteum
- Ovarian neoplasm

TREATMENT

- Observation may be appropriate in patients with minimal symptoms who do not desire fertility.
- Medical treatment improves pelvic pain and reduces lesion size but does not enhance fertility. Medical treatment options are outlined in Table 46–1.
  - Progestins and oral contraceptives (which can be taken continuously or cyclically) cause atrophy of endometrial glands and stroma.
  - GnRH agonists cause temporary medical castration, which makes endometriosis regress. Bone loss limits the length of time they can be used, unless "add-back therapy" with low dose estrogen, progestins, or bisphosphonates is given.
  - Danazol, a relatively expensive androgen, is rarely used due to its androgenic side effects.
- Surgical treatment is appropriate in many patients and can be accomplished at the time of diagnostic laparoscopy. Figure 46–3 shows the laparoscopic appearance of endometriosis on the ovary and Fig. 46–4 shows endometriosis on the rectosigmoid.
- Laparoscopy has replaced laparotomy in most cases.
- Surgery attempts to destroy or excise all endometriosis, lyse adhesions, and restore normal anatomy.
- Laparoscopic surgery is clearly the preferred treatment for patients with infertility and has been shown to improve pregnancy rates.
- Large endometriomas also can be resected at laparoscopy, thereby preserving the ovaries and fertility.
- Endometriosis can recur after medical and conservative surgical therapy. After conservative surgery, reported recurrence rates vary greatly but usually exceed 10 percent in 3 years and 35 percent in 5 years.

- Hysterectomy and bilateral salpingo-oophorectomy, with excision of other implants, are indicated in women who do not desire further childbearing or who have severe symptoms.
- Medical therapy may be indicated after surgery if the endometriotic lesions are not completely resected and to prevent recurrences.

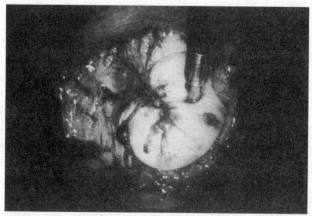

FIG. 46-3 Laparoscopic appearance of endometriosis on the ovary. Lesions are blue-black in color.

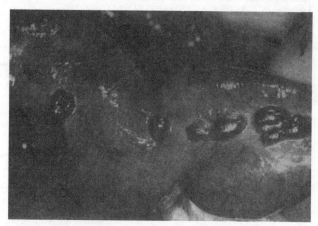

FIG. 46-4 Laparoscopic appearance of red lesions of endometriosis on the rectosigmoid.

TABLE 46-1   Medical Therapy for Endometriosis

CATEGORY OF DRUG	SPECIFIC AGENTS	DOSE	FREQUENCY
Progestins	Medroxyprogesterone acetate	10–30 mg PO	daily
	Depot medroxyprogesterone acetate	150 mg IM	every 90 days
	Norethindrone acetate	5 mg PO	daily
Combination oral contraceptives	Low-dose combination pill	one tablet	daily
GnRH agonists[a]	Leuprolide acetate	3.75 mg IM	every 4 weeks × 6 months
	Nafarelin acetate	200 mg intranasal	twice daily × 6 months
Danazol		200 mg PO	1–4 times daily

[a]Treatment longer than 6 months leads to significant bone loss unless estrogen or progestin add-back therapy is given.

- Laparotomy is indicated if endometriosis involves the bowel, bladder, or rectovaginal septum.
- Assisted reproductive techniques (ART) such as superovulation and intrauterine insemination or in vitro fertilization may be needed to treat infertility associated with endometriosis. Fecundity rates are similar to those reported for other diagnoses.

BIBLIOGRAPHY

American College of Obstetricians and Gynecologists. Medical management of endometriosis. *ACOG Tech Bull* No. 11, December 1999.

Ho HN, Wu MY, Yang YS. Peritoneal cellular immunity and endometriosis. *Am J Reprod Immunol* 1997;38(6):400–412.

Sanghaghpeykar H, Poindexter AN III. Epidemiology of endometriosis among parous women. *Obstet Gynecol* 1995;5:983–992.

Winkel CA. Evaluation and management of women with endometriosis. *Obstet Gynecol* 2003;102(2):397–408.

47 URINARY INCONTINENCE

John D. Davis

DEFINITION AND EPIDEMIOLOGY

- Urinary incontinence is a condition in which involuntary loss of urine is both a social and hygienic problem and can be objectively demonstrated.
- Urinary incontinence affects approximately 25 percent of noninstitutionalized women over the age of 60; 50 percent of nursing home residents are incontinent.
- Risk factors associated with urinary incontinence are listed in Table 47-1.
- Less than half of women who suffer from urinary incontinence seek help for the problem (because of embarrassment, denial, or unawareness of treatment options).

FORMS OF URINARY INCONTINENCE

- The three most common forms of incontinence are **stress urinary incontinence** (SUI), detrusor overactivity, and mixed incontinence (a combination of SUI and detrusor overactivity), which occur in approximately 45, 20, and 30 percent of incontinent women respectively.

TABLE 47-1   Risk Factors Associated with Incontinence

Immobility/chronic degenerative disease
Impaired cognition
Medications, including diuretics
Obesity
Smoking
Fecal impaction
Delirium
Low fluid intake
Environmental barriers
High-impact physical activities
Diabetes
Stroke
Estrogen depletion
Pelvic muscle weakness
Childhood nocturnal enuresis
Pregnancy/vaginal delivery/episiotomy

Adapted from Fantl JA, Newman DK, Colling J, et al. *Urinary Incontinence in Adults: Acute and Chronic Management.* Clinical Practice Guideline no. 2, 1996 update. AHCPR publication no. 96-0682. Rockville, MD: Agency for Health Care Policy and Research, U.S. Department of Health and Human Services, Public Health Service, March 1996.

- SUI is the loss of urine associated with physical exertion such as coughing, sneezing, running, lifting, and jumping.
- SUI is caused by displacement of the urethrovesical junction out of the abdominal cavity, leading to unequal transmission of abdominal pressure to the bladder and proximal urethra.
- The classic patient with SUI has delivered at least one child vaginally, leaks small amounts of urine coincident with increases in abdominal pressure, and does not experience irritative bladder symptoms. Pelvic examination of such a patient will usually show evidence of pelvic relaxation and urethral hypermobility.
- An important subtype of SUI is **intrinsic sphincter deficiency** (ISD), where the urethra lacks sufficient tone to maintain continence. Such patients often have continuous urine loss or leak with only small increases in abdominal pressure.
- Women with detrusor overactivity leak urine due to uncontrolled bladder contractions. Such patients experience irritative bladder symptoms, may leak larger amounts of urine due to uncontrolled bladder contractions, and have the urge to void just before the incontinent episode.
- Idiopathic detrusor overactivity is called **detrusor instability** (DI); detrusor overactivity secondary to neurologic conditions (such as multiple sclerosis or a stroke) is termed **detrusor hyperreflexia**.
- Less common but still important causes of urinary incontinence are overflow incontinence (involuntary urine loss due to overdistention of the bladder), true incontinence (due to urinary tract fistulas), functional incontinence (where physical or cognitive

TABLE 47-2   Transient Causes of Urinary Incontinence (mnemonic DIAPPERS)

Delirium
Infection (of the urinary tract)
Atrophic vaginitis
Pharmacologic (eg, diuretics, alpha blockers)
Psychologic
Endocrine (diabetes mellitus or insipidus)
Restricted mobility
Stool impaction

impairment prevents someone from reaching the bathroom before experiencing urine loss), and transient or reversible causes of incontinence. Transient causes of incontinence are listed in Table 47-2.

BASIC EVALUATION

- All patients with urinary incontinence should undergo a basic evaluation including history, physical examination, urinalysis, and measurement of **postvoid residual** (PVR) volume.
- Important components of the history of incontinent patients include duration, characteristics, and frequency of urine loss; precipitating risk factors and associated symptoms; medication use; previous therapy for incontinence; and expectations of treatment.
- During the pelvic examination, the vagina should be examined for signs of hypoestrogenism and the presence of a fistula. The adequacy of pelvic support should be noted. A brief neurologic screen, including assessment of the bulbocavernosus reflex and anal wink, should be done. Pelvic tone should be assessed and a rectal examination should be done to rule out impaction.
- Abnormalities on urinalysis (including evidence of infection or other urinary tract abnormality) should be evaluated and treated before proceeding with any further incontinence evaluation.
- A PVR of greater than 100 mL is abnormal and may be indicative of urethral obstruction and/or poor bladder contractility.

URODYNAMIC TESTING

- When the basic evaluation strongly suggests SUI or DI as the cause of a woman's incontinence, she may be treated accordingly without further workup. When the basic evaluation fails to identify the etiology of the patient's uncontrolled urinary loss (or if the patient is over age 50, has symptoms of mixed incontinence, or has had previous anti-incontinence surgery), additional testing is indicated.
- Urodynamic tests—including simple **cystometrogram** (CMG), multichannel CMG, and **urethral pressure profilometry** (UPP)—are used to evaluate the functional status of the bladder and urethra.
- A simple CMG measures intravesical pressure versus the volume of fluid in the bladder.
- A simple CMG, or single-channel cystometry, may be done in the office by placing a urethral catheter with an attached 60-mL syringe into the bladder and slowly filling the bladder with saline. Involuntary detrusor contractions can be identified by noting a rise in the fluid level in the syringe; first sensation and bladder capacity can also be determined.
- Multichannel CMG requires more sophisticated equipment and more advanced training to perform than the simple CMG. During multichannel CMG, pressure transducers are placed into the bladder and also into the vagina or rectum (to measure intraabdominal pressure). The bladder is filled with saline and the recorded intraabdominal pressure is subtracted from the recorded total bladder pressure to determine the true detrusor pressure. This form of testing is more accurate in identifying true detrusor overactivity than simple CMG.
- During multichannel testing, the **abdominal leak point pressure** (ALPP) can be determined. The ALPP is the abdominal or vesical pressure required to overcome urethral resistance and cause urine loss.
  - A normal ALPP is greater than 90 cmH$_2$O; an ALPP of 60 to 90 cmH$_2$O is a borderline result.
  - An ALPP of less than 60 cmH$_2$O is abnormal and may be associated with ISD.
- **Urethral pressure profilometry** is a test where a pressure transducer is slowly withdrawn through the urethra to determine the resting urethral tone. Normal urethral tone is greater than 50 cmH$_2$O, while measurements between 20 and 50 cmH$_2$O are considered borderline. A maximum urethral closure pressure of less than 20 cmH$_2$O may be indicative of ISD.

THERAPY

DETRUSOR INSTABILITY

- Patients with DI should first have any reversible causes of incontinence addressed. Urinary tract infection, caffeine (a bladder irritant) intake, and certain medications (eg, diuretics) all may cause DI. Antibiotic therapy, discontinuation of caffeine, or substitution of alternative medications alone may alleviate the patient's problem.

- Bladder retraining, analogous to toilet training, is a safe, inexpensive, and effective treatment of DI. Patients are asked to void only at progressively longer timed intervals (usually starting at 30-min intervals and increasing the voiding interval by 30 min weekly, to a maximum interval of 2 to 3 h) and to suppress any detrusor contractions with Kegel exercises and deep breathing (see below).
- Patients with DI who fail to respond to the above may benefit from drug treatment. Anticholinergic agents (eg, oxybutynin) are the most commonly used class of medications to treat DI. The usual starting dose of extended-release oxybutynin is 5 mg once daily. The most common side effect of anticholinergic medications is dry mouth.

STRESS URINARY INCONTINENCE

- Patients with mild-to-moderate SUI may benefit from Kegel exercises (contracting the pelvic floor muscles as if they were trying to stop their urinary stream). Patients should be asked to contract their muscles for 10 s 10 to 20 times at least 3 times a day.
- Patients who have difficulty doing Kegel exercises properly may benefit from biofeedback. During biofeedback, a physical therapist places a pressure transducer in the vagina and the patient receives visual or auditory feedback when she is contracting her pelvic floor musculature properly.
- Patients with more severe SUI or those who fail to respond to pelvic floor exercises may require surgical therapy.
- The "gold standard" for anti-incontinence surgery has been the Burch retropubic urethropexy. During this procedure, the prevesical space is opened and two to three sutures are placed in the endopelvic fascia lateral to the urethra from the urethrovesical junction to the level of the midurethra. These sutures are anchored superiorly to Cooper's ligament to suspend the proximal urethra intraabdominally, thereby equalizing the transmission of abdominal pressure to the bladder and proximal urethra, preventing urinary loss.
- The Burch retropubic urethropexy has a 5-year success rate of approximately 80 percent.
- A newer treatment for SUI is **tension-free vaginal tape** (TVT), a Prolene mesh placed suburethrally to create a support upon which the urethra can close during episodes of increased abdominal pressure.
- Compared to the retropubic urethropexy, the TVT is approximately 90 percent effective, can be done in

one-half to one-third the time, and can be performed under local anesthesia on an outpatient basis.

INTRINSIC SPHINCTER DEFICIENCY

- A Burch retropubic urethropexy is usually not adequate treatment for patients with ISD and a hypermobile urethra. Such patients usually require a suburethral sling or TVT.
- Patients with ISD and a fixed urethra may be treated with periurethral bulking agents (collagen) to increase urethral tone.

BIBLIOGRAPHY

Agency for Health Care Policy and Research. *Urinary Incontinence in Adults: Acute and Chronic Management.* Clinical Practice Guideline no. 2, 1996 update. AHCPR Publication No. 96-0682. Rockville, MD: U.S. Department of Health and Human Services, March 1996.

American College of Obstetricians and Gynecologists. Urinary and fecal incontinence. In: *Precis, Gynecology: An update in obstetrics and gynecology,* 2nd ed. Washington, DC: ACOG, 2001:54–73.

 48 PRE- AND POSTOPERATIVE CARE

John D. Davis

PREOPERATIVE ASSESSMENT

- All patients undergoing gynecologic surgery must have a thorough history taken and undergo a complete physical examination. The purpose of the history and physical examination is to confirm the presence of a gynecologic disorder, verify that the gynecologic disorder requires surgical treatment, and identify factors that could place the patient at higher risk for perioperative complications.
- The extent of preoperative testing should be based on the patient's disease process, her general medical condition, as well as the complexity of the planned surgical procedure.
- Most medical centers require that patients have a complete blood count preoperatively.
- A urinalysis is required only in symptomatic patients.

- A preoperative pregnancy test is advisable for all patients at risk for pregnancy.
- Serum electrolytes should be measured in patients with renal or cardiac disease, those taking diuretics, and the elderly.
- Assessment of clotting function is indicated only in patients in whom a bleeding diathesis is suspected.
- A determination of blood type and a screen for antibodies should be obtained in patients at risk for significant bleeding.
- An electrocardiogram should be obtained preoperatively in patients 50 years of age and older as well as those with known cardiac disease.
- A chest radiograph is indicated for elderly patients and those with known pulmonary or cardiac disease.
- A preoperative imaging study of the urinary tract (intravenous pyelogram or computed tomography) to rule out preexisting damage to the ureters is advisable if a patient has undergone a previous difficult gynecologic procedure, has a congenital anomaly of the reproductive tract, or has a very large pelvic mass.

PROPHYLACTIC ANTIBIOTICS

- Wound infection and pelvic cellulitis are common causes of morbidity related to gynecologic surgery.
- All patients undergoing vaginal hysterectomy—regardless of age, menopausal status, or presence or absence of other risk factors—have a decreased incidence of pelvic cellulitis when prophylactic antibiotics are administered.
- In low-risk patients (middle to upper socioeconomic status, uncomplicated procedure) undergoing abdominal hysterectomy, prophylactic antibiotics do not consistently decrease the incidence of pelvic cellulitis or wound infection because the baseline incidence of infection is so low.
- In high-risk patients (low socioeconomic status, extended duration of surgery, excessive intraoperative blood loss) undergoing abdominal hysterectomy, prophylactic antibiotics decrease the incidence of both pelvic cellulitis and wound infection and thus shorten the duration and expense of hospitalization.
- The most appropriate choice of antibiotic for prophylaxis is cefazolin (1 g), a relatively broad-spectrum, inexpensive, first-generation cephalosporin. If the patient is allergic to beta-lactam antibiotics, doxycycline (100 mg) is a reasonable alternative.
- Prophylactic antibiotics should be administered 30 min before the procedure begins so as to ensure adequate tissue levels at the surgical site. An additional dose of medication should be given if the surgical procedure is prolonged or blood loss is excessive.

PREVENTION OF VENOUS THROMBOSIS

- The incidence of venous thrombosis in patients undergoing gynecologic surgery is 15 percent, with a range of 5 to 45 percent, depending on the procedure performed and associated risk factors. Pulmonary embolism accounts for 40 percent of all deaths following gynecologic surgery.
- Risk factors for the development of **venous thromboembolism** (VTE) in gynecologic surgical patients are listed in Table 48-1.
- Unfractionated heparin, low-molecular-weight heparin, and intermittent pneumatic compression stockings are all effective in reducing the incidence of thromboembolic complications of gynecologic surgery.
- An appropriate dose of unfractionated heparin would be 5000 to 7500 U (depending on the patient's weight) SQ twice daily, beginning prior to surgery and continuing until the patient is fully ambulatory.
- The appropriate dose of a low-molecular-weight heparin (enoxaparin, Lovenox®) is 40 mg SQ once daily, beginning 2 h prior to surgery and continuing for 7 to 10 days.
- Patients should be encouraged to ambulate as soon as possible postoperatively in order to limit venous stasis and reduce the incidence of thromboembolism.

GASTROINTESTINAL TRACT

- The majority of patients undergoing gynecologic surgery do not require mechanical preparation of the bowel.
- Patients at risk for entry into the bowel during their surgical procedure (known extensive intraabdominal adhesions, previous bowel resection, possible malignancy) should undergo bowel preparation preoperatively.
- A common method of preparing the bowel the day before surgery is to administer GOLYTELY

TABLE 48-1   Risk Factors for Venous Thromboembolism in Patients Undergoing Gynecologic Surgery

Age > 40 years
Obesity
Perioperative immobility
Trauma (eg, radical pelvic surgery)
Malignancy
Prior radiation therapy
Medical conditions including
  Diabetes mellitus
  Cardiac disease, heart failure
  Severe varicose veins
  Previous venous thrombosis with or without embolization
  Chronic pulmonary disease
  Antithrombin III, protein C, or protein S deficiency

(polyethylene glycol in a balanced salt solution) 1.5 L/h until the effluent is clear. Some authorities also recommend giving neomycin (1 g) and erythromycin base (1 g) orally at 2 p.m., 4 p.m., and 10 p.m. the day before surgery.

CARDIOVASCULAR DISEASE

- Patients with poorly controlled congestive heart failure, poorly controlled hypertension (diastolic blood pressure above 110 mmHg), unstable angina, or a history of a myocardial infarction within the preceding 6 months are at high risk for a perioperative cardiovascular complications. Such patients should be evaluated by a cardiologist before proceeding with elective gynecologic surgery.
- Perioperative administration of beta blockers reduces the risk of cardiac death and nonfatal myocardial infarction in patients at high risk for cardiovascular complications.
- An appropriate beta blocker for such high-risk patients is metoprolol (Lopressor 50 mg twice daily) beginning 1 week before surgery and continued for at least 4 weeks postoperatively.
- Cardiac conditions associated with an increased risk of bacterial endocarditis are listed in Table 48-2. Perioperative endocarditis prophylaxis is recommended for patients in the high- and moderate-risk categories. Prophylactic regimens for patients

TABLE 48-2 Cardiac Conditions Associated with Endocarditis

High-risk category
  Prosthetic cardiac valves, including bioprosthetic and homograft valves
  Previous bacterial endocarditis
  Complex cyanotic congenital heart disease (eg, single ventricle states, transposition of the great arteries, tetralogy of Fallot)
  Surgically constructed systemic pulmonary shunts or conduits
Moderate-risk category
  Most other congenital cardiac malformations (other than above and below)
  Acquired valvular dysfunction (eg, rheumatic heart disease)
  Hypertrophic cardiomyopathy
  Mitral valve prolapse with valvular regurgitation and/or thickened leaflets
Negligible-risk category (no greater risk than the general population)
  Isolated secundum atrial septal defect
  Surgical repair of atrial septal defect, ventricular septal defect, or patent ductus arteriosus (without residua beyond 6 mo)
  Previous coronary artery bypass graft surgery
  Mitral valve prolapse without valvular regurgitation
  Physiologic, functional, or innocent heart murmurs
  Previous Kawasaki's disease without valvular dysfunction
  Previous rheumatic fever without valvular dysfunction
  Cardiac pacemakers (intravascular and epicardial) and implanted defibrillators

undergoing genitourinary procedures are listed in Table 48-3.

RESPIRATORY SYSTEM

- Pulmonary complications, including atelectasis and pneumonia, occur frequently after gynecologic surgery.
- Risk factors for postoperative pulmonary complications are listed in Table 48-4.
- Methods aimed at reducing the incidence of postoperative pulmonary complications are listed in Table 48-5.
- Women who smoke are at a fourfold increased risk of postoperative pulmonary complications. Smokers should be strongly encouraged to stop smoking before undergoing elective gynecologic surgery.

POSTOPERATIVE FLUID MANAGEMENT

- The average woman loses approximately 2500 mL of water per day. Insensible loss (perspiration, respiration) accounts for approximately 1000 mL of lost fluid, while urine output accounts for the rest.
- Postoperative patients who are not able to drink or eat must have this fluid replaced intravenously. In addition, postoperative patients should receive 100 to 140 meq of sodium and 40 to 60 meq of potassium daily.
- In healthy patients, these requirements are commonly met by administering 3 L of half-normal saline with 20 meq of potassium chloride added to each liter of intravenous fluid (1/2 NS with 20 meq KCl/L administered at 125 mL/h).
- Patients who are febrile, who have a nasogastric tube in place, or who have diarrhea require additional replacement of fluid and electrolytes.

POSTOPERATIVE PAIN MANAGEMENT

- Moderate-to-severe postoperative pain usually is treated with narcotic analgesics. Narcotics may be administered by **patient-controlled analgesic** (PCA) systems and by epidural catheters.
- Advantages of PCA systems include the following:
  ○ Uniform level of analgesic, leading to better pain relief
  ○ Patient control of medication administration with secondary reduction in patient anxiety
  ○ Requirement for minimal nursing support

TABLE 48-3　Prophylactic Regimens for Genitourinary Procedures

SITUATION	AGENTS	REGIMEN
High-risk patients	Ampicillin plus gentamicin	Adults: ampicillin 2.0 g IM or IV plus gentamicin 1.5 mg/kg (not to exceed 120 mg) within 30 min of starting the procedure: 6 h later, ampicillin 1 g IM/IV or amoxicillin 1 g orally
		Children: ampicillin 50 mg/kg IM or IV (not to exceed 2.0 g) plus gentamicin 1.5 mg/kg within 30 min of starting the procedure: 6 h later, ampicillin 25 mg/kg IM/IV or amoxicillin 25 mg/kg orally
High-risk patients allergic to ampicillin/amoxicillin	Vancomycin plus gentamicin	Adults: vancomycin 1.0 g IV over 1–2 h plus gentamicin 1.5 mg/kg IV/IM (not to exceed 120 mg); complete injection/infusion within 30 min of starting the procedure
		Children: vancomycin 20 mg/kg IV over 1–2 h plus gentamicin 1.5 mg/kg IV/IM: complete injection/infusion within 30 min of starting the procedure
Moderate-risk patients	Amoxicillin or ampicillin	Adults: amoxicillin 2.0 g orally 1 h before procedure, or ampicillin 2.0 g IM/IV within 30 min of starting the procedure
		Children: amoxicillin 50 mg/kg orally 1 h before procedure, or ampicillin 50 mg/kg IM/IV within 30 of starting the procdure
Moderate-risk patients allergic to ampicillin/amoxicillin	Vancomycin	Adults: vancomycin 1.0 g IV over 1–2 h: complete infusion within 30 min of starting the procedure
		Children: vancomycin 20 mg/kg IV over 1–2 h: complete infusion within 30 min of starting the procedure

TABLE 48-4　Risk Factors for Postoperative Pulmonary Complications

Chronic obstructive pulmonary disease
Asthma
Productive cough
Cigarette smoking
Age > 60 years
Obesity
Malnutrition (including alcoholism)
Anesthesia time > 3 h
Thoracic or upper abdominal surgery

TABLE 48-5　Methods of Reducing Pulmonary Complications

Preoperative
　Cessation of smoking
　Aggressive treatment of chronic obstructive pulmonary disease or asthma with bronchodilators and steroids
　Chest physiotherapy
　Patient education in use of incentive spirometry
　Antibiotics for respiratory infection
Postoperative
　Bronchodilators
　Chest physiotherapy
　Incentive spirometry
　Early ambulation
　Heparin or intermittent pneumatic compression stockings

POSTOPERATIVE CARE OF THE GASTROINTESTINAL TRACT

- Postoperatively, a clear liquid diet may be started when a patient is alert and has no nausea, vomiting, or abdominal distention.

- The routine use of nasogastric tubes postoperatively, even in patients who have undergone bowel surgery, is unnecessary. Nasogastric tubes cause significant discomfort and, when used on a routine basis, do not provide significant benefit for patients.
- Adynamic ileus is relatively common after major gynecologic surgery. Minor to moderate degrees of ileus usually respond to restriction of oral intake. More severe degrees of ileus may require decompression with a nasogastric tube.
- The characteristics that distinguish an ileus from a mechanical small bowel obstruction are listed in Table 48-6.

CARE OF THE BLADDER

- Bladder atony is common after major pelvic surgery. Therefore a Foley catheter should routinely be placed in the bladder intraoperatively to allow drainage of urine and to measure urine output accurately.
- The catheter usually can be removed the day following surgery as long as the patient is ambulatory. Patients who undergo surgical procedures on the bladder or urethra (eg, an anterior colporrhaphy or an anti-incontinence procedure) may require a longer period of catheter drainage.
- Patients who experience urinary retention after the removal of the catheter may be treated with intermittent self-catheterization. Self-catheterization may be

TABLE 48-6 Distinguishing Features of Ileus and Obstruction

CLINICAL FEATURE	POSTOPERATIVE ILEUS	POSTOPERATIVE OBSTRUCTION
Abdominal pain	Discomfort from distention but no cramping pains	Cramping progressively severe
Relation to previous surgery	Usually within 48–72 h of surgery	Usually delayed 5–7 days from surgery
Nausea and vomiting	Present	Present
Distention	Present	Present
Bowel sounds	Absent or hypoactive	Borborygmi with peristaltic rushes and high-pitched tinkles
Fever	Only if related to associated peritonitis	Rarely present unless bowel becomes gangrenous
Abdominal radiographs	Distended loops of small and large bowel; gas usually present in colon	Single or multiple loops of distended bowel (usually small bowel) with air-fluid levels
Treatment	Conservative, with nasogastric suction, enemas, cholinergic stimulation	Conservative, with nasogastric decompression Surgical exploration

discontinued once the postvoid residual volume of urine is less than 100 mL.

- Women with catheters draining into a closed system develop urinary tract infections (UTI) at a rate of approximately 5 percent per 24 h.
- Symptoms of a catheter-related UTI usually develop 24 to 48 h after catheter removal. Patients with postcatheter infections should be treated with short courses (3 to 10 days, depending on the severity of the infection and the patient's previous history of recurrent UTIs) of oral antibiotics such as nitrofunantoin monohydrate macrocrystals (Macrobid, 100 mg twice daily) or double strength trimethoprim/sulfamethoxazole (Bactrim or Septra, twice daily).

BIBLIOGRAPHY

American College of Obstetricians and Gynecologists. Perioperative care. In: Precis, *Gynecology:* An update in obstetrics and gynecology, 2nd ed. Washington, DC: ACOG, 2001:21–27.

Dajani AS, Taubert KA, Wilson W, et al. Prevention of bacterial endocarditis. Recommendations by the American Heart Association. *JAMA* 1997;277(22):1794–1801.

Rock JA, Thompson JD. *TeLinde's Operative Gynecology,* 8th ed. Philadelphia: Lippincott-Raven, 1997, chap 9.

Stenchever MA, Droegemueller W, Herbst AL, Mishell DR Jr. *Comprehensive Gynecology.* St. Louis: Mosby, 2001, chap 24.

49 PRECOCIOUS PUBERTY

Alice Rhoton-Vlasak

NORMAL PUBERTY

- Puberty is the process by which sexually immature persons develop secondary sexual characteristics and become capable of reproduction.
- Changes usually occur between the ages of 10 and 16.
- The somatic changes of puberty were first standardized by Marshall and Tanner. Table 49-1 outlines the Tanner classification of breast and pubic hair development.
- The Tanner classification can be used to assess girls with precocious or delayed puberty.

TABLE 49-1   Tanner Staging of Breast and Pubic Hair Development

Breast Development

Stage 1:	Preadolescent; elevation of the papilla only
Stage 2:	Breast bud stage; elevation of breast and papilla as a small mound, enlargement of areolar diameter
Stage 3:	Further enlargement and elevation of breast and areola with no separation of their contours
Stage 4:	Projection of areola and papilla to form a secondary mound above the level of the breast
Stage 5:	Mature stage, projection of papilla only caused by recession of the areola to the general contour of the breast

Pubic Hair

Stage 1:	Preadolescent; no visible pubic hair
Stage 2:	Sparse growth of long, slightly pigmented downy hair, straight or curled, primarily along labia
Stage 3:	Considerably darker, coarser, and more curled; hair spreads sparsely over mons
Stage 4:	Hair now adult-type, but area covered is still considerably smaller than in the adult; no spread to medial surface of thighs
Stage 5:	Adult appearance in quantity and type with classic female distribution and spread to medial aspect of thighs

- The sequence of developmental events is as follows:
  - Growth acceleration
  - Thelarche (mean age 9 to 11 years)—breast development
  - Pubarche/adrenarche—development of pubic and axillary hair
  - Maximal growth velocity
  - Menarche (mean age 12.8 years)
  - Ovulation (mean age 14.5 years)
- Regular ovulatory cycles occur approximately 20 months after menarche and mark the end of pubertal changes.

DEFINITION OF PRECOCIOUS PUBERTY

- Precocious puberty is the development of sexual maturation at an age greater than 2.5 standard deviations below the mean, or the appearance of any secondary sexual characteristics before 8 years of age or onset of menarche before 10 years of age.
- The incidence is 1:10,000 children in North America and is more common in girls than boys.

ETIOLOGY

- The classification of precocious puberty is outlined in Table 49-2.
- GnRH-dependent precocious puberty is caused by the premature activation of the hypothalamic-pituitary axis, leading to normal pubertal development at an earlier age.
- GnRH-independent precocious puberty results from an independent source of sex steroids rather than central maturation.

TABLE 49-2   Classification of Precocious Puberty

GnRH-dependent (true precocity)
  Idiopathic—most common cause
  CNS disorders
      Hypothalamic hamartomas
      CNS tumor (craniopharyngioma, glioma, astrocytoma, neuroblastoma)
      CNS infection (abscess, encephalitis, meningitis)
      Head trauma
      Hydrocephalus
      Cranial irradiation
GnRH-independent (precocious pseudopuberty)
  Endogenous estrogen production
  Ovarian cyst or tumor
  Other hormone-producing tumors
  McCune-Albright syndrome
  Exogenous estrogens

- McCune-Albright syndrome is caused by an activating mutation of the gene coding for the stimulatory G protein of glycoprotein hormone receptors. It causes endocrine dysfunction, polyostotic fibrous dysplasia, and café au lait spots. Children affected with McCune-Albright syndrome tend to present at an earlier age, often with a very early onset of vaginal bleeding. The diagnosis is established by identification of skin lesions, bone lesions, or pathologic fractures. The prognosis is not as good as with other causes because of limited potential for adult height and possible infertility. Few treatments are available.

PSEUDO–PRECOCIOUS PUBERTY (ISOLATED PRECOCIOUS DEVELOPMENT)

- Premature thelarche is the isolated development of breast tissue prior to age 8. Usually it is self-limited and requires no therapy. Bone age is usually normal. Close surveillance is important to rule out progression to true precocious puberty.
- Premature adrenarche is the isolated development of pubic or axillary hair before 8 years of age. It is usually idiopathic, but evaluation for an enzyme deficiency or tumor is indicated. This condition is more common in Hispanic or African-American girls.
- Premature menarche is the appearance of cyclic vaginal bleeding in children in the absence of secondary sexual development. The evaluation for this condition should include an assessment for infection, foreign body, abuse, trauma, and neoplasm. The prognosis for normal adult height and fertility is good.

DIAGNOSTIC EVALUATION

- A detailed history should be obtained, documenting age of onset, duration, and course of progression.
- The physical examination should focus specifically on:
  - General changes and review of the growth curve
  - Assessment of the skin
  - Breast examination and documentation of Tanner stage II or greater
  - Examination of the genitalia to assess Tanner stage and degree of estrogenization
- Laboratory evaluation helps differentiate central from peripheral precocious puberty and aids in directing therapy.
- All patients should have the following laboratory tests:
  - Thyroid-stimulating hormone (TSH)
  - Follicle-stimulating hormone (FSH)
  - Luteinizing hormone (LH)
  - GnRH stimulation test
- Selected patients may need specialized tests such as these:
  - Human chorionic gonadotropin (hCG)
  - Dehydroepiandrosterone sulfate (DHEAS)
  - Testosterone
  - Estradiol
  - 17 hydroxy-progesterone
- Radiologic evaluation should include the following:
  - Bone age
  - Head MRI or CT scan
  - Pelvic/abdominal ultrasound

MANAGEMENT

- The main treatment goals are to:
  - Diagnose intracranial lesions
  - Maximize adult height
  - Arrest sexual maturation
  - Facilitate regression of secondary sexual characteristics
  - Minimize emotional and psychologic issues related to precocious development.
- GnRH-dependent precocious puberty should be treated with GnRH agonists, which suppresses gonadotropin and sex-steroid production to prepubertal levels.
- Chronic administration of GnRH agonists is safe and effective for both males and females. Within 6 to 18 months, there will usually be a regression in secondary sexual characteristics, a deceleration in skeletal maturation, and cessation of menses.

- Treatment should be continued until puberty is appropriate, based on age, height, height potential, and emotional maturity.
- Treatment for other causes of precocious puberty is directed at the specific etiology. For example, in the case of a brain tumor, the patient should have surgery to excise the mass.

BIBLIOGRAPHY

American College of Obstetrics and Gynecology. Precis: An update in obstetrics and gynecology. Abnormalities of puberty. *Reproductive Endocrinology,* 2nd ed. Washington, DC: ACOG, 2002:42–50.

Sun SS, Schubert CM, Chumlea WC, et al. Natinal estimates of the timing of sexual maturation and racial differences among U.S. children. *Pediatrics* 2002;110 (5):911–919.

Traggiai C, Stanhope R. Disorders of pubertal development: Best practice and research. *Clin Obstet Gynecol* 2003; 17(1):41–56.

50 DEVELOPMENTAL ANOMALIES OF THE FEMALE GENITAL TRACT

Alice Rhoton-Vlasak

OVERVIEW

- Female urogenital anomalies account for 10 percent of all congenital malformations.
- Congenital abnormalities may be caused by genetic error, teratogenesis, or multifactorial influences.
- Abnormalities may occur in the perineum, vagina, cervix, uterus, fallopian tubes, and ovaries.
- Minor abnormalities may be of little consequence, but major abnormalities may lead to severe impairment of menstrual and reproductive function. Proper treatment can ameliorate the effects of many abnormalities.

EMBRYOLOGY

- Genital development will occur as female unless the Y chromosome is present. The Y chromosome contains the testis determining gene, which directs differentiation

toward a testis. The testis, in turn, makes hormones that direct the development of male genital ducts.
- Normal ovarian embryologic development begins at 4 weeks. The genital ridge develops at 4 to 5 weeks.
- Figure 50-1 depicts follicle growth, ovulation, and fertilization.
- Primordial germ cells from the hindgut endoderm migrate to the genital ridge by 8 weeks. If a Y chromosome is absent, definitive ovarian characteristics develop by 12 to 16 weeks.
- Primordial germ cells replicate by mitosis from 8 weeks until term, forming oogonia.
- Follicles first can be seen at about 20 weeks. The follicles contain germ cells with surrounding granulosa and theca cells.
- The oogonia enter prophase of the first meiotic division and are called primary oocytes. Meiosis I will be completed at the time of ovulation and meiosis II at the time of fertilization.
- In the absence of testicular determinants, the paramesonephric (müllerian) ducts persist. Normal feminization or masculinization of the external genitalia is the result of the absence or presence of androgens.

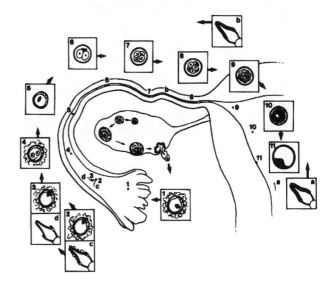

Diagrammatic representation of follicle growth, ovulation, sperm migration and maturation, fertilization, and preimplantation. *a-d,* Demonstrate sperm during migration through female tract accomplishing capacitation and acrosome reaction. *1,* Egg in meiosis enters fallopian tube after ovulating. *2,* Capacitated sperm penetrates cumulus cells and zona pellucida. *3,* Fertilization occurs; second meiotic division is complete. *4,* Male and female pronuclei are seen within the cytoplasm of egg; both polar bodies are present beneath the zona pellucida. *5,* First mitotic division takes place. *6,* Cleavage is complete. *7,* Four-cell stage. *8,* Eight-cell stage. *9,* Morula. *10,* Early blastocyst formation. *11,* Blastocyst formation; implantation occurs.

FIG. 50-1 Representation of follicle growth, fertilization, and preimplantation. (From Droegmueller W, Herbst AZ, Mishell DR, Sterchever MA. *Comprehensive Gynecology.* St. Louis: Mosby–Year Book, 1992:8. With permission.)

- Genetic sex is determined at fertilization, but the embryonic gonad is bipotential, capable of differentiating into either an ovary or testis.
- Differentiation occurs in an orderly sequence of events during gestation (Fig. 50-2). At puberty, secondary sexual characteristics develop, again in an orderly sequence of events, culminating in the ability to reproduce.
- Table 50-1 describes the male and female embryonic structures and their derivatives.
- The next sections outline various anomalies that can occur at different locations in the female genital tract, as well as disorders of sexual differentiation.

DISORDERS OF SEXUAL DIFFERENTIATION

- A rare but serious disorder of sexual differentiation is the presentation of a newborn with ambiguous genitalia.
- Abnormal sexual differentiation can be classified into conditions of excessive masculinization of subjects with a 46 XX chromosome complement (female pseudohermaphrodite), or under masculinization of individuals with a 46 XY chromosome complement (male pseudohermaphrodite).

- A true hermaphrodite has varying degrees of ambiguous genitalia and both ovarian follicles and testicular tissue.
- Causes of **ambiguous genitalia** in a neonate with a 46 XX karyotype include the following:
  ○ Congenital adrenal hyperplasia (CAH)
  ○ Excessive maternal androgens
  ○ 46 XX gonadal dysgenesis
  ○ 46 XX true hermaphroditism
  ○ Adrenal or ovarian tumors
- The most common cause of **female pseudohermaphroditism** is CAH (Fig. 50-3). The most common cause of CAH is 21-hydroxylase deficiency. The salt-wasting form of 21-hydroxylase deficiency is life-threatening and therefore is the most critical condition to be excluded in the differential diagnosis of ambiguous genitalia.
- In the adrenal enzyme deficiency states, masculinization of the female fetus occurs secondary to high levels of androgenic precursors produced by the adrenal gland.
- In the male pseudohermaphrodite, undermasculinization occurs due to inadequate testosterone or dihydrotestosterone production or lack of androgen responsiveness in target tissues. Causes include the following:
  ○ Mixed gonadal dysgenesis (45X, 46 XY)
  ○ LH receptor defects

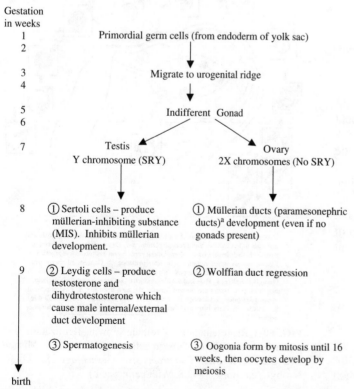

Gestation in weeks

1, 2	Primordial germ cells (from endoderm of yolk sac)
3, 4	Migrate to urogenital ridge
5, 6	Indifferent Gonad
7	Testis — Y chromosome (SRY) Ovary — 2X chromosomes (No SRY)

8   ① Sertoli cells – produce müllerian-inhibiting substance (MIS). Inhibits müllerian development.

① Müllerian ducts (paramesonephric ducts)[a] development (even if no gonads present)

9   ② Leydig cells – produce testosterone and dihydrotestosterone which cause male internal/external duct development

② Wolffian duct regression

③ Spermatogenesis

③ Oogonia form by mitosis until 16 weeks, then oocytes develop by meiosis

birth

[a] Normal uterine development requires fusion of the paired paramesonephric ducts, septal resorption, elongation, and canalization.

FIG. 50-2 Embryologic development of the gonads and genital tract.

TABLE 50-1   Male and Female Derivatives of Embryonic Urogenital Structures

EMBRYONIC STRUCTURE	MALE	FEMALE
Labioscrotal swellings	Scrotum	Labia majora
Urogenital folds	Ventral portion of penis	Labia minora
Phallus	Penis	Clitoris
	Glans, corpora cavernosa penis, and corpus spongiosum	Glans, corpora cavernosa, bulb of the vestibule
Urogenital sinus	Urinary bladder	Urinary bladder
	Prostate gland	Urethral and paraurethral glands
	Prostatic utricle	Vagina
	Bulbourethral glands	Greater vestibular glands
	Seminal colliculus	Hymen
Paramesonephric duct	Appendix of testes	Hydatid of Morgagni
		Uterus and cervix
		Fallopian tubes
Mesonephric duct	Appendix of epididymis	Appendix vesiculosus
	Ductus epididymis	Duct of epoöphoron
	Ductus deferens	Gartner's duct
	Ejaculatory duct and seminal vesicle	—
Metanephric duct	Ureter, renal pelvis, calyces, and collecting system	Ureter, renal pelvis, cycles, and collecting system
Mesonephric tubules	Ductuli efferentes	Epoöphoron
	Paradidymis	Paroöphoron
Undifferentiated gonad	Testis	Ovary
Cortex	Seminiferous tubules	Ovarian follicles
Medulla	—	Medulla
	—	Rete ovarii
Gubernaculum	Gubernaculum testis	Round ligament of uterus

Source: From Droegemueller W, Herbst AL, Mishell DR, Stenchever MA. *Comprehensive Gynecology*. St. Louis: Mosby–Year Book, 1992:14. With permission.

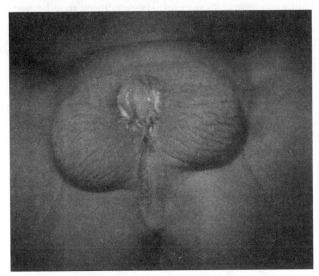

FIG. 50-3 Newborn female with ambiguous genitalia diagnosed with congenital adrenal hyperplasia. (Photograph courtesy of Simon Kiperzstok, MD.)

○ 17-hydroxylase deficiency
○ 5 alpha reductase deficiency
○ Incomplete or partial androgen insensitivity

- In cases of **androgen insensitivity** (AI), the external genital abnormalities can be highly variable, ranging from phenotypic female to phenotypic male.
- Androgen insensitivity is an X-linked condition caused by a testosterone receptor defect in a 46 XY individual with testes and normal male testosterone levels. Affected individuals exhibit female genitalia and normal intraabdominal or inguinal testes. The uterus is absent. The diagnosis is often made at puberty, when females present with primary amenorrhea, normal breast development, and a blind vaginal pouch. The testes should be removed because they may undergo malignant change.
- Evaluation of an infant with ambiguous genitalia should include the following:
  ○ Physical examination in the delivery room
  ○ Serum electrolytes
  ○ Serum concentration of 17-hydroxyprogesterone
  ○ Karyotype
  ○ If a Y chromosome is detected, serum testosterone and dihydrotestosterone concentrations should be assessed
- Physical examination should assess for
  ○ Presence of palpable gonads

○ Length of the phallus
○ Position of the urethral meatus
○ Degree of labioscrotal fusion
○ Presence of a vagina, vaginal pouch, or urogenital sinus

• Therapy depends on the underlying condition. Determination of the sex of rearing depends on the genital findings and the potential for sexual functioning as an adult. Genetic females with ambiguity should undergo corrective surgery. Y-containing gonads should be removed to prevent malignant degeneration.

• 46 XY individuals with female external genitalia related to complete defects of masculinization include
○ Complete androgen insensitivity
○ Swyer's syndrome
○ Complete testosterone biosynthesis defects

• The sex of rearing is female, and these individuals do not require corrective surgery. The gonads should be removed. Estrogen replacement is needed to develop/maintain female secondary sexual characteristics, protect the bones, and stimulate menses in those with a uterus.

• Swyer's syndrome is 46 XY gonadal dysgenesis. Affected individuals present with
○ Hypergonadotropic hypogonadism ($\uparrow$FSH)
○ Lack of secondary sexual development
○ Normal infantile female external genitalia
○ Normal uterus and fallopian tubes
○ Normal or above average height

• The most common cause of gonadal dysgenesis (resulting in hypergonadotropic hypogonadism) is Turner's syndrome (45 X). The condition is covered in detail in Chap. 51, on delayed puberty.

CONGENITAL MALFORMATIONS OF THE FEMALE GENITAL TRACT

• Major abnormalities may lead to severe impairment of menstrual, psychologic, and reproductive function. These individuals often present at the time of adolescence or puberty.

• A multidisciplinary approach may be needed to ensure the correct diagnosis and surgical therapy.

• Many congenital malformations include associated disorders of other organ systems that must be identified.

• An extremely careful assessment of the psychologic status of the patient is imperative to assess the ability to understand the necessary treatments and long-term implications of the diagnosis.

• Table 50-2 outlines possible congenital malformations of the female genital tract according to the site within the genital system. Fallopian tube and cervical abnormalities are extremely rare.

TABLE 50-2   Congenital Malformations of the Female Genital Tract

ANATOMIC SITE	DISORDERS
Vulva	Clitorimegaly
	Bifid clitoris
	Ambiguous genitalia
	Labial fusion
Vagina	Remant cysts—müllerian remnant or epidermal inclusion
	Obstructive outflow disorders
	Imperforate hymen
	Transverse vaginal septum
	Longitudinal vaginal septum
	Vaginal agenesis
Uterus	Agenesis of uterus and vagina (Mayer-Rokitansky-Küster-Hauser syndrome)
	Uterine anomalies:
	Arcuate
	Bicornuate
	Septate
	Unicornuate
	Didelphic
Cervix	Agenesis
Fallopian tube	Duplication
	Unilateral agenesis

DISORDERS OF THE CERVIX AND VULVA

• The clinical presentation of congenital absence of the cervix includes cyclic abdominal pain presenting in the presence of amenorrhea and normal secondary sexual characteristics. The diagnosis is made by ultrasound when the cervix is noted to be absent and there is a hematometra present. Hysterectomy may be necessary to treat this condition.

• Abnormalities of vulvar development include clitoromegaly, labial fusion, and ambiguous genitalia. These disorders can result from excess androgens due to congenital adrenal hyperplasia, late-onset congenital adrenal hyperplasia, or an androgen-secreting tumor of the ovary or adrenal gland.

• Treatment of congenital adrenal hyperplasia consists primarily of cortical replacement. Treatment of an androgen-secreting tumor requires surgical removal of the tumor.

• Surgical reconstruction of the vulvovaginal area may be needed to create an anatomically acceptable and functional vulva and vagina. The use of dilators may be required. Clitoral resection may be necessary, although this procedure may lead to problems with normal sexual function.

DISORDERS OF THE VAGINA

• Vaginal cysts are usually located on the lateral or posterior vaginal walls. The cysts may be asymptomatic or may present with swelling in the vagina or with

dyspareunia. Generally, vaginal cysts should be managed by excision.
- Obstructive outflow tract disorders of the vagina usually are identified at the time of menarche because of obstruction to the flow of menstrual blood. These conditions present with primary amenorrhea in association with increasing dysmenorrhea.
- Disorders causing these symptoms include
  - Imperforate hymen
  - Transverse vaginal septum
  - Cervical agenesis
- The hymen is a thin mucous membrane that forms at the junction of the sinovaginal bulbs with the urogenital sinus. It is usually perforated during fetal life. Failure of perforation results in the imperforate hymen.
- Imperforate hymen usually presents with a mass arising from the pelvis that is palpable abdominally. Inspection of the vulva by separation of the labia demonstrates a membrane through which menstrual blood may be seen and that appears as a dark-blue mass. The treatment is surgical, involving a cruciate incision in the membrane from 2 o'clock to 8 o'clock and 10 o'clock to 4 o'clock. No attempt should be made to evacuate the vagina at the time of surgery. Reproductive function following this treatment is usually normal.
- A transverse vaginal septum occurs when the area of canalization between the müllerian tubercle and sinovaginal bulbs is not complete. The septum may be partial or complete and usually lies at the junction of the upper third and lower two-thirds of the vagina. The incidence is about 1 per 75,000 females.
- A vaginal septum can occur at any point in the vagina; the most common location is in the lower vagina. This anomaly may be associated with other congenital malformations of the genital tract, urinary tract, or rectum. The presentation is similar to that for the imperforate hymen.
- Treatment of a transverse vaginal septum is surgical, ranging from simple excision to complete vaginal reconstruction.
- A longitudinal vaginal septum develops if the two lateral müllerian ducts fail to fuse at their lower border. Usually two uterine horns and two cervices will be present, with each cervix leading into a hemivagina. The septum that divides these vaginas may be partial or complete.
- Some patients with a longitudinal vaginal septum may be asymptomatic. Others may experience pain during intercourse or difficulty inserting tampons. Treatment usually requires removing the septum.
- Vaginal agenesis usually presents with total absence of the vagina in association with uterine agenesis or hypoplasia. The condition also has been called the

Mayer-Rokitansky-Küster-Hauser (MRKH) syndrome. The incidence of this syndrome is 1 in 5000 live births.
  - Affected patients are usually identified in early adolescence, when they have primary amenorrhea in association with normal secondary sexual characteristics. Ovarian function is normal, and the karyotype is 46 XX.
  - The inheritance pattern of MRKH is polygenic and multifactorial. This disorder may be associated with renal, otic, and skeletal abnormalities.
  - All patients should have an intravenous pyelogram or renal ultrasound.
  - Patients with MRKH should receive counseling about the condition and its reproductive implications. They should be reassured that they can have genetically related children through oocyte retrieval and use of a gestational surrogate.
  - Creation of a vagina may be undertaken with passive dilation of the vaginal dimple using graduated dilators. Satisfactory vaginal length for intercourse has been achieved in approximately 85 percent of cases. Surgical management should be reserved for patients who fail to achieve a functional vagina with passive dilation. A neovagina may be created by a McIndoe-Reed skin graft, vulvovaginoplasty, bowel vaginoplasty, or Vecchieti's procedure. The most common procedure used in the United States is the McIndoe-Reed technique, with the use of split thickness skin grafts taken from the buttocks.
- Patients with complete androgen insensitivity may present in a similar fashion at adolescence with normal secondary sexual characteristics, primary amenorrhea, and a blind vaginal pouch. Unlike patients with congenital absence of the uterus, they have no ovaries, an elevated serum concentration of testosterone, and a 46 XY karyotype. These women require removal of the gonads.
- Multiple congenital uterine anomalies may occur. The uterus, cervix, and upper third of the vagina are derived from the paramesonephric (müllerian) ducts, the caudal ends of which fuse medially to form the uterovaginal primordium. Various steps in the process can be altered, resulting in
  - Complete or partial failure of one or both ducts to form.
  - Lack of complete fusion of the lower segments of the paired ducts.
  - Failure of development after successful formation.
- Complete agenesis of the uterus is rare and usually associated with MRKH syndrome.
- Multiple uterine anomalies have been described and are outlined in Fig. 50-4. Many of the described anomalies will be asymptomatic.
- The rudimentary uterine horn with functioning endometrium may present in teenagers at the time

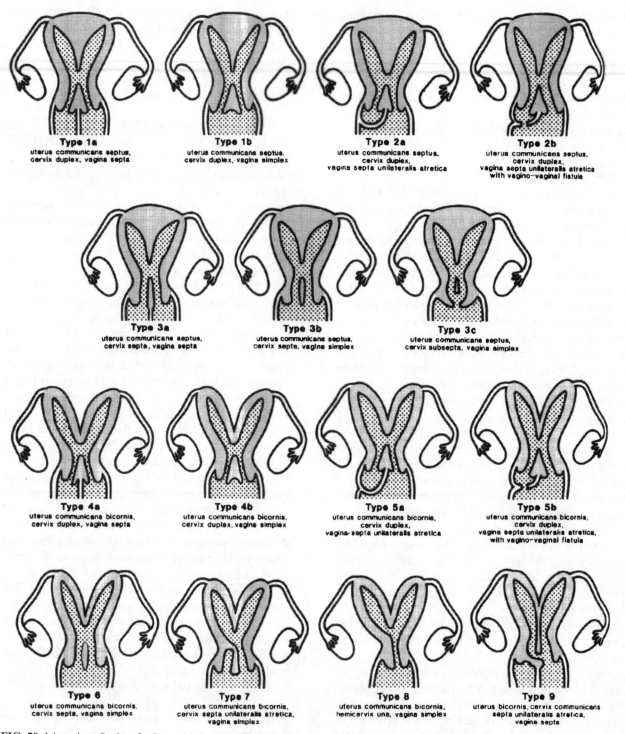

FIG. 50-4 American Society for Reproductive Medicine Classification System for Congenital Uterine Anomalies. (From Toaff ME, Lev-Toaff AS, Toaff R. Communicating uteri: Review and classification with introduction of two previously unreported types. *Fertil Steril* 1984;41(5):661–679. With permission.)

of menarche because it causes increasingly severe dysmenorrhea and hematometra. Treatment requires excision of the rudimentary horn and reconstruc-

tion of the uterus. Figure 50-5 demonstrates an asymmetric rudimentary horn of a unicornuate uterus seen at laparoscopy. Figure 50-6 is a hys-

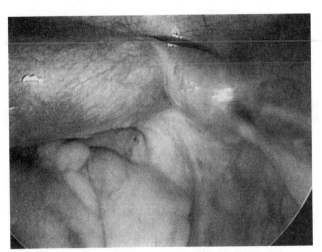

FIG. 50-5 Laparoscopic view of a unicornuate left uterine horn and rudimentary, nonfunctional right uterine horn.

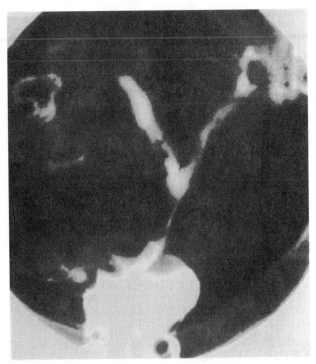

FIG. 50-7 Hysterosalpingogram demonstrating a septate or bicornuate uterus. Hysteroscopy revealed a large uterine septum that was resected.

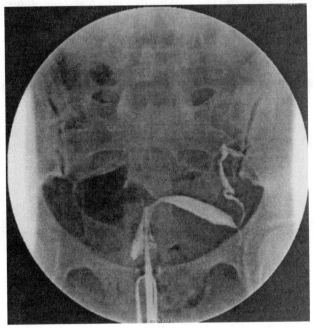

FIG. 50-6 Hysterosalpingogram view of a unicornuate uterus (same as that seen in Fig. 50-5).

terosalpingogram of the unicornuate uterus seen in Fig. 50-5.

- The septate uterus has been associated with recurrent miscarriages and fetal malpresentation. Treatment generally consists of hysteroscopic excision of the septum. Other obstetric problems that are more common in women with uterine anomalies include abnormal labor, abnormal presentations, and preterm labor.
- The diagnosis of a uterine anomaly is usually made by hysterosalpingography or a combination of hys-

teroscopy and laparoscopy. Figs. 50-6 and 50-7 demonstrate several uterine anomalies in patients with infertility and recurrent spontaneous abortions.

- ○ For patients with nonobstructive uterine anomalies, treatment is usually not indicated, but they should be evaluated for renal abnormalities.
- ○ Septate uteri usually require correction, either by endoscopy or laparotomy.
- ○ In the past, septa were often treated with wedge excision of the septum and reunification of the cavity (Strassman procedure) or cone resection of the septum (Jones procedure).
- ○ Fifteen to 20 percent of women with a history of recurrent abortion may have anomalies of the uterus, so a workup should include an investigation for these abnormalities.

BIBLIOGRAPHY

American Congress of Obstetricians and Gynecologists. Precise: An update in obstetrics and gynecology. Sexual development and puberty. *Reproductive Endocrinology*, 2nd ed. Washington DC: ACOG, 2002:32–51.

Arulkumaran S. Human sex differentiation and its abnormalities, congenital malformations of the genital tract and their management. *Clin Obstet Gynecol* 2003;17(1):1–40.

Breech LL, Laufer MR. Obstructive anomalies of the female reproductive tract. *J Reprod Med* 1999;44(3):233–240.

Folch M, Pigem I, Konje JC. Mullerian agenesis: Etiology, diagnosis, and management. *Obstet Gynecol Surv* 2000; 55(10): 644–649.

Lin PC, Bhatnagar KP, Nettleton S, Nakajima ST. Female genital anomalies affecting reproduction. *Fertil Steril* 2002;78(5):899–915.

Reindollar RH, McDonough PG. The child with ambiguous genitalia. In: Lavery JP, Sanfilippo JS, eds. *Pediatric and Adolescent Obstetrics and Gynecology*. New York: Springer-Verlag, 1985:38–60.

51 DELAYED PUBERTY

Alice Rhoton-Vlasak

EPIDEMIOLOGY

- Delayed puberty is defined as the absence of normal pubertal events at an age 2.5 standard deviations greater than the mean.
- An investigation is warranted in the absence of thelarche (breast development) by age 13 and the absence of menarche (onset of menses) by age 15. Patients who present with normal thelarche but no further progression of sexual maturation also should be evaluated.
- The classification of delayed puberty is summarized in Table 51-1.
- The purpose of evaluating a girl with this disorder is to assess whether spontaneous but delayed puberty will occur or if there is a disorder that will lead to sexual infantilism in the absence of treatment.
- Primary amenorrhea (or normal breast development and absent menarche) is in Chap. 52. Etiologies include anatomic genital abnormalities, inappropriate positive feedback, and androgen insensitivity syndrome.

CAUSES OF DELAYED PUBERTY

- This condition is more common in girls than boys.
- Affected patients have normal health and nutritional status but their physical growth is at or below the third percentile.
- Consitutional delay of puberty may occur in a familial pattern.
- Bone age is lower than chronological age. When a bone age of 11 to 12 years is obtained, breast budding and the growth spurt will usually ensue.
- Once puberty is attained, however, these patients often do not reach their targeted adult height.

TABLE 51-1 Classification of Patients with Delayed Puberty

TYPE	SERUM GONADOTROPIN CONCENTRATIONS	SERUM ESTROGEN CONCENTRATIONS
Constitutional delay	Low	Low
Hypogonadotropic hypogonadism	Low	Low
Central nervous system abnormalities		
Tumors		
Postirradiation		
Postinfectious		
Developmental anomalies		
Isolated gonadotropin deficiencies		
Kallmann's syndrome		
Idiopathic		
Multiple pituitary hormone deficiency		
Temporary gonadotropin deficiency		
Chronic illness		
Anorexia nervosa		
Malnutrition		
Excessive physical training		
Psychiatric illness		
Hypothyroidism		
Hypergonadotropic hypogonadism	High	Low
Turner's syndrome (gonadal dysgenesis)		
XX and XY gonadal dysgenesis		
Autoimmune oophoritis		
Radiation and chemotherapy		
Galactosemia		
Noonan's syndrome		

- A prolonged delay in puberty may be associated with malnutrition, anorexia nervosa, or chronic diseases.

HYPOGONADOTROPIC HYPOGONADISM

- In patients with this condition, pubertal delay results from a temporary or permanent inability to secrete GnRH or pituitary gonadotropins (FSH, LH).
- The abnormality may be caused the failure of GnRH transport from the hypothalamus to the pituitary or by lack of target-organ response secondary to GnRH receptor mutations.
- Affected patients usually have undetectable or low levels of pituitary gonadotropins.

HYPERGONADOTROPIC HYPOGONADISM

- In patients with this condition, the defect is due to a gonadal abnormality, which results in a lack of sex steroid secretion. Affected patients have elevated serum concentrations of gonadotropins.
- Many affected patients have a karyotype abnormality.
- Turner's syndrome is the most common form of primary gonadal failure. The characteristics of Turner's syndrome are summarized in Table 51-2.

EVALUATION OF DELAYED PUBERTY

- Evaluation is needed if breast budding has not occurred by age 13, menarche has not occurred by age 15, or pubertal progression is slow. Figure 51-1 demonstrates a 19-year-old with delayed puberty due to 46 XY gonadal dysgenesis (Swyer's syndrome).
- The basic evaluation includes the following:
  ○ Detailed history of the mother's pregnancy and the patient's childhood.
  ○ Physical examination assessing growth curve, neurologic development, and Tanner stages of breast development.

TABLE 51-2 Principal Characteristics of Turner's Syndrome

Prevalence—1:2000–2500 live-born females
Usual karyotype—45 X
Streak gonads
Short stature
Sexual infantilism
Facial abnormalities
Shield chest
Skeletal, renal, and cardiac anomalies

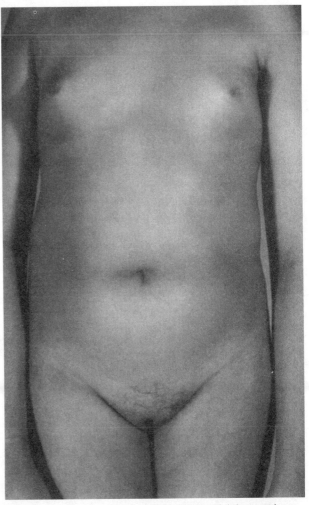

FIG. 51-1 A 19-year-old girl with 46 XY gonadal dysgenesis, normal stature, sexual infantilism, primary amenorrhea, and gonadoblastoma. (Photograph courtesy of Simon Kiperzstok, MD.)

  ○ Laboratory testing for FSH, LH, TSH, prolactin, and estradiol.
  ○ A karyotype should be performed if the LH and FSH are elevated.
  ○ A GnRH stimulation test also should be obtained.
  ○ Adrenal or ovarian androgen secretion should be evaluated if virilization is present.
  ○ Imaging studies should include a bone age and MRI or CT scan of the head.
- The diagnosis of a constitutional delay of puberty is established when other abnormalities have been excluded.

TREATMENT

- Counseling with the patient and family is important.
- Underlying conditions such as a hypothalamic or pituitary tumor or medical complications should be treated.

- Therapy with estrogen replacement or recombinant growth hormone is indicated to initiate secondary sexual characteristics and induce a pubertal growth spurt. Estrogen replacement should begin with an agent such as conjugated equine estrogen, 0.3 mg/day for 6 months. The dose then should be increased to 0.625 to 1.25 mg/day. The patient should also receive a progestin such as medroxyprogesterone acetate, 2.5 mg orally, for 12 days of each month. Oral contraceptives may be used in place of the estrogen-progestin regimen.
- If a Y chromosome is found in an otherwise normal-phenotype female, the gonads should be removed to prevent development of a gonadal tumor.

BIBLIOGRAPHY

American College of Obstetricians and Gynecologists. Abnormalities of puberty: Precis: An update in obstetrics and gynecology. *Reproductive Endocrinology*, 2nd ed. Washington, DC:ACOG, 2002:42–50.

Kingensmith GH. Delayed puberty. In: Schlaff WD, Rock JA, eds. *Decision Making in Reproductive Endocrinology.* Boston: Blackwell, 1993:11–17.

Reiter EO, Lee PA. Delayed puberty. *Adolesc Med* 2002; 13(1):101–118, viii.

52 AMENORRHEA

Alice Rhoton-Vlasak

DEFINITION

- **Primary amenorrhea** is defined as the absence of menstrual cycles by age 16 in a female with normal secondary sexual characteristics or by age 14 in the absence of secondary sexual characteristics. The incidence is 2.5 percent.
- **Secondary amenorrhea** is defined as the absence of menses for 3 months or more in a woman with past menses. The incidence varies and may approach almost 100 percent under conditions of extreme physical or emotional distress.
- Amenorrhea indicates either failure of the hypothalamic-pituitary-gonadal axis to induce cyclic changes in the endometrium, the absence of end organs or end-organ response, or obstruction of the outflow tract.

- Amenorrhea should be recognized and evaluated because it may be associated with infertility, osteoporosis, genital atrophy, and social or sexual dysfunction.

ETIOLOGY OF PRIMARY AMENORRHEA

- The major causes of primary amenorrhea are summarized in Table 52-1.
- Patients with primary amenorrhea and **hypergonadotropic hypogonadism** (high FSH and low estradiol levels) often have abnormal chromosomes, typically 45 X (Turner's syndrome).
- If a Y chromosome is present, the patient has mixed gonadal dysgenesis (ie, 45 X/46 XY). The presence of a Y chromosome and streak gonads predisposes 30 percent of these patients to gonadal ridge tumors. Therefore the gonads should be removed as soon as the diagnosis is made.
- Patients with 46 XY gonadal dysgenesis (Swyer's syndrome) have testicular development arrested early

TABLE 52-1   Causes of Primary Amenorrhea

Amenorrhea with lack of secondary sexual characteristics (hypogonadal)
  Hypogonadotropic hypogonadism
    Physiologic delay
    Kallmann's syndrome (GnRH deficiency)
    Central nervous system tumor
    Hypothalamic/pituitary dysfunction
      Anorexia and weight loss
      Excessive exercise
      Systemic disease
    Hypothyroidism
    Hyperprolactinemia
  Hypergonadotropic hypogonadism
    Gonadal dysgenesis (45 XO, 46 XX, or 46 XY)
    Pure gonadal dysgenesis.
    Sex chromosome mosaicism
    Ovarian failure (due to radiation of chemotherapy)
    Gonadotropin resistance (Savage or Jones syndrome)
    galactosemia enzyme deficiencies.
    17-hydroxylase deficiency in XX or XY individual
Amenorrhea associated with the presence of secondary sexual characteristics
  Müllerian abnormalities (anatomic)
    Imperforate hymen
    Transverse vaginal septum
    Müllerian agenesis
  Androgen insensitivity
  True hermaphroditism
  Absent endometrium
  Ovarian failure
    Chromosomal
    Iatrogenic (radiation, chemotherapy, or surgery)
    Galactosemia
    Autoimmune disease
    Idiopathic
    Polycystic ovary syndrome

in fetal development. They lack testosterone and müllerian inhibiting factor, so they develop female internal and external genitalia but do not have pubertal development. The dysgenetic gonads should be removed.

- **Hypogonadotropic hypogonadism** results from hypothalamic failure to secrete GnRH or from pituitary disease.
  ○ Physiologic delay is one of the most common etiologies.
  ○ GnRH deficiency (Kallmann's syndrome) is the second most common cause and is associated with anosmia and midline facial defects.
- The most common etiology of primary amenorrhea in the presence of normal secondary sexual characteristics is müllerian agenesis (Rokitansky's syndrome). The frequency of this condition is 1:4000 females.
- Features of müllerian agenesis include:
  ○ Normal breast development
  ○ Absence of müllerian structures (no uterus, cervix, fallopian tubes, or upper vagina)
  ○ Normal serum testosterone concentration
  ○ Normal pubic hair
- In patients with müllerian agenesis, an ultrasound or intravenous pyelogram should be obtained to detect associated renal anomalies. Vertebral, cardiac, and other congenital anomalies also are increased in frequency in affected patients.
- Androgen insensitivity presents in a similar fashion to müllerian agenesis. Affected girls have primary amenorrhea, breast development, and a lack of menses. No müllerian structures are present, and patients have an absent or blind vaginal pouch. Androgens are aromatized to estrogen, causing breast development. A lack of androgen receptor in target tissue causes the defect. The Y-containing gonads must be removed after puberty.

CLINICAL EVALUATION

- The workup should include a careful developmental, prenatal, neonatal, and pubertal history.
- A detailed physical examination should be performed, with assessment of Tanner stages, height, weight, and growth curves.
- Pertinent laboratory tests may include the following:
  ○ Prolactin
  ○ Thyroid stimulating hormone (TSH)
  ○ FSH
  ○ LH
  ○ Bone age
  ○ Karyotype
  ○ Serum androgen concentrations

○ GnRH challenge test
○ Progestin challenge test (see discussion of secondary amenorrhea)
- If the serum FSH concentration is low or normal, an MRI or CT of the head is indicated to assess for intracranial disease.
- Appropriate referrals should be made to a specialist for evaluation and treatment.

TREATMENT OF PRIMARY AMENORRHEA

- Hypergonadotropic hypogonadal patients require estrogen replacement (with low doses initially) and then either combination/cyclic hormone replacement or oral contraceptives to initiate or complete puberty and preserve bone development.
- Y-containing or dysgenetic gonads should be removed surgically.
- Patients lacking vaginal development (eg, müllerian agenesis or androgen-insensitivity syndrome) may be able to create a functional vagina by daily use of vaginal dilators. If this intervention is unsuccessful or they cannot use dilators, surgery may be necessary.
- Hypogonadotropic hypogonadal patients will need careful assessment of diet, exercise, and stress factors. Ovulation induction may be needed to achieve a pregnancy. Estrogen replacement is necessary to stimulate pubertal development, growth, and menses. It should be given in a similar fashion as to patients with delayed puberty (see Chap. 51).

ETIOLOGY OF SECONDARY AMENORRHEA

- The major causes of secondary amenorrhea are summarized in Table 52-2.
- The most common cause of secondary amenorrhea is pregnancy.

CLINICAL EVALUATION

- The most important aspect of the evaluation is the history and physical examination.
- The clinical evaluation of patients with secondary amenorrhea is summarized in Fig. 52-1.
- The physical examination should focus on the following:
  ○ Body dimensions and habitus
  ○ Distribution and extent of terminal hair
  ○ Tanner staging of the breasts and genitalia as well as the presence of breast secretions

TABLE 52-2   Causes of Secondary Amenorrhea

Common
  Pregnancy
  Hypothalamic disorders
  Stress or exercise induced
  Anorexia nervosa
  Idiopathic
  Chronic disease
  Anovulation
  Polycystic ovary syndrome
  Congenital adrenal hyperplasia
  Hyperprolactinemia
  Hyper- or hypothyroidism
Less common
  Premature ovarian failure (<40 years old)
  Asherman's syndrome (intrauterine adhesions)
  Pituitary failure (Sheehan's syndrome) or tumors
Rare
  Cushing's disease or syndrome
  Adrenal tumor
  Diabetes
  Radiation or chemotherapy
  Surgery
  Malnutrition
  Cirrhosis of the liver

○ External and internal genitalia, with a focus on exposure to androgens and estrogens

• The progestin challenge test is used to assess estrogen status and aid in the clinical diagnosis. Either medroxyprogesterone acetate (10 mg orally for 10 days) or progesterone in oil (100 to 200 mg intramuscularly in a single dose) can be given. Any genital bleeding within 10 days is considered a positive result and indicates that the endometrium has been primed appropriately by estrogen and that the outflow tract is patent.

• If the progestin challenge test is negative (suggesting low levels of endogenous estrogen), then estrogen and progesterone together should induce bleeding if the endometrium is normal and the outflow tract is patent. Conjugated estrogen, 2.5 mg orally daily for 25 days, plus medroxyprogesterone acetate, 10 mg orally on days 16 through 25, are used. Patients with Asherman's syndrome may not bleed following this regimen.

• All patients should have a pregnancy test, thyroid-stimulating hormone (TSH), and prolactin. Figure 52-1

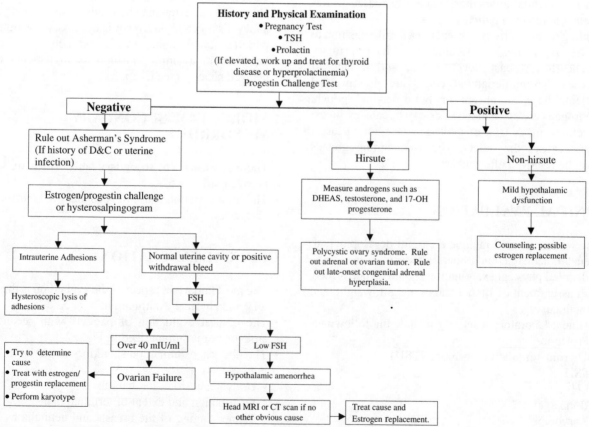

FIG. 52-1   Evaluation of secondary amenorrhea.

outlines other laboratory tests for the evaluation of patients with secondary amenorrhea.

TREATMENT

- Once the etiology of secondary amenorrhea has been determined, treatment should be based on the etiologic factor and the patient's reproductive desires.
- Patients with normal estrogen concentrations (ie, withdrawal to progestin challenge) require cycling with a progestational agent (medroxyprogesterone acetate 10 mg orally 10 to 12 days/month) or daily oral contraceptives to prevent endometrial hyperplasia and carcinoma.
- Hypoestrogenic patients—such as those with hypothalamic amenorrhea, ovarian failure, or hyperprolactinemia—who are not candidates for ovulation induction require hormone replacement therapy to prevent symptoms of estrogen deficiency and protect the bones.
- In patients desiring pregnancy, ovulation may be induced with bromocriptine (if hyperprolactinemia is present) or with clomiphene citrate or gonadotropins (if the patient has hypothalamic failure or polycystic ovary syndrome). Patients with ovarian failure will require the use of donor eggs.

BIBLIOGRAPHY

American College of Obstetrics and Gynecology. Disorders of ovulation and menstruation. Precis: An update in obstetrics and gynecology. *Reproductive Endocrinology,* 2nd ed. 2002. Washington, DC: ACOG, 2002:57–99.

Aydinel SA, Simon JA, Padilla SL. Secondary amenorrhea. In: Schlaff WD, Rock JA, eds. *Decision Making in Reproductive Endocrinology.* Boston: Blackwell, 1993:55–64.

Padilla SL. Primary amenorrhea. In: Schlaff WD, Rock JA, eds. *Decision Making in Reproductive Endocrinology.* Boston: Blackwell, 1993:49–54.

Timreck LS, Reindollar RH. Contemporary issues in primary amenorrhea. *Obstet Gynecol Clin North Am* 2003; 30(2):287–302.

53 DYSMENORRHEA

Alice Rhoton-Vlasak

EPIDEMIOLOGY

- Dysmenorrhea affects 50 to 70 percent of reproductive-age women and is severe in 10 percent.

- The peak age of occurrence is 20 to 24 years.
- Dysmenorrhea is the single greatest source of lost productivity in women.
- Table 53-1 lists the principal causes of dysmenorrhea.

DEFINITIONS

- **Primary dysmenorrhea**: painful menstrual cramps with no identifiable organic etiology.
- **Secondary dysmenorrhea**: painful menstrual cramps due to a clinically recognized cause.

PATHOGENESIS OF PRIMARY DYSMENORRHEA

- Primary dysmenorrhea is a feature of ovulatory cycles and often occurs within 12 months of menarche.
- Excess prostaglandin F2α activity in the endometrium leads to intense uterine contractions as well as nausea, vomiting, and diarrhea.
- Primary dysmenorrhea has a genetic predisposition.

CLINICAL FEATURES OF PRIMARY DYSMENORRHEA

- Ninety percent of patients experience symptoms within the first 2 years of menarche.
- Symptoms begin within a few hours of the onset of menstrual flow and last 48 to 72 h.
- Pain is described as cramp-like and may radiate to the back or legs.
- Associated symptoms include nausea and vomiting, fatigue, diarrhea, and low backache.
- The physical examination usually is normal.

TREATMENT OF PRIMARY DYSMENORRHEA

- Therapy is directed at reducing prostaglandin production and action.

TABLE 53-1 Principal Causes of Dysmenorrhea

Primary dysmenorrhea
Elevated prostaglandin activity
Secondary dysmenorrhea
Endometriosis
Pelvic adhesions
Pelvic inflammation
Uterine fibroids
Uterine polyps
Uterine malformations
Cervical stenosis
Pelvic congestion syndrome

- Nonsteroidal anti-inflammatory drugs (NSAIDs) such as ibuprofen, naproxen, celecoxib, and rofecoxib provide effective treatment in approximately 80 percent of patients. There is no clear advantage of one drug over another.
- Oral contraceptives or progestins, such as medroxyprogesterone acetate and norethindrone, can be used either alone or in conjunction with NSAIDs to treat dysmenorrhea.
- Nonmedical interventions include a low-fat diet and exercise.
- Surgery should be used only in cases where an anatomic abnormality is suspected or the patient has failed medical management.
- Table 53-2 outlines treatment options for primary dysmenorrhea.

CLINICAL FEATURES OF SECONDARY DYSMENORRHEA

- The evaluation should include a careful history of age of onset of pain, character, location, radiation, exacerbating factors, and relation to menstrual flow.
- Physical examination is directed at detecting possible causes such as leiomyomata (fibroids), adenomyosis, endometriosis, adhesions, or infection.
- Diagnostic testing may include cervical cultures, pelvic ultrasound, and sonohysterography (instillation of saline into the uterine cavity). Laparoscopy may be useful, especially when endometriosis is suspected.
- Secondary dysmenorrhea often develops in older women with associated symptoms such as dyspareunia, infertility, or abnormal bleeding. Figure 53-1 demonstrates an intramural fibroid diagnosed at laparoscopy in a patient with new onset of secondary dysmenorrhea.
- Management consists of treatment of the underlying disease.

TABLE 53-2   Treatment of Dysmenorrhea

Reassurance and explanation
Antiprostaglandins
  Ibuprofen
  Naproxen
  Mefenamic acid
  Celecoxib
Progestins
  Rofecoxib
  Medroxyprogesterone acetate
  Norethindrone
Nonmedical interventions
Low fat diet
Exercise
  Heat therapy
Surgery
  Transcutaneous electrical nerve stimulation
  Presacral neurectomy
  Laparoscopic uterosacral nerve division
  Hysterectomy

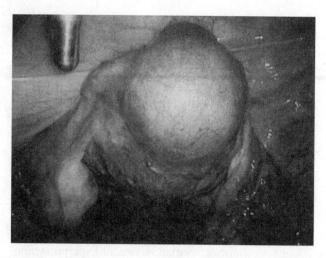

FIG. 53-1 Laparoscopic view of an intramural fibroid associated with a new onset of severe secondary dysmenorrhea.

BIBLIOGRAPHY

American Congress of Obstretrics and Gynecology. Dysmenorrhea. Precis: An update in obstetrics and gynecology. *Reproductive Endocrinology,* 2nd ed. Washington, DC: ACOG, 2002:115–116.

Harel Z. A contemporary approach to dysmenorrhea in adolescents. *Paeditr Drugs* 2002;4(12):797–805.

54   DYSFUNCTIONAL UTERINE BLEEDING

Alice Rhoton-Vlasak

DEFINITION

- **Dysfunctional uterine bleeding** (DUB) is defined as abnormal uterine bleeding unrelated to anatomic lesions of the uterus. It is a diagnosis of exclusion.
- The underlying cause is unknown, but it is likely due to aberrations in the hypothalamic-pituitary-ovarian axis, leading to anovulation and excessive estrogenic stimulation of the endometrium.
- DUB may occur with ovulatory cycles but usually is associated with anovulatory cycles.
- Bleeding patterns vary and could encompass any of the patterns outlined in Chap. 37, on abnormal uterine bleeding.
- Endometrial histology generally reveals proliferative, mixed, or even hyperplastic endometrium. The

abnormalities are associated with alterations in endometrial vascular homeostasis.
- Treatments that result in a conversion from a proliferative to secretory endometrium will correct most bleeding problems.

EPIDEMIOLOGY

- DUB occurs most often at the extremes of reproductive age, with 20 percent of cases in adolescents and 40 percent in patients over age 40.
- Management depends on the age of the patient.

DIAGNOSIS

- A detailed history should include information about menstrual history, reproductive history, weight changes, hirsutism, galactorrhea, infertility, medications, and course of bleeding.
- A complete physical examination should be performed.
- At the time of physical examination, cervical cytology should be performed. An endometrial biopsy

should be performed in any patient over 35 years of age (once pregnancy has been excluded) and younger women who are obese.
- Patients with untreated DUB are at increased risk for endometrial hyperplasia and neoplasia due to unopposed estrogenic stimulation of the endometrium.
- Laboratory tests that may be useful are outlined in Table 54-1.
- Other tests, such as pelvic ultrasound or hysteroscopy, may be necessary to rule out other anatomic causes of abnormal uterine bleeding.

TREATMENT

- The objective of management is to relieve heavy bleeding and restore the menstrual cycle to a universal synchronous event.
- Management generally employs medical therapy once anatomic causes and cancer are excluded. If an underlying disease, such as hypothyroidism is detected, it should be treated, and the abnormal bleeding usually will resolve.
- Multiple medical therapies are available to treat DUB including the following:
  - Progestins
  - Oral contraceptives
  - Estrogen
  - Antiprostaglandins
  - GnRH agonists
  - Progestin IUD
- Table 54-2 summarizes medical therapies for nonacute DUB.
- For patients with more acute bleeding and anemia, more aggressive are therapies available to stop bleeding

TABLE 54-1 Laboratory Evaluation of Dysfunctional Uterine Bleeding

Complete blood count (CBC)
Coagulation studies
   Prothrombin time and partial thromboplastin time
   Platelet count
Quantitative human chorionic gonadotropin
Prolactin
Thyroid function tests
Liver function tests
Cervical cultures
Platelet function tests

TABLE 54-2 Treatment of Dysfunctional Uterine Bleeding

DRUG CLASS	DRUG	ROUTE	DOSE
Progestins	Medroxyprogesterone acetate[a]	Oral	5–10 mg daily
	Norethindrone acetate[a]	Oral	2.5–5.0 mg daily
	Norethindrone[a]	Oral	0.7–1.0 mg daily
Contraceptive formulations	Low-dose combinations OCs	Oral	Once daily
	Contraceptive patch	Transdermal	Change weekly
	Contraceptive vaginal ring	Intravaginal	Change every 3 weeks
	Depo-medroxyprogesterone acetate	Intramuscular	150 mg every 12 weeks
	Levonorgestrel intrauterine device	Intrauterine	Effective 5 years
GnRH agonist	Leuprolide acetate	Intramuscular	Every 1–6 months
	Naferelin acetate	Intranasal	Daily
Antiprostaglandins	Ibuprofen	Oral	600–800 mg 3×1 day
	Naproxen	Oral	250–500 mg 2–4×1 day
	Mefenamic acid	Oral	250–500 mg 3×1 day

[a]Usually prescribed 10 to 14 days per month but can be given daily to achieve amenorrhea.

TABLE 54-3   Treatment Options for Acute Bleeding[a]

Conjugated equine estrogen (Premarin), 25 mg IV q 4 h until bleeding stops or for 24 h followed by 10 mg daily oral conjugated estrogen for 28 days[b]

Conjugated equine estrogen, 10 mg Po 4× daily for 24 h

Low-dose monophasic oral contraceptive 2 to 4 times daily for 1 week, followed by 1 pill daily[c]

[a]If bleeding is not controlled within 24 to 48 h, consider an organic cause or surgical intervention with D&C or hysterectomy.
[b]Add medroxyprogesterone acetate, 10 mg daily for the last 10 days.
[c]Should be used only in women who do not smoke and have no contraindication to the administration of oral contraceptives.

immediately. Treatment options are outlined in Table 54-3.

- For patients whose bleeding cannot be controlled with hormones, whose lifestyle is compromised, or who are symptomatically anemic, a dilation and curettage (D&C) may temporarily stop the bleeding.
- Persistent/recurrent bleeding may require intervention with abdominal or vaginal hysterectomy.
- Endometrial ablation may be used in patients opposed to hysterectomy or with contraindications to hysterectomy. Multiple hysteroscopic and nonhysteroscopic techniques now exist to perform an endometrial ablation. The cure rate with ablation ranges from 60 to 90 percent. The outcome is better if patients are pretreated with GnRH agonists or progestins.
- The most important step in diagnosis and management of patients with abnormal uterine bleeding is to rule out cancer as the cause.

BIBLIOGRAPHY

Abbot J, Hawe J, Hunter D, Garry R. A double-blind randomized trial comparing Cavaterm and the Novasure endometrial ablation systems for the treatment of dysfunctional uterine bleeding. *Fertil Steril* 2003;80(1):203–208.

Munro MG. Dysfunctional uterine bleeding: Advances in diagnosis and treatment. *Curr Opin Obstet Gynecol* 2001;13(5):475–489.

Rimsza ME. Dysfunctional uterine bleeding. *Pediatr Rev* 2002;27(7):227–233.

Speroff L. Dysfunctional uterine bleeding. In: Speroff L, Glass RH, Kase NG, eds. *Clinical Gynecologic Endocrinology and Infertility,* 6th ed. Philadelphia: Lippincott Williams & Wilkins, 1999:575–593.

55 GALACTORRHEA
Alice Rhoton-Vlasak

OVERVIEW

- **Galactorrhea** is a benign condition in which there is milky secretion of fluid from the breast unrelated to pregnancy or nursing (Fig. 55-1). Microscopic evaluation of the discharge demonstrates fat globules of varying size.
- Approximately 20 percent of patients with galactorrhea have hyperprolactinemia, whereas 50 percent of patients with hyperprolactinemia have galactorrhea.
- Prolactin is an anterior pituitary hormone secreted by the lactotroph cells. It is also produced by decidualized endometrium, myometrium, and leiomyomata.
- The normal serum concentration of prolactin is <20 ng/mL.
- Serum concentrations of prolactin vary during the menstrual cycle, with the highest levels occurring after ovulation. Pregnancy is associated with serum prolactin concentrations of 200 to 400 ng/mL at term.
- Serum prolactin concentrations are normally under the inhibitory control of the neurotransmitter dopamine.
- Galactorrhea results from an increase in autonomous prolactin production or a reduced secretion of prolactin-inhibitory factor (PIF, dopamine).
- The clinical presentation of hyperprolactinemia may include menstrual dysfunction, galactorrhea, infertility, headaches, or visual disturbances.

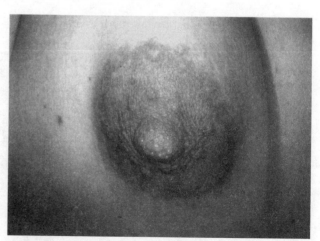

FIG. 55-1   Milk-like secretion from the nipple.

ETIOLOGY

- The four principal causes of hyperprolactinemia/galactorrhea are as follows:
  - Idiopathic hyperprolactinemia
  - Pituitary adenoma
  - Hypothyroidism
  - Drug intake
- Physiologic causes of hyperprolactinemia include the following:
  - Stress
  - Diet
  - Exercise
  - Nipple stimulation
  - Pregnancy
  - Hypoglycemia
- Table 55-1 outlines the differential diagnosis of galactorrhea-hyperprolactinemia.
- A hypothalamic craniopharyngioma is the nonpituitary tumor most commonly associated with hyperprolactinemia. The tumor arises from epithelial remnants of Rathke's pouch. Hyperprolactinemia occurs because the tumor interferes with dopamine transport.
- Empty sella syndrome is caused by congenital weakness in the diaphragma sella, which enables cerebrospinal fluid to escape into the pituitary fossa. This syndrome is an unusual cause of hyperprolactinemia-galactorrhea.

TABLE 55-1 Differential Diagnosis of Galactorrhea-Hyperprolactinemia

Central nervous system
  Trauma
  Tumor or cysts
  Infections
  Granulomas
  Pseudotumor cerebri
Pituitary
  Prolactinomas
    Microadenomas ($<$10 mm)
    Macroadenomas ($>$10 mm)
  Trauma
  Tumors
  Pituitary stalk section
  Empty sella syndrome
Thyroid
  Hypothyroidism
Drug-induced
  Antipsychotics
  Tranquilizers
  Antidepressants
  Antihypertensives
  Estrogens
Peripheral Neural Stimulation
  Chest wall stimulation (surgery or trauma)
  Nipple stimulation
  Spinal cord lesions
  Herpes zoster
Ectopic production
  Lung or renal tumor
Medical illness
  Renal failure
Idiopathic

DIAGNOSIS

- Ideally, serum prolactin concentrations should be measured fasting at 8 a.m. when the patient is in the follicular phase of the cycle. If the serum prolactin concentration is mildly elevated ($>$20 ng/mL $<$50 ng/mL), the test should be repeated.
- Patients with regular menses, mild galactorrhea, and a normal serum prolactin are at low risk for a pituitary adenoma. This situation is common in women who have previously nursed their children.
- Pituitary adenomas are more common with prolactin levels $>$100 ng/mL. A visual field examination is generally unnecessary except in patients with macroadenomas (tumors $>$1 cm).
- Macroadenomas produce superior, bitemporal hemianopsia in approximately 70 percent of patients.
- The diagnostic evaluation should include a history, physical examination, laboratory testing, and possibly radiographic imaging. Figure 55-2 outlines the diagnostic algorithm.
- The ideal pituitary imaging technique is a head MRI with gadolinium contrast. It will detect both small tumors and mass lesions that could cause hyperprolactinemia (Figs. 55-3 and 55-4).

TREATMENT

- The treatment of hyperprolactinemia and galactorrhea depends on multiple factors:
  - Symptoms
  - Desire for pregnancy
  - Presence and type of tumor
  - Degree of estrogen deficiency
- Indications for treatment include socially embarrassing galactorrhea, infertility, and amenorrhea.
- The recommended forms of management are periodic observation, drug therapy, surgery, and, very rarely, radiation therapy.
- Observation is indicated in menstruating women with galactorrhea and normal prolactin levels or idiopathic hyperprolactinemia.

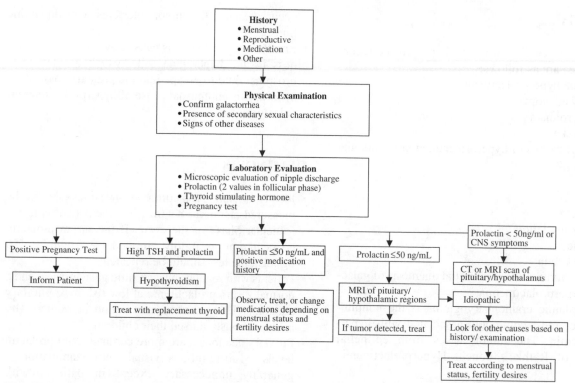

FIG. 55-2   Algorithm for the evaluation of galactorrhea-hyperprolactinemia.

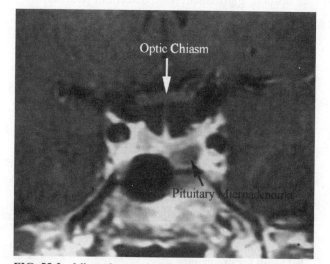

FIG. 55-3   Microadenoma in left side of pituitary gland.

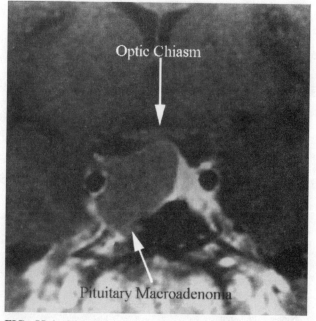

FIG. 55-4   Macroadenoma in right side of pituitary gland, extending cephalad to compress the optic chiasm.

• In approximately one-third of patients, the prolactin level will return to normal within 5 years even if no treatment is provided. Patients may need treatment if hypoestrogenism develops.

• The mainstays of medical treatment of hyperprolactinemia are the dopamine agonists (Table 55-2).

• Adverse side effects of dopamine agonists can be minimized by administering the drug in the evening and by starting the medicine at the lowest dose and increasing it gradually over several weeks.

• Dopamine agonists are indicated for excessive galactorrhea, microadenomas with hypoestrogenism, macroadenomas, and in the case of patients desiring pregnancy.

TABLE 55-2   Dopamine Agonists for Hyperprolactinemia

DRUG	DOSE	ROUTE	SIDE EFFECTS
Bromocriptine	2.5–15 mg/day	Oral	Nausea, nasal congestion, lethargy, orthostatic hypotension
Cabergoline	0.25–1.0 mg twice weekly	Oral	Same as bromocriptine but less severe

TABLE 55-3   Indications for Surgery in Patients with Hyperprolactinemia

Pituitary hemorrhage
Macroadenoma
Intolerance of medication
Resistance to medication
Symptomatic enlargement during pregnancy—no response to medication

- Dopamine agonists are effective in restoring menses in 80 percent and eliminating galactorrhea in 57 to 100 percent of patients.
- Patients who desire pregnancy should be treated with dopamine agonists until conception occurs. Macroadenomas may require therapy even during pregnancy.
- Dopamine agonists do not cause an increased incidence of congenital anomalies or miscarriages.
- Patients with idiopathic hyperprolactinemia or microadenomas who are not hypoestrogenic may be treated with cyclic progestins or oral contraceptives. Periodic assessment of prolactin levels and menstrual status should be performed. Periodic pituitary imaging is necessary for any pituitary tumor.
- Hyperprolactinemic patients who are amenorrheic and hypoestrogenic who do not desire pregnancy can be treated with dopamine agonists, oral contraceptives, or hormone replacement therapy.
- A macroadenoma can generally be managed with dopamine agonists indefinitely. Lesions that do not respond to dopamine agonists are best treated with surgery or radiation therapy. Indications for pituitary surgery are outlined in Table 55-3.
- Complications of pituitary surgery include pituitary insufficiency, diabetes insipidus, cerebral spinal fluid leak, carotid artery injury, and infection. Therefore surgery should be the last resort for treatment of pituitary adenomas.

BIBLIOGRAPHY

American College of Obstetrics and Gynecology. Hyperprolactinemia and other pituitary disorders. Precis: An update in obstetrics and gynecology. *Reproductive Endocrinology,* 2nd ed. Washington, DC: ACOG, 2002:79–81.

Billier BM. Guidelines for the diagnosis and treatment of hyperprolactinemia. *J Reprod Med* 1999;44(12 suppl):1075.

Zacur HA. Indications for surgery in the treatment of hyperprolactinemia. *J Reprod Med* 1999;44:1127–1131.

56   ANDROGEN EXCESS

Alice Rhoton-Vlasak

DEFINITIONS

- Androgen excess disorders usually present with hirsutism, acne, alopecia, and even virilization, amenorrhea, and infertility.
- **Hirsutism** is defined as excessive growth of androgen-dependent sexual hair. It is most often manifest as increased hair on the upper lip, chin, ears, cheeks, lower abdomen, back, chest, and proximal limbs.
- Hirsutism should be viewed as a sign rather than a diagnosis.
- **Virilization** is a more severe state of hyperandrogenism, resulting in masculinization and hirsutism. Virilization is never idiopathic and may be due to a malignant androgen-producing neoplasm.
- Physical changes associated with virilization include alopecia (balding), deepening of the voice, acne, severe hirsutism, clitoromegaly, and increased muscle mass.
- Androgen excess disorders result from either excess production or excess effect of androgens.
- Potential sources of increased androgens include the ovaries, the adrenal glands, medications, or exogenous hormones.

PHYSIOLOGY OF ANDROGEN EXCESS

- **Androgens** represent a class of steroid hormones structurally related to estrogens and progestins. All steroid hormone production begins with the conversion of cholesterol to pregnenolone. Figure 56-1 outlines the steroid biosynthesis pathways.
- The rate-limiting step in androgen formation is the regulation of $P450_C17$ gene expression, which is dependent on the concentrations of luteinzing hormone (LH) in the ovary and adrenocotricotropic hormone (ACTH) in the adrenal gland.
- The most important androgens are testosterone, dihydrotestosterone, androstenedione, dehydroepiandrosterone (DHEA), and dehydroepiandrosterone-sulfate (DHEA-S).

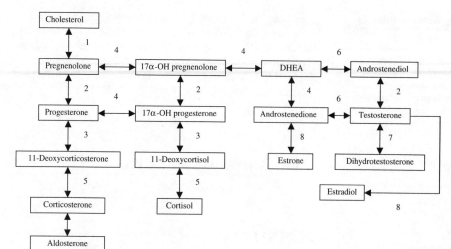

FIG. 56-1 Diagram of steroid biosynthesis. Enzymes in pathway: (1) Side chain cleavage; (2) 3-B hydroxysteroid reductase; (3) 21 hydroxylase (21 hydroxylase deficiency is the most common cause of congenital adrenal hyperplasia); (4) 17 hydroxylase, 17; 20 lyase; (5) 11 B hydroxysteroid reductase; (6) 17B hydroxysteroid reductase; (7) 5α-reductase; (8) aromatose hydroxylase.

- The adrenal gland preferentially secretes weak androgens, such as DHEA or DHEA-S.
- The ovary is the preferential source of testosterone, with approximately 75 percent of circulating testosterone coming from the ovary, either directly or indirectly by peripheral conversion from estrogen.
- Androstenedione, which has only 10 percent of the androgenic potency of testosterone, is of both ovarian (50 percent) and adrenal (50 percent) origin.
- Testosterone is converted within the cells of the skin to dihydrotesterone, which is the most potent androgen. The enzyme responsible for the conversion is 5α-reductase.
- After secretion by the ovaries or adrenals, most androgens are bound to protein and are biologically inactive. The active or nonprotein bound fraction represents only about 1 percent of the total circulating testosterone.

PHYSIOLOGY OF THE HAIR FOLLICLE

- **The pilosebaceous unit** in the skin consists of hair follicles and sebaceous glands. Both are sensitive to androgens. The pilosebaceous units are found everywhere on the body except the palms of the hands, the lips, and the soles of the feet.
- Hair follicle development begins at 2 months' gestation; by birth, all units have developed. Before puberty, the body hair is a fine, unpigmented vellus hair.
- During puberty, as ovarian and adrenal androgens increase, vellus hair is converted to terminal hair. Terminal hair (or sexual hair, found in the pubic area, axillae, lower abdomen, thighs, legs, arms, chest, and face) is coarse, long, and more pigmented.
- Table 56-1 outlines the stages of hair growth. The length of each hair is determined by the length of the

TABLE 56-1   Phases of Hair Growth

Anagen phase	Growth—initiated with the shedding of old hair and new growth
Catagen phase	Rapid involution—shaft ceases to grow, root moves up and hair bulb shrivels
Telogen phase	Inactivity—resting until a new cycle begins

anagen and telogen phase. Each hair follicle has its own growth cycle independent of the adjacent hair follicle.

- The growth and development of the hair follicle may be influenced by sex hormones, genetic factors, and racial and ethnic differences.
- Estrogens retard hair growth, whereas androgens initiate and stimulate hair growth and pigmentation.
- Hirsutism results when androgens stimulate transformation of vellus into terminal hair.
- Androgens have the opposite effect on the hair follicles of the scalp, causing hair loss and thinning, particularly in the crown region of the head.

EVALUATION

- The history should include information about age of menarche; menstrual regularity; age of onset and rapidity of development of hirsutism; associated problems such as acne, infertility, galactorrhea, weight change; family history; and evidence of virilization.
- Physical examination should focus on the findings listed in Table 56-2. The modified Ferriman-Gallway scale has been developed for use as a pictoral clinical scale to assess the extent and distribution of hirsutism (Fig 56-2).

TABLE 56-2   **Physical Findings in Hirsute Patients**

ANATOMIC SITE	PHYSICAL FINDINGS
General	Central obesity, deepening of the voice
Skin	Acne, hirsutism, acanthosis nigricans, balding, violaceous abdominal striae or moon face
Cardiovascular	Hypertension
Pelvis	Clitoromegaly, vaginal atrophy, pelvic mass

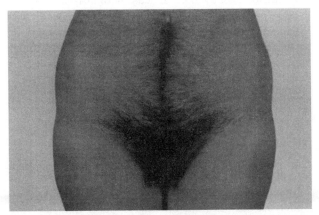

FIG. 56-2   Male pattern escutcheon in a patient with polycystic ovary syndrome.

- Laboratory evaluation depends on the rapidity of onset, age of onset, and associated physical findings. The tests should help to identify life-threatening conditions associated with hyperandrogenism, such as Cushing's syndrome, congenital adrenal hyperplasia, and ovarian or adrenal tumors.
- Laboratory tests may include the following:
  - Serum testosterone concentration: values less than 200 ng/dL will rule out almost all tumors.
  - DHEA-S values: >700 ng/dL should be viewed as highly suspicious for an adrenal tumor.
  - Serum concentration of 17-hydroxyprogesterone: values >200 ng/dL require further evaluation for congenital adrenal hyperplasia. Further evaluation should include ACTH stimulation testing.
  - TSH and prolactin: indicated if patient has irregular menstrual cycles.
  - If Cushing's syndrome is suspected, an overnight dexamethasone suppression test or 24-h urinary cortisol is required.
  - Pelvic ultrasound may be used to assess for an ovarian tumor if serum testosterone concentrations are elevated. Adrenal CT or MRI is used to assess for adrenal tumors.

DIFFERENTIAL DIAGNOSIS OF HIRSUTISM

IDIOPATHIC HIRSUTISM (FAMILIAL)

- This condition is characterized by hirsutism in eumenorrheic women with normal circulating androgens.
- It is a diagnosis of exclusion and may be identified in about 50 percent of patients.

OVARIAN CAUSES OF HIRSUTISM

- Polycystic ovary syndrome (PCOS) occurs in 4 to 6 percent of reproductive-age women and is the most common cause of pathologic hirsutism. The hallmark features of this condition are as follows:
  - Hyperandrogenism
  - Oligoovulation
  - Anabolic changes
  - Exclusion of other pathologic causes, such as congenital adrenal hyperplasia (CAH), hyperprolactinemia, Cushing's syndrome, and androgen-secreting tumors.
- PCOS is a heterogenous disorder of unknown etiology, with the most common manifestations being hirsutism (90 percent), menstrual irregularity (90 percent), infertility (75 percent), and obesity. Insulin resistance is now recognized as one of the key abnormalities in patients with PCOS.
- Stromal hyperthecosis is a severe form of PCOS caused by proliferation of ovarian stroma, with foci of luteinized theca cells. It may result in virilization, obesity, hypertension, and altered glucose metabolism.
- Ovarian androgen-producing tumors are rare and usually present with rapidly developing hirsutism, amenorrhea, and virilization. Serum testosterone concentrations will be >200 ng/dL, and a unilateral mass often is palpable on pelvic examination. Table 56-3 outlines the possible ovarian causes of hirsutism, including potential neoplasms.

ADRENAL CAUSES OF HIRSUTISM

- **Late-onset congenital adrenal hyperplasia** (CAH) may be present in 1 to 2 percent of U.S. women. CAH is inherited as an autosomal recessive disorder resulting from mutations in enzymes required for adrenal steroidogenesis. The enzyme defects cause precursors to cortisol to become elevated and shifted into biosynthetic pathways for androgens. Serum concentrations of testosterone and androstenedione become elevated and cause hirsutism. The most common enzyme

TABLE 56-3   Differential Diagnosis of Hirsutism

Idiopathic
Nonneoplastic ovarian causes
   Polycystic ovary syndrome
   Stromal hyperthecosis
   HAIR-AN: hyperandrogenism, acanthosis nigricans, insulin resistance
Ovarian tumors
   Sertoli-Leydig cell tumors
   Hylar cell tumors
   Germ cell tumors
   Granulosa cell tumors
   Gynandroblastomas
   Gonadoblastomas
   Brenner tumors
Adrenal causes
   Congenital adrenal hyperplasia
   Cushing's syndrome
   Adrenal tumors
Iatrogenic causes
   Anabolic steroids
   Methyl testosterone
   Danazol

defect is 21-hydroxylase, followed by 11-B hydroxylase and 3-B hydroxysteroid dehydrogenase. Treatment usually consists of steroid replacement with dexamethasone or prednisone.

- **Cushing's syndrome** results from hypercortisolism due to one of three etiologies: (1) adrenal tumor, (2) ectopic production of ACTH by a nonpituitary tumor, or (3) excess production of ACTH by the pituitary (Cushing's disease). Excess serum concentrations of cortisol and its precursors are the cause of hirsutism. Physical findings typically include moon facies, buffalo hump, abdominal striae, centripetal fat distribution, and hypertension.

- Cortisol excess can be identified with a 24-h urine test for free cortisol (normal values <100 mg/24 h) or a 1-h overnight dexamethasone suppression test. If initial screening tests are abnormal, extended suppression tests, ACTH stimulation tests, or radiologic studies are indicated.

- Adrenal tumors are a rare cause of hirsutism. The main androgen detected is DHEA-S (>700 to 800 ng/dL). This cutoff has poor sensitivity. If an adrenal tumor is suspected, a CT scan or MRI should be obtained.

TREATMENT

- The selection of therapy for hirsutism depends on physical and laboratory findings as well as the patient's desire for childbearing.
- If an ovarian or adrenal tumor exists, surgical removal of the tumor is indicated.

- Congenital adrenal hyperplasia is treated by the administration of prednisone, which replaces deficient cortisol and provides sufficient negative feedback to restore normal ACTH secretion.
- Cushing's syndrome should be treated by surgical removal of the source of excess cortisol or ACTH.
- Women with idiopathic hirsutism or hirsutism due to PCOS or stromal hyperthecosis (who desire childbearing) should receive medication to suppress adrenal or ovarian androgen production or drugs that block the peripheral effect of androgen. The latter medications may take at least 4 to 6 months to be effective. Mechanical hair removal can control hirsutism and is often a front-line treatment used by women. Electrolysis or laser therapy of hair follicles is the only way to remove excessive hair permanently. All other medical therapies only convert hair from a dark terminal hair to a fine vellus hair.

MEDICAL THERAPY

- Oral contraceptives are the mainstay of treatment of hirsutism. They inhibit ovarian steroid production and increase sex hormone binding globulin, thus lowering bioavailable testosterone. GnRH agonists have a similar effect on lowering ovarian androgen production.
- An advantage of oral contraceptives is the additional contraceptive effect, reduction in acne, and induction of regular menses, which protects the endometrium from unopposed estrogen.
- There are four androgen receptor antagonists currently available to treat hirsutism. Despite proven efficacy, none of the drugs are specifically approved by the U.S. Food and Drug Administration (FDA) to treat hirsutism.
  - Spironolactone is an aldosterone antagonist that acts by competitive androgen receptor blockade and decreases 5α-reductase activity. The daily dosage is 100 to 200 mg. Side effects may include mild diuresis when first taken, fatigue, breast tenderness, and menstrual changes.
  - Finasteride is a selective type 2 5α-reductase inhibitor given in doses of 5 mg/day.
  - Flutamide is a potent, highly specific nonsteroidal antiandrogen that inhibits target tissue androgen receptor sites. The daily dose is 250 mg one to three times per day. Side effects include decreased appetite, amenorrhea, decreased libido, and, rarely, hepatotoxicity. Flutamide should be reserved for resistant cases of hirsutism, and liver enzymes must be monitored.
  - Cyproterone acetate is an androgen receptor antagonist that is widely used in Europe but is not available in the United States.

- All women on androgen therapy should use effective contraception due to the potential for teratogenic effects on a male fetus conceived during therapy.
- One topical therapy has been approved by the FDA for removal of unwanted facial hair: eflornithine hydrochloride (Vaniqua). This drug is an ornithine decarboxylase inhibitor that works by inhibiting the growth of hair follicles. Daily dosage consists of 13.9 percent cream applied to the affected area twice a day for a minimal of 4 h with each application. It is pregnancy category C and appears to be well tolerated.

PROGNOSIS

- Treatment should be individualized, and progress can be monitored on a clinical basis. The patient should receive detailed counseling so that her expectations about the effects of therapy are realistic. Adjunctive therapy is almost always needed.

BIBLIOGRAPHY

American College of Obstetricians and Gynecologists. Polycystic ovary syndrome, hirsutism, and other androgen excess disorders: Precis. *Reproductive Endocrinology,* 2nd ed. Washington, DC: ACOG, 2002:83–99.

Azziz R. The evaluation and management of hirsutism. *Obstet Gynecol* 2003;101(5 Pt 1):995–1007.

Azziz R, DeWailly D, Owerbach D. Clinical review 56: Nonclassic adrenal hyperplasia: Current concepts. *J Clin Endocrinol Metab* 1994;78:810–815.

Carmina E. Anti-androgens for treatment of hirsutism. *Expert Opin Invest Drugs* 2002; 11(3):357–363.

Fruzzeti F, Bersi C, Parrini D, Ricci C, Genazzani AR. Treatment of hirsutism: Comparisons between different antiandrogens with central and peripheral effects. *Fertil Steril* 1999;71:445–451.

57 PREMENSTRUAL SYNDROME

Alice Rhoton-Vlasak

DEFINITIONS

- **Premenstrual syndrome** (PMS) is the cyclic, repetitive disorder occurring during the luteal phase of the menstrual cycle; it comprises distressing physical, psychologic, and behavioral changes that disappear with the onset of menstrual flow.

- PMS is entered as a genitourinary disorder in the International Statistical Classification of Diseases and Related Health Problems-10th revision (ICD-10).
- The ICD-10 defines PMS as a condition with:
  ○ Mild psychologic discomfort
  ○ Also physical symptoms of bloating, weight gain, breast tenderness, swelling of the hands and feet, various aches and pains, poor concentration, sleep disturbance, and change in appetite. Table 57-1 lists the most common symptoms.
    ▪ Symptoms must occur in the luteal phase and abate with menses.
    ▪ Only one symptom is required to establish the diagnosis.
- **Premenstrual dysphoric disorder** (PMDD) is a moderate to severe form of PMS in which there are a multitude of symptoms that impair daily living.
- PMDD is defined by the American Psychiatric Association and recognized as a diagnosable and treatable psychiatric disorder.

PREVALENCE

- Seventy-five percent of women experience some recurrent PMS symptoms.
- Severe symptoms are experienced by 5 to 10 percent of women.
- The highest incidence occurs in women in their late twenties to early thirties.

ETIOLOGY

- Many theories have been presented, but none is completely supported by medical evidence.
- Current and past theories include the following:
  ○ Progesterone deficiency
  ○ Estrogen excess
  ○ Increased activity of the aldosterone/renin system
  ○ Vitamin B_6 deficiency
  ○ Serotonergic dysregulation
  ○ Luteal reduction in endogenous opiate activity

TABLE 57-1 Principal Clinical Manifestations of Premenstrual Syndrome

TYPE	MANIFESTATIONS
Affective	Depression, anger, irritability, anxiety, confusion, sadness, crying easily, nervous tension
Physical	Breast tenderness, bloating, swelling, headache, skin problems, aches
Behavioral	Increased appetite, food craving, decreased concentration, decreased motivation, avoidance of activities

DIAGNOSIS

- The diagnosis is based primarily on the patient's medical, psychiatric, psychosocial, and family history.
- Forty to 60 percent of women seeking treatment for PMS have underlying psychiatric disorders rather than PMS.
- A complete physical examination should be performed to exclude other treatable conditions.
- Laboratory testing should be very limited and dependent on presenting symptoms.
- A daily rating scale (or a menstrual diary) is the accepted method of diagnosing PMS. Figure 57-1 shows a typical menstrual symptom diary.
- The patient should chart her symptoms for two cycles.

- Symptoms must be present in the luteal phase, and there must be a symptom-free period of at least 7 days in the first half of the cycle.
- If the symptoms persist in the follicular phase, another diagnosis is more likely.
- Symptoms should increase by >30 to 50 percent during the luteal phase. Increases by 60 to 75 percent suggest PMDD.

DIFFERENTIAL DIAGNOSIS

- Psychiatric conditions such as major depression, anxiety disorder, personality disorder, substance abuse, and eating disorders must be considered in the differential.

GRADING OF MENSES

0-NONE
1-slight
2-moderate
3-heavy
4-heavy and clots

GRADING OF SYMPTOMS(COMPLAINTS)

0-NONE
1-mild-present but does not interfere with activities
2-moderate-present and interferes with activities but not disabling
3-severe-disabling. Unable to function

Day of cycle	1	2	3	4	5	6	7	8	9	10	11	12	13	14	15	16	17	18	19	20	21	22	23	24	25	26	27	29	29	30	31	32	33	34	35
Date																																			
Menses																																			
PMT-A																																			
Nervous tension																																			
Mood swings																																			
Irritability																																			
Anxiety																																			
PMT-H																																			
Weight gain																																			
Swelling of extremities																																			
Breast tenderness																																			
Abdominal bloating																																			
PMT-C																																			
Headache																																			
Craving for sweets																																			
Increased appetite																																			
Heart pounding																																			
Fatigue																																			
Dizziness																																			
PMT-D																																			
Depression																																			
Forgetfulness																																			
Crying																																			
Confusion																																			
Insomnia																																			
DYSMENORRHEA-PAIN																																			
Cramps (low abdominal)																																			
Backache																																			
General aches/pains																																			
Basal weight in lbs.																																			
Basal body temperature																																			
Treatment																																			

NOTES:

FIG. 57-1 A typical menstrual symptom diary used to prospectively chart symptoms to make a diagnosis of PMS.

- Medical conditions such as the following must also be considered:
  - Seizure disorder
  - Chronic fatigue syndrome
  - Migraine
  - Asthma
  - Hypothyroidism
  - Diabetes mellitus
  - Adrenal disease

TREATMENT

- Once the diagnosis of PMS or PMDD is made, treatment should be based on the patient's desire for an improvement in her symptoms. The treatment should be tailored to the patient's most prominent symptoms and to their severity.
- Nonpharmacologic treatment is recommended for mild symptoms of short duration, reserving medical management for severe symptoms. Table 57-2 outlines nonpharmacologic treatment options.
- There are numerous pharmacologic interventions.
- A selective serotonin reuptake inhibitor (SSRI) is the initial drug of choice for severe PMS. Fluoxetine is the best studied of this group.
- Table 57-3 outlines treatment options for PMS. Some patients with severe PMS may fail medical therapy and require surgical treatment.
  - Surgical treatment consists of bilateral oophorectomy, possibly with hysterectomy.
  - Surgery should be preceded by a trial of medical oophorectomy with a GnRH agonist.
  - Postoperative estrogen replacement generally does not cause a recurrence of symptoms.

TABLE 57-2 Nonpharmacologic Treatment of PMS

Dietary changes
Caffeine restriction
High carbohydrate diet
Limit alcohol, tobacco, chocolate
Sodium restriction
Dietary supplementation
Calcium carbonate 1000 mg/day
Magnesium 200–400 mg
Vitamin E 400 IU daily
Exercise
20- to 40-min aerobic workout four times a week
Supportive therapy
Stress reduction
Relaxation techniques
Behavior modification

BIBLIOGRAPHY

American College of Obstetricians and Gynecologists. Premenstrual syndrome: Clinical management guidelines for obstetricians and gynecologists. *ACOG Pract Bull* No. 15, 2003.

TABLE 57-3 Pharmacologic Treatments for Premenstrual Syndrome

MEDICATION	DOSAGE	INDICATION	SIDE EFFECTS
NSAIDs	Luteal phase	Pain	Gastrointestinal upset, rash, renal toxicity
Diuretics	Spironolactone 25–50 mg 2× daily in luteal phase	Fluid retention	Fatigue, headaches, dehydration, weakness
Fluoxetine[a]	10–20 mg daily luteal phase	Altered mood	Anxiety/nervousness, insomnia, nausea, sexual dysfunction
Sertraline	50–100 mg daily or in luteal phase	Altered mood	Same as fluoxetine
Proxetine	10–30 mg daily or in luteal phase	Altered mood	Same as fluoxetine
Nefazodone	100–600 mg/day	Altered mood	Same as fluoxetine
Venlafaxine	25 mg bid	Altered mood	Mild increase in BP
Alprazolam	0.25 mg daily to 0.25 mg 4× daily in luteal phase	Anxiety, depression	Abuse potential, sedation, tolerance
Buspirone	15–30 mg daily in luteal phase	Anxiety	Dizziness, nausea, headache
Oral contraceptives[b]	One daily	Physical symptoms	Nausea, breast tenderness, mood alterations
GnRH agonists	Leuprolide acetate 3.75 mg monthly	Suppression of ovulation	Vasomotor symptoms, headache, vaginal dryness, bone loss

[a]Studies have demonstrated limited effectiveness in PMS, but may work for physical symptoms.
[b]Only drug FDA-approved for the treatment of PMS.

American College of Obstetricians and Gynecologists. Premenstrual syndrome. Precis: An update in obstetrics and gynecology. *Reproductive Endocrinology,* 2nd ed. Washington, DC: ACOG, 2002: 61–67.

Gianetto-Berruti A, Feyles V. Premenstrual syndrome. *Minerva Gynecol* 2002;54(2):85–95.

58   POLYCYSTIC OVARY SYNDROME

Alice Rhoton-Vlasak

INTRODUCTION

- **Polycystic ovary syndrome** (PCOS) is one of the most common endocrine disorders in reproductive-age women. It affects 5 to 10 percent of women and is a common cause of androgen excess and hirsutism.
- PCOS first was described in 1935 by Stein and Leventhal, who noted an association between amenorrhea, obesity, hirsutism, and polycystic ovaries. Histologic changes noted in the ovary include a thickened ovarian capsule and numerous follicular cysts surrounded by a hyperplastic, luteinized theca interna.
- Studies have demonstrated that PCOS is a complex, heterogeneous disorder of unknown etiology that has diverse clinical and biochemical features.
- There is no consensus opinion on the definition of PCOS, but the diagnostic criteria published in 1990 by the National Institute of Child Health and Human Development are of value in identifying affected patients:
  - Hyperandrogenism and/or hyperandrogenemia
  - Oligoovulation
  - Exclusion of other known disorders such as congenital adrenal hyperplasia, Cushing's syndrome, hyperprolactinemia, or an androgen-secreting tumor
- The presence of polycystic ovaries on ultrasound was noted as a possible inclusion criterion, although it is controversial, because 25 percent of women with no features of PCOS may have an ultrasound appearance of polycystic ovaries.

BIOCHEMICAL AND METABOLIC FEATURES

- Alterations in multiple body systems may contribute to the development of PCOS. The interactions of these systems lead to a vicious cycle whereby the initiation of PCOS and hyperandrogenism lead to its perpetuation.

- Alterations in the hypothalamic-pituitary unit lead to inappropriate gonadotropin secretion, manifest by an elevated LH-to-FSH ratio. Altered GnRH secretion also affects LH and FSH levels.
- An elevated serum concentration of LH causes LH-dependent hyperplasia of ovarian theca cells, which then secrete excess ovarian androgens. Androgen excess leads to inhibition of sex hormone–binding globulin (SHBG) production, which causes increased serum concentration of free androgen and estrogen. Excess androgens are aromatized to estrogens in peripheral sites, causing perpetuation of the cycle and increased risk for abnormal uterine bleeding.
- Insulin resistance affects 25 to 60 percent of women with PCOS. The insulin resistance causes compensatory hyperinsulinemia, which contributes to androgen excess by stimulating androgen production in the adrenal glands and ovaries.
- Overall, the metabolic derangements predispose affected women to an increased risk of cardiovascular disease and type II diabetes.

CLINICAL FEATURES

- PCOS tends to develop shortly after menarche and persists throughout reproductive life. The most common presenting symptoms are outlined in Table 58-1.
- Findings on physical examination may include hirsutism, acne, bilateral ovarian enlargement, and acanthosis nigricans.
- Acanthosis nigricans is a dermatologic manifestation of chronic hyperinsulinemia consisting of localized areas of velvety gray-brown hyperpigmentation usually in the skin folds of the arms, legs, or neck. Skin tags often are found in or near areas of acanthosis. **HAIR-AN syndrome** (hyperandrogenism, insulin resistance, and acanthosis nigricans) is a variant of PCOS.
- The ultrasound appearance of polycystic ovaries typically shows multiple 2- to 8-mm subcapsular preantral follicles forming a black "pearl necklace" sign (Fig. 58-1).

TABLE 58-1   Clinical Manifestations of Polycystic Ovary Syndrome

Hirsutism
Obesity
Acne
Infertility
Oligomenorrhea or amenorrhea
Abnormal uterine bleeding
Virilization

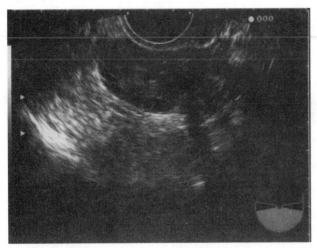

FIG. 58-1 Transvaginal ultrasound picture of the polycystic ovary with multiple small, subcapsular follicles with a "string of pearls" appearance.

TABLE 58-2   Laboratory Testing to Evaluate in Polycystic Ovary Syndrome

BLOOD TESTS (NORMAL RANGE)	USUAL RESULTS IN PCOS
Total testosterone[a] (<60 ng/dL)	Normal or slightly elevated
DHEA-S[a] (<400 ng/dL)	Normal or slightly elevated
Prolactin (<20 ng/mL)	Normal or slightly elevated
Lipid profile	Elevated
Cholesterol (<200 ng/dL)	
LDL (<130 ng/dL)	
Triglycerides (<200 ng/dL)	
Fasting insulin (<20 mIU/mL)	Normal to elevated
Fasting glucose or	Glucose-intolerant
2-h glucose test (<110 mg/dL)	
Glucose-to-insulin ratio (>4.5)	Abnormal <4.5
Thyroid-stimulating hormone	Normal or elevated

[a]Rarely needed unless more severe signs of androgen excess or acute onset.

- Long-term health sequelae of PCOS include an increased risk of endometrial cancer, type II diabetes, and cardiovascular disease.

DIAGNOSTIC AND LABORATORY TESTING

- The diagnosis is based on clinical findings, after excluding other disorders of androgen excess as outlined in Chap. 56.
- Symptoms usually are gradual in onset and consist of those outlined in Table 58-1.
- Laboratory evaluation should be limited if PCOS. FSH to LH ratios usually are not necessary. Table 58-2 outlines laboratory tests that may be of value in confirming the diagnosis.
- Optional tests to consider include the following:
  ○ Transvaginal ultrasound to assess ovarian morphology
  ○ Determination of serum gonadotropin concentrations

TREATMENT

- Treatment depends on the predominant clinical findings and the patient's desires concerning contraception and childbearing. Table 58-3 outlines treatment options.
- All women with PCOS should be screened for cardiovascular risk factors by determination of body mass index (BMI: weight in kilograms divided by height in square meters) and measurement of serum lipids. A normal BMI is <25 kg/m^2. Regular exercise and weight loss should be part of any treatment program.
- Infertility associated with PCOS is treated with ovulation induction with clomiphene citrate, beginning with a dose of 50 mg on days 5 to 9 of the menstrual cycle. Clomiphene citrate is an orally administered nonsteroidal drug. Up to 80 percent of women with PCOS will ovulate on clomiphene, and about 60 percent will conceive. Most pregnancies occur within the first 6 months; thereafter, an alternative treatment should be used. Documentation of ovulation is needed to confirm ovulatory cycles on clomiphene. The main risks of clomiphene are a 5 to 7 percent incidence of multiple pregnancy and very low risk of **ovarian hyperstimulation syndrome (OHSS)**.
- Alternate options for ovulation induction in women failing clomiphene treatment include metformin, gonadotropin therapy, and ovarian drilling.
  ○ Metformin, either alone or as adjunctive treatment to clomiphene or gonadotropins in hyperinsulinemic PCOS patients, has been used to improve ovulatory rates. Metformin has a small risk of causing lactic acidosis. It also may cause gastrointestinal symptoms such as bloating, diarrhea, nausea, and vomiting. Weight loss frequently occurs while a patient is taking metformin, which also improves ovulation rates.
  ○ Gonadotropin therapy, with subcutaneous injections of FSH or FSH/LH, is used to induce ovulation in cases of clomiphene failure. Patients should be monitored with serum estrogen levels and pelvic ultrasounds to assess follicular growth. The main risks are a 20 percent rate of multiple pregnancy

TABLE 58-3   Treatment Options in Patients with PCOS

MEDICATION	INDICATION IN PCOS	DOSE
Low-dose combination oral contraceptives	Hirsutism: suppress androgen secretion	1 pill orally daily
	Menstrual regulation: prevention of endometrial hyperplasia	
Progestins	Menstrual regulation:	
Medroxyprogesterone acetate (MPA)	prevention of endometrial hyperplasia	10 mg orally for 10 days/month
Norethindrone acetate		2.5 mg orally for 10 days/month
Antiandrogens[a,b]	Androgen-receptor blocker,	
Spironolactone	inhibition of steroidogenesis, and 5α-reductase inhibitor (used as diuretic and aldosterone antagonist)	100 mg orally 1 or 2 times per day
Flutamide[c]	Androgen receptor agonist	250 mg orally daily
Finasteride	5α-reductase inhibitor	1 or 5 mg orally daily
Clomiphene citrate	Ovulation induction	50–250 mg orally days 5–9 of cycle
Insulin-sensitizing agents	Decreases insulin to allow	
Metformin	ovulation and improvement of menstrual regularity	500 mg orally tid
Gonadotropins		
Recombinant FSH	Ovulation induction if clomiphene citrate failed	Low-dose daily starting at 75 U SQ as directed
Highly purified FSH	Ovulation induction if clomiphene citrate failed	Low-dose daily starting at 75 U SQ as directed
Eflornithine decarboxylase	Hirsutism	19.9% cream twice daily to affected areas for a minimum of 4 h daily

[a]None were developed specifically to treat hyperandrogenism in women and none are FDA-approved.
[b]The antiandrogens are class D or X in pregnancy and should be prescribed only to women with adequate, effective contraception (ideally birth-control pills).
[c]May cause hepatitis, therefore rarely used.

and an increased risk of OHSS. The goal of therapy is unifollicular development.

○ Laparoscopic ovarian drilling is available to patients who fail to ovulate with clomiphene and do not wish to incur the expense and risks of gonadotropin therapy. Randomized studies have found no difference in pregnancy or miscarriage rates between ovarian drilling and gonadotropins, but there is a reduction in multiple pregnancy rates with the former treatment.

• Dysfunctional uterine bleeding (DUB) in patients with PCOS is due to anovulation. Patients also may develop amenorrhea or oligomenorrhea.

• Treatment with cyclic progestins or oral contraceptives is recommended to reduce the risk of endometrial hyperplasia/carcinoma. It is important to perform endometrial biopsies even in young women who present with PCOS and abnormal bleeding. Obesity further increases the risk of endometrial abnormalities. Pregnancy must be ruled out before performing an endometrial biopsy.

• Diet, weight loss, and exercise are beneficial in all obese PCOS patients. Reduction in weight reduces androgen levels and insulin resistance and may help restore ovulatory cycles.

BIBLIOGRAPHY

American College of Obstetrics and Gynecology. *ACOG Pract Bull* #41, Polycystic ovary syndrome. December 2002.

Bradshaw KD, Carr BR. Polycystic ovary syndrome in decision making. In: Schlaff WD, Rock JA, eds. *Reproductive Endocrinology.* Boston: Blackwell, 1993:283–289.

Dunaif A. Insulin resistance and the polycystic ovary syndrome mechanism and implications for potogenesis. *Endocrinol Rev* 1997;83:774–800.

59 EVALUATION AND TREATMENT OF THE INFERTILE COUPLE

Alice Rhoton-Vlasak

BACKGROUND

• Infertility is a common condition that affects at least 14 percent of American couples. Most couples experience

infertility as a life crisis in which they feel isolated and powerless. Recent delays in childbearing have increased the incidence of infertility secondary to age-related declines in fertility.
- The organization of the infertility evaluation requires consideration of all aspects of reproduction (male, ovulatory, pelvic, tubal, cervical), taking into account the expense, invasiveness, and risks of each procedure.
- Both partners in a couple contribute to potential fertility, and both may be subfertile.
- The initial assessment is followed by the basic diagnostic workup, which determines further testing and treatment options.

DEFINITIONS

- **Infertility** is the inability to conceive after 12 months of unprotected intercourse. There is a 20 percent monthly probability of pregnancy in a normal couple. Eighty-five percent of normal couples conceive within 1 year.
- **Sterility** implies an inability to achieve a pregnancy.
- **Fecundability** is the probability of achieving a pregnancy within one menstrual cycle.
- **Fecundity** is the ability to achieve a live birth in one menstrual cycle.
- An inverse relationship exists between a fecundabilty and the woman's age. The decline begins in the early thirties and progresses rapidly in the early forties.
- Several events are necessary for conception to occur. An egg must be released from the ovary. The egg must then be picked up by the fallopian tube and fertilized by sperm in the tube. Infertility results when a problem develops in one or more steps in the process.
- Incidence of etiologies:
  ○ Male: 40 percent
  ○ Ovulatory: 15 to 20 percent
  ○ Tubal: 30 percent
  ○ Cervical/uterine: 5 to 10 percent
  ○ Peritoneal and endometriosis: 40 percent
  ○ Unexplained: 5 to 10 percent

DIAGNOSTIC EVALUATION

- The history should be taken with both partners present. The woman should be questioned about her menstrual history, galactorrhea, weight changes, hirsutism, pelvic pain, dyspareunia, dysmenorrhea, and history of pelvic infections.
- A sexual and pregnancy history also should be obtained from both partners. Information about exposures to toxins or previous surgery, previous infertility history, workup, and treatment should be reviewed.

- The workup should not be delayed, especially in patients over age 35.
- A careful physical examination of the female partner should be performed. The major findings to note are outlined in Table 59-1.
- Table 59-2 outlines laboratory, radiologic, and surgical diagnostic testing.
- The initial basic evaluation can be performed within 6 to 8 weeks.
- A tentative schedule of testing should be planned and then an estimate of costs determined.
- Frequently, the initial history will indicate a probable cause of infertility, but it is important to complete a basic evaluation of all the major factors so that a secondary diagnosis will not be ignored.
- The initial approach should focus on the least invasive methods for detecting the most common causes of infertility.

MALE-FACTOR INFERTILITY

- This condition is usually diagnosed by a semen analysis obtained after 48 h of abstinence. The specimen

TABLE 59-1   Physical Examination of the Infertile Female

Weight and body mass index
Signs of systemic illness
Thyroid enlargement or nodules
Skin examination with attention to presence of acne, hirsutism, and acanthosis nigricans
Presence of breast secretions
Pelvic or abdominal tenderness
Vaginal/cervical discharge or abnormality
Uterine size, shape, tenderness
Adnexal or cul-de-sac mass or tenderness

TABLE 59-2   Basic Infertility Evaluation

TEST	TIMING[a]	CONDITION TESTED
Semen analysis	After 48 h of abstinence	Male-factor infertility
Thyroid-stimulating hormone (TSH)	Any	Ovulatory infertility
Prolactin	Follicular phase	Ovulatory infertility
Progesterone	~Day 21 or 7 days post-LH surge	Ovulatory infertility
Hysterosalpingogram[b] (HSG)	Days 5-12 of cycle	Tubal/uterine factor
Postcoital test	Midcycle 4-12 h after coitus	Cervical infertility
Laparoscopy[c]	Follicular phase	Endometriosis/tubal infertility
Clomid challenge test	Days 3 and 10	Ovarian reserve testing

[a]Timing based on day 1 of cycle being the first day of menstrual flow.
[b]Radiologic test done under fluoroscopy.
[c]Outpatient surgical procedure.

should be delivered to the laboratory within 30 min of collection.

- At least two semen analyses, 2 to 4 weeks apart, are recommended if an abnormality is found. Values for a normal semen analysis are reviewed in Table 59-3.
- There are many causes of male infertility, including disorders of spermatogenesis, obstruction of the spermatic duct, disorders of sperm motility, and sexual dysfunction.
- Possible treatments include the following:
  ○ Intrauterine insemination
  ○ In vitro fertilization (IVF) with intracytoplasmic sperm injection (ICSI)
  ○ Donor sperm
- Cytogenetic abnormalities in the male may contribute to infertility in cases of a severe male factor. Therefore a karyotype, including identification of microdeletions of the Y chromosome, and testing for cystic fibrosis should be offered.

OVULATORY FACTOR

- If menstrual cycles are regular and the patient clearly has premenstrual symptoms, further testing to confirm ovulation is probably unnecessary.
- If cycles are irregular with or without evidence of androgen excess, testing for TSH, prolactin, and androgens should be performed.
- **Basal body temperature** (BBT) charting requires the patient to obtain her temperature daily before rising from bed in the morning. In ovulatory cycles, the BBT typically rises 1 to 3 days after the midcycle LH surge. BBTs are hard to interpret and may be very subjective.
- A midluteal serum progesterone concentration can be used to confirm ovulation. Values from 3 to 10 ng/mL are consistent with ovulation. An ovulation predictor kit can be used to detect an LH surge, and the progesterone assay should be obtained 7 days after the LH surge.
- If menstrual cycles are irregular or ovulation is not confirmed by other methods, treatment is needed for ovulation induction. Clomiphene citrate or injectable

gonadotropins can be used for this in cases of polycystic ovary syndrome or idiopathic anovulation.

- Other causes of anovulation identified by a workup, such as hypothyroidism or hyperprolactinemia, should be treated appropriately.

TUBAL OR UTERINE-FACTOR INFERTILITY

- Patent and functional tubes are necessary for conception.
- Infertility may result from the complete blockage of the distal end of the tube (hydrosalpinx) due to infection, surgery, or endometriosis. Proximal tubal obstruction may result from salpingitis isthmica nodosa, infection, or idiopathic causes.
- Abnormalities of the uterus are a rare cause of infertility but can cause failure of implantation. Factors that have been implicated include congenital anomalies, leiomyomas, and intrauterine synechiae.
- **Hysterosalpingography** (HSG) and laparoscopy with chromopertubation (injection of dye) may be used to evaluate tubal patency. HSG has the additional advantage of being able to evaluate the uterine cavity.
- The HSG should be done in the proliferative phase of the cycle after menses have ceased. It utilizes an iodinated dye injected transcervically. Figure 59-1 and Fig. 59-2 demonstrate a normal and abnormal HSG, respectively.
- The procedure is contraindicated in women with a pelvic mass, pelvic tenderness, or allergy to contrast or iodine.
- Complications of an HSG include the following:
  ○ Pain
  ○ Dye allergy

TABLE 59-3   Normal Semen Analysis Values

VARIABLE	VALUE
Volume	2-5.0 mL
pH	>7.2
Sperm concentration	>20 million/mL
Sperm motility (%)	>50%
Sperm antibodies	Negative
White blood cells	<0.5 million/mL
Morphology	
Standard	>50% normal
Kruger	>14% normal

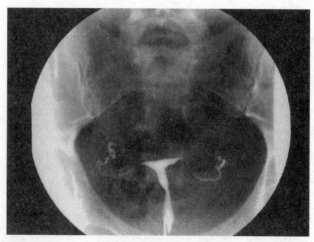

FIG. 59-1   Hysterosalpingogram demonstrating a normal uterine cavity and normal, patent fallopian tubes.

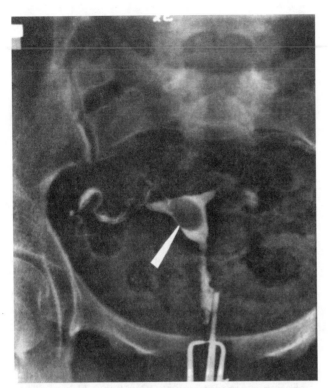

FIG. 59-2 Hysterosalpingogram demonstrating a large intrauterine filling defect (arrow). The filling defect was found to be a submucosal myoma. The fallopian tubes are patent.

- ○ Dye embolization
- ○ Salpingitis
- Cervical cultures should be performed before HSG. Patients who test positive for gonorrhea or chlamydial infection should be treated with appropriate antibiotics.
- HSG can detect uterine abnormalities such as:
  - ○ Submucous leiomyoma
  - ○ Congenital anomaly—eg, unicornuate or bicornuate uterus, uterine didelphys, uterine septum
  - ○ Polyps
  - ○ Intrauterine synechiae (Asherman's syndrome)
- Many intrauterine abnormalities can be treated with hysteroscopic resection.
- HSG also can identify tubal abnormalities such as the following:
  - ○ Salpingitis isthmica nodosa (tubal diverticulitis)
  - ○ Tubal tuberculosis (rare in the United States)
  - ○ Proximal or distal occlusion
  - ○ Pelvic adhesions
- HSG is a good screening tool but may miss 20 to 30 percent of abnormalities detected at laparoscopy.
- Any abnormality found on HSG should be evaluated by laparoscopy or hysteroscopy.
- Treatment options may include tubal surgery, tubal reconstruction, or **in vitro fertilization** (IVF). In the case of severely damaged tubes, IVF is the best option.

CERVICAL FACTOR

- Conditions within the cervix, leading to abnormal cervical mucus, can contribute to infertility, but they are rarely the sole cause.
- **The postcoital test** (PCT) is used to determine whether there is a cervical factor.
- The PCT is done by collecting cervical mucus 4 to 12 h after midcycle intercourse. The quality, quantity, and clarity of the cervical mucus are assessed. At least five forwardly motile sperm should be seen.
- Many specialists do not routinely perform the PCT because its value in guiding treatment has not been proven.

PELVIC FACTOR/ENDOMETRIOSIS

- A history suggesting endometriosis includes pelvic pain, dyspareunia, dysmenorrhea, and infertility.
- Forty percent of women with infertility and no other symptoms will have endometriosis at laparoscopy.
- Laparoscopy, with direct visual examination of the pelvis, is the only method available for specific diagnosis.
- Treatment of endometriosis should occur at the time of laparoscopy, even if only minimal disease is observed.
- Improved pregnancy rates with **assisted reproductive technologies** (ART) are noted when endometriosis is treated at the time of laparoscopy.
- The extent of tubal disease should be assessed at laparoscopy and a decision made as to whether treatment should be offered with **superovulation and intrauterine insemination** (SO/IUI) or IVF.

MATERNAL AGE AND OVARIAN RESERVE

- An age-related decline in fertility begins many years prior to menopause, despite continued regular cycles. Since many women delay childbearing into their thirties and forties, this problem has become increasingly evident.
- Ovarian reserve testing assesses a women's reproductive potential with respect to ovarian follicle number and oocyte quality.
- Testing is performed by measuring the serum concentration of FSH on day three of the cycle or by **clomid challenge testing** (CCT). The following patients should be screened:
  - ○ Age≥30 years
  - ○ Unexplained infertility

- Patients who respond poorly to initial treatment
- History of failed IVF
- Prior to IVF
- If results are abnormal, the best treatment is use of donor oocytes. The chance of conceiving with SO/IUI or IVF is only 5 percent.
- Fifteen percent of couples will have a negative work-up and be diagnosed with unexplained infertility. Treatment options include SO/IUI, IVF, or adoption.

TREATMENT OPTIONS

- Male-factor infertility may require consultation with a urologist. Other treatment options include the following:
  - Timed intrauterine insemination
  - Superovulation with gonadotropins and intrauterine insemination
  - Donor sperm insemination
  - IVF with or without the use of **intracytoplasmic sperm injection** (ICSI)
- IVF and ICSI are used in the case of a severe male factor. With ICSI, only one viable sperm for each egg is necessary.
- First-line therapy for ovulatory infertility is administration of ovulation-enhancing medications such as clomiphene citrate, human menopausal gonadotropins, or recombinant gonadotropins.
- **Clomiphene citrate** (CC) is an orally active antiestrogen that inhibits the negative feedback of endogenous estrogen on the hypothalamus, thus causing a rise in FSH and stimulation of follicular maturation.

Table 59-4 outlines the use of CC and other fertility medications.

- Eighty percent of anovulatory women will ovulate on CC, but only 60 percent will become pregnant. In women with polycystic ovary syndrome and hyperinsulinemia, metformin, 500 mg orally three times daily, may be added to improve the rate of ovulation.
- Women with anovulation due to hypothalamic amenorrhea, thyroid disease, or hyperprolactinemia require treatment of their underlying condition.
- Contraindications to CC include pregnancy, liver disease, and a history of visual changes with previous use.
- If patients fail to ovulate with CC or if they require superovulation and intrauterine insemination, gonadotropins should be used to induce ovulation.
- Gonadotropins are given at low doses in anovulatory patients to cause only one follicle to develop. In patients with other causes of infertility, slightly higher doses are administered to try to achieve multifollicular development.
- Gonadotropin cycles should be monitored with serial blood estradiol levels and transvaginal ultrasound. When follicles reach a size of 18 to 20 mm, human chorionic gonadotropin (hCG) 10,000 U is given to induce ovulation. Timed intercourse or washed intrauterine insemination follows. Pregnancy rates of 15 to 20 percent are usually possible.
- The two most frequent complications of infertility treatment are multiple pregnancy and **ovarian hyperstimulation syndrome** (OHSS). Couples must be counseled about the risks before treatment. Figure 59-3 demonstrates a transvaginal ultrasound view of 6-week twin gestational sacs resulting from IVF.

TABLE 59-4   Medications Used to Treat Infertility

MEDICATION	DOSING/ROUTE	RISKS	INDICATION
Clomiphene citrate (CC)	50 mg orally, days 3–7 or days 5–9 (max dose 250 mg)	5–10% multiple pregnancy <5% risk of ovarian hyperstimulation (OHSS)	Anovulation
Gonadotropins hMG—human menopausal gonadotropins (contain LH/FSH)	75-IU vials given IM or SQ	15–40% multiple pregnancy 10% risk of OHSS	Anovulation— failed CC Superovulation and intrauterine insemination for unexplained endometriosis, mild male factor, tubal factor
Recombinant FSH	75 IU vials/ampules given SQ (max dose—6 ampules/day)	<1% chance of severe OHSS	IVF
Pulsatile gonadotropin-releasing hormone (GnRH)	Intravenous pump	Infection Failure to ovulate	Anovulation Hypothalamic dysfunction
Human chorionic gonadotropin	10,000 U SQ		Trigger ovulation or oocyte maturation in IVF

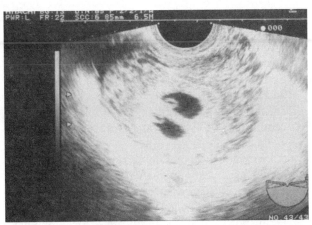

FIG. 59-3 A transvaginal ultrasound image with twin intrauterine gestational sacs resulting from in vitro fertilization.

- OHSS is characterized by ovarian enlargement and increased capillary permeability. Usually, OHSS is mild and self-limited, but it may be severe, resulting in hospitalization with ascites, pleural effusions, thromboembolic complications, adult respiratory distress syndrome, and even death. Cycles should be closely monitored to prevent this complication. Treatment depends on severity. Figure 59-4 illustrates ovarian hyperstimulation.

ASSISTED REPRODUCTIVE TECHNOLOGIES (ART)

- Assisted reproductive technologies are procedures that involve the handling of oocytes and embryos outside the body, with gametes or embryos replaced into the body to establish pregnancy.

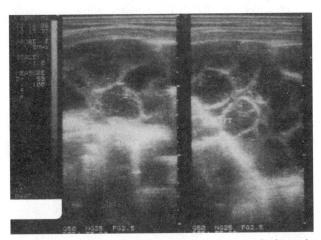

FIG. 59-4 Transvaginal ultrasound shows marked cystic enlargement of ovary following ovulation induction.

- IVF is the most frequently used procedure. It requires:
  - Ovarian stimulation with gonadotropins
  - Close monitoring with ultrasound and estradiol levels
  - Use of hCG to trigger oocyte maturation with 18- to 20-mm follicles
  - Transvaginal ultrasound-guided oocyte retrieval
  - Fertilization in the laboratory with standard insemination or ICSI
  - Transcervical embryo transfer 3 to 5 days after oocyte retrieval
- Indications for IVF include the following:
  - Tubal infertility
  - Endometriosis
  - Male infertility
  - Unexplained infertility
  - Failure to conceive with ovulation induction
- Pregnancy rates vary with age, with the best chances of conception being *about* 40 percent for women under 35 years of age.
- Complications of IVF include the following:
  - Infection
  - OHSS
  - Multiple pregnancy
  - Ectopic pregnancy
  - Increased risk of spontaneous abortion
- Other disadvantages of IVF are the high cost ($5,000 to $10,000 per cycle) and the great commitment of time and emotion.
- Women with diminished ovarian reserve or advanced reproductive age (>42 years) should be offered treatment with anonymous or nonanonymous oocyte donation. Pregnancy rates with any treatment other than oocyte donation are less than 5 percent per cycle.
- Conventional therapies result in conception in 50 to 60 percent of infertile couples. Despite the advances, not all couples will conceive.
- Participation in infertility evaluation and treatment can be among the most stressful and devastating experiences in a couple's life. Professional counseling should be offered to all infertility patients.

BIBLIOGRAPHY

American College of Obstetricians and Gynecologists. Infertility. Precis: An update in obstetrics and gynecology. *Reproductive Endocrinology,* 2nd ed. Washington, DC: ACOG, 2002:124–156.

Arul Kumaran S, ed. The management of subfertility. *Clin Obstet Gynecol* 2003;17(2):4,169–367.

Marcoux S, Maheux R, Berube S. Laparoscopic surgery in infertile women with minimal or mild endometriosis. Canadian Collaborative Group on Endometriosis. *N Engl J Med* 1997; 337:217–222.

60 MENOPAUSE

Alice Rhoton-Vlasak

DEFINITIONS

- **Physiologic menopause** is the cessation of menses for a minimum of 12 months due to cessation of follicular development. The median age of menopause is 51 years.
- **Perimenopause** is the period of time (approximately 4 years) between the onset of menopausal symptoms through the first year after cessation of menses.
- **Induced/surgical menopause** is the cessation of ovarian function brought about by surgical removal of the ovaries, radiation therapy, or chemotherapy.
- **Premature menopause (ovarian failure)** is the spontaneous cessation of menses before age 40. It occurs in 9.9 percent of women in the United States.
- **Postmenopause** is the phase of life that follows the menopause. Women in the United States are expected to live 35 years after they enter menopause.
- The **climacteric** is the phase of the aging process during which a woman passes from the reproductive to the nonreproductive stage of adulthood.

PHYSIOLOGY OF MENOPAUSE

- Menopause occurs due to the depletion of follicles from the ovary and a loss of oocyte responsiveness to gonadotropins.
- Human fetal ovaries develop by mitosis. There are 7 million oogonia by 20 weeks of gestation. Oocyte atresia begins before birth and continues throughout reproductive life, so that only 400 to 500 oocytes are actually ovulated. Menopause occurs when the oocytes are depleted and the ovaries are no longer responsive to pituitary gonadotropins.
- Typically, when women reach their forties, menstrual cycles begin to lengthen. The perimenopausal transition usually lasts 4 years. The median age of onset of the transition is 47.5 years.
- Hormonal changes associated with the transition include the following:
  - Increased serum concentration of follicle-stimulating hormone (FSH).
  - Increased serum concentration luteinizing hormone (LH).
  - Decreased ovarian production of inhibin.
  - Decreased ovarian production of estradiol.
  - Serum concentrations of estrone may increase as androstenedione from the ovary or adrenal gland is converted in peripheral fat to estrone. Serum concentrations of estrone are correlated with body weight.
  - Anovulation becomes more common in the perimenopausal years. Menstrual cycles become irregular, with occasional heavy menses and an increased risk of endometrial hyperplasia or cancer.
  - Perimenopausal women still are at risk for unexpected/unplanned pregnancy as fluctuations in ovarian function can occur.
  - The age of menopause is not influenced by marital status, height, weight, age of childbearing, or prolonged use of oral contraceptives. The age of menopause *is* affected by smoking.

CLINICAL CONSEQUENCES OF ESTROGEN LOSS

- Many symptoms occur as a result of estrogen loss in menopause. Estrogen deficiency also is associated with an increased risk of adverse changes such as osteoporosis (bone loss), cardiovascular disease, and Alzheimer's disease. Table 60-1 lists common clinical symptoms and consequences of estrogen loss in menopausal women.
  - Vasomotor symptoms occur in 80 percent of women and typically diminish in 1 to 2 years. The onset and severity of hot flashes is related to the rate of estrogen decline. Figure 60-1 outlines the events of the hot flash.
  - Menstrual disturbances are common in the perimenopausal and early postmenopausal years. Anovulation may lead to dysfunctional uterine bleeding that may be very heavy. Specific causes must be ruled out. Hormonal therapy (HT) should

TABLE 60-1 Clinical Symptoms Associated with Menopause

- Hot flashes/vasomotor symptoms
- Insomnia
- Anxiety/irritability
- Vaginal bleeding
- Poor concentration
- Mood changes
- Dyspareunia
- Vaginal dryness
- Loss of libido

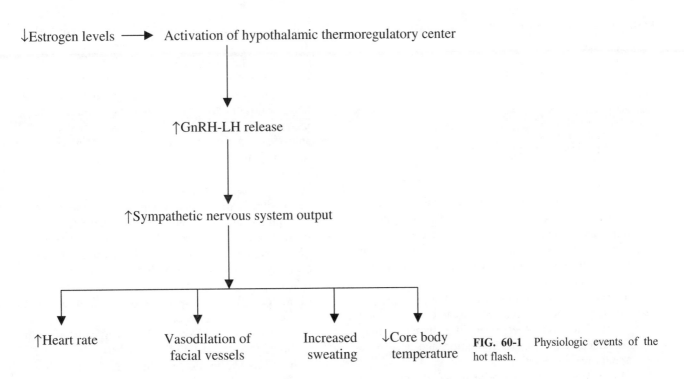

↓Estrogen levels ⟶ Activation of hypothalamic thermoregulatory center

↑GnRH-LH release

↑Sympathetic nervous system output

↑Heart rate   Vasodilation of facial vessels   Increased sweating   ↓Core body temperature

FIG. 60-1 Physiologic events of the hot flash.

not be given until the workup is complete. HT itself may cause abnormal bleeding.

○ Urogenital atrophy (vagina, urethra, and bladder trigone) may occur, leading to dyspareunia, vaginal irritation or dryness, or urinary incontinence. Urogenital atrophy responds well to oral, transdermal, or vaginal estrogen replacement therapy.

○ Osteoporosis.

■ Bone loss begins at age 28 and accelerates after menopause.

■ Osteoporosis is a systemic skeletal disease characterized by microarchitectural deterioration of bone tissue, which leads to reduced bone mass and enhanced bone fragility. Osteoporosis is responsible for 1.5 million fractures that occur in women over 50 years of age.

■ The most common fracture sites are as follows:
□ Lumbar vertebrae
□ Distal radius
□ Femoral neck

■ Osteoporotic fractures represent a major public health expenditure due to morbidity and mortality (16 percent in the first 3 to 4 months). Table 60-2 lists the risk factors for osteoporosis.

■ The best method to assess bone density is a **dual-energy x-ray absorptiometry** (DEXA) scan of the lumbar spine and dominant hip.

■ The World Health Organization has created a useful definition of osteoporosis based on bone den-

TABLE 60-2 Risk Factors for Osteoporosis

- Genetic (family history)
- Caucasian or Asian race
- Early menopause
- Chronic steroid use
- Dietary calcium and vitamin D deficiency
- Underweight
- Sedentary lifestyle
- Tobacco use
- Alcohol abuse

sity measurements. Bone density results are reported as T and Z scores. The T score is the number of standard deviations above or below age- and race-matched young controls. The Z score compares the patient with a population adjusted for age, gender, and race.

■ Normal bone mineral density is defined as a T score above −1.0 SD. Osteopenia is defined as a T score between −1.0 and −2.5 SD below the mean. Osteoporosis is defined as a T score less than −2.5 SD.

■ Oral and transdermal HT as well as bisphosphonates are effective for the prevention and treatment of osteoporosis.

• Cardiovascular disease

○ Cardiovascular disease, specifically coronary artery disease, is the most frequent cause of death in American women over age 50.

TABLE 60-3   Cardiovascular Effects of Estrogen

Lipid dependent:
- Increase high-density lipoprotein (HDL)
- Decrease low-density lipoprotein (LD)
- Decrease lipoprotein A
- Decrease LDL oxidation

Lipid independent:
- Retard atherosclerosis
- Restore vascular reactivity

○ Estrogen has both lipid-dependent and lipid-independent cardiovascular benefits. Table 60-3 outlines some cardioprotective effects of estrogen.
○ Adverse effects of menopause on cardiovascular risk are strongly correlated with weight gained during the menopausal transition.
○ Central nervous system and cognition
  - Estrogen has beneficial effects on cerebral blood flow. The loss of estrogen in menopause may enhance senile plaque formation and accelerate cognitive dysfunction.
  - Research indicates estrogen may influence areas of the brain important for memory. Studies continue to assess whether estrogens have a protective role in the prevention of dementia or of Alzheimer's disease.
  - Mood alterations include irritability, dysphoria, nervousness, and depression. Hypoestrogenism and social or psychological stresses may contribute to these changes.

EVALUATION

- Laboratory evaluation—such as determination of the serum concentrations of FSH, LH, and estradiol—usually is not indicated.
- Assessment of endometrial thickness or histology may be indicated in women with abnormal uterine bleeding.
- Routine care should include the following:
  ○ Yearly history and examination
  ○ Pap smear
  ○ Colon cancer screening with colonoscopy or flexible sigmoidoscopy
  ○ Breast cancer screening with mammography
  ○ Lipid assessment
  ○ TSH
  ○ DEXA scan for women at risk for osteoporosis

TREATMENT

- Many women will not require any treatment in the perimenopausal or menopausal period. Every woman with menopausal symptoms should be counseled about the physiologic nature of her symptoms.
- Typically, as long as regular uterine bleeding occurs, no treatment is usually required. If women complain of hot flashes while still having menstrual periods and there are no contraindications, treatment with low-dose oral contraceptive pills can be initiated.
- Before considering treatment, it is important to determine the magnitude of the patient's symptoms and her family history.
- Once a decision has been made to treat a postmenopausal patient, it is important to consider the risks and benefits of hormonal therapy, the route of administration, and whether other treatment options are available. Risks of HT (estrogen/progesterone used in a woman with a uterus) include the following:
  ○ Endometrial hyperplasia/cancer if on unopposed estrogen (20 percent per year).
  ○ Breast cancer—long-term use is associated with mildly increased risk (RR 1.2 to 1.5).
  ○ Thromboembolic disease is increased two to three-fold.
  ○ Gallbladder disease.
  ○ Exacerbation of liver disease.
  ○ Possible increased risk of heart attacks/strokes.
  ○ Abnormal bleeding.
  ○ Hypertriglyceridemia.
- Current indications for use of HT include the following:
  ○ Vasomotor symptoms
  ○ Urogenital atrophy
  ○ Prevention and treatment of osteoporosis
- Contraindications to HT include the following:
  ○ Vaginal bleeding of unknown cause
  ○ Suspected/known breast cancer
  ○ Endometrial cancer
  ○ History of thromboembolism
  ○ Chronic liver disease
  ○ Hypertriglyceridemia
- The benefits of HT include the following:
  ○ Relief of vasomotor symptoms
  ○ Prevention/treatment of osteoporosis
  ○ Relief of urogenital atrophy
  ○ Reduction in colon cancer risk
  ○ Reduction in macular degeneration and tooth loss
  ○ Possible prevention of Alzheimer's
- Women who have had a hysterectomy require treatment with estrogen replacement (ERT) only. Progestin is added only to protect the endometrium from unopposed estrogen.
- The contraindications to ERT and HT are the same. The Women's Health Initiative (a large multicenter U.S. trial on combination HT) suggests that the risks of heart attack, stroke, and breast cancer may be increased in women on combination HT.

- Women should receive the lowest possible doses of estrogen to relieve symptoms and prevent bone loss. Estrogen can be administered orally, transdermally, or intravaginally. Intravaginal estrogen is used to treat symptoms of urogenital atrophy.
- Side effects of estrogen may include breast tenderness, nausea, headache, and bloating.
- Progestin-induced side effects include breast tenderness, weight gain, bloating, and mood changes.
- Vaginal bleeding may occur with combination HT. It is more likely to occur with cyclic than continuous HT regimens. Evaluation should be undertaken if it is excessive or occurs at unexpected intervals.

TREATMENT REGIMENS

- Possible dosing schedules for combination HT include
  - Cyclic with estrogen days 1 to 25 and at least 12 days of progestin
  - Cyclic with daily estrogen and at least 12 days of progestin
- Options for endometrial protection include the following:
  - Cyclic progestin 10 to 12 days/month
  - Continuous daily progestin in combination with estrogen
  - Intermittent progestin every 3 to 4 days
  - Intrauterine progestin
  - Vaginal progesterone cream
- Table 60-4 outlines options for progestin use in combination with cyclic or continuous HT. Table 60-5 outlines options for use of estrogen in combination with progestins or alone in women without a uterus.
- Options for combination therapy for women desiring only one pill per day include the following:
  - Conjugated equine estrogen (CEE), 0.625 mg daily, and medroxyprogesterone acetate (MPA), 2.5 or 5 mg, daily

TABLE 60-5   Estrogens Available for Use Alone or in Combination with Progestin[a,b]

DRUG	ROUTE	DOSE
Conjugated equine estrogen	Oral	0.3, 0.625, 0.9, 1.5, and 2.5 mg
Piperazine estrone sulfate	Oral	0.625, 1.25, 2.5 mg
Micronized esterified	Oral	0.5, 1, 2 mg
Esterified	Oral	0.3, 0.625, 0.9, 1.25, 2.5 mg
Estradiol patch	Transdermal[c]	0.025, 0.0375, 0.05, 0.75, 0.1 mg/day
Conjugated equine estrogen cream (0.0625%)	Intravaginal	6-week course
Estradiol cream (0.01%)	Intravaginal	6-week course
Estradiol ring, 2 mg	Intravaginal	
Vaginal tablets	25 ng intravaginal	6-week course

[a] All except vaginal therapy will protect bone and relieve vasomotor symptoms.
[b] Unopposed daily estrogen should be used only in women without a uterus.
[c] Patch changed once or twice a week.

  - CEE (0.4 mg) and MPA (1.5 mg)
  - Estradiol (1 mg) and norethindrone acetate (0.9 mg) daily
  - Estradiol (1 mg) and norethindrone acetate (0.5 mg) daily
- A combination patch with estradiol (0.05 mg) and norethindrone acetate (140 or 250 mg) is also available
- All menopausal patients should be counseled about HT, but not every woman will choose to use hormones.
- If a patient does elect to start HT she should be seen for follow-up in 2 to 3 months. Therapy should be individualized for each woman.
- Menopausal patients also should be counseled about healthy lifestyle and should receive 1200 mg/day of calcium with vitamin D.
- In women with known osteopenia or osteoporosis, HT has been shown to increase BMD in the spine and hip.

TABLE 60-4   Progestin Dosing for Combination Hormonal Therapy

DRUG	ROUTE	CONTINUOUS DOSING	CYCLIC DOSING[a]
Medroxyprogesterone acetate (Provera)	Oral	2.5–5 mg daily	5–10 mg
Micronized[b] progesterone	Oral	100 mg daily	200–400 mg
Norethindrone	Oral	0.35 mg daily	0.35–0.70 mg
Norethindrone acetate	Oral	2.5 mg	2.5 mg daily
Progesterone gel 4–8%	Vaginal		4% gel twice weekly/vagina
Levonorgestrel intrauterine device (Mirena)	Intrauterine		Used for 5 years
Transdermal[c] norethindrone acetate	Skin patch		Patch changed twice weekly

[a] Administered 10–12 days/month
[b] Do not use in patients with peanut allergy. May cause somnolence.
[c] Available only in combination patch with estrogen.

- Alternatives to ERT for bone treatment or protection in women who will not or cannot take it include the following:
  - Bisphosphonates are antiresorptive agents. Alendronate and risidronate are available and can be administered once weekly. Both have been shown to reduce the incidence of spine and hip fractures.
  - Raloxifene is a selective estrogen receptor modulator. It has an estrogenic effect on bone, while having antiestrogenc effects on the uterus and breast. Raloxifene will worsen vasomotor symptoms.
- Alternative approaches for treatment of menopausal symptoms include the following:
  - Antidepressants such as venlafaxine or sertraline have been used to treat vasomotor symptoms.
  - Phytoestrogens, which are plant-derived estrogens, also have been used. Isoflavones are the most commonly used and are derived from soybeans and flax seed. Limited data show a possible improvement in vasomotor symptoms.

BIBLIOGRAPHY

American College of Obstetricians and Gynecologists. Menopause. Precis: *Reproductive Endocrinology,* 2nd ed. Washington, DC:ACOG, 2002:169–188.

Speroff L. *Managing Menopause: A Clinician's Guidebook.* Montvale, NJ: Thompson Medical Economics, 2002:1–155.

Women's Health Initiative Investigators. Risks and benefits of estrogen plus progestin in healthy postmenopausal women. Principal results from the Women's Health Initiative Randomized Controlled Trial. *JAMA* 2002;288: 321–333.

61 CERVICAL CANCER

John D. Davis

EPIDEMIOLOGY

- In the United States, cervical cancer is the third most common malignancy of the female genital tract. In 2003, approximately 12,100 women were expected to be diagnosed with cervical cancer, and approximately 4100 of these were expected to die from the disease.
- Well-established risk factors for the development of cervical cancer include early onset of sexual activity, multiple sexual partners, human papillomavirus (HPV) infection, immunosupression (including infection with human immunodeficiency virus), and smoking.
- The incidence of invasive cervical cancer has steadily declined over the past half-century due to Papanicolaou screening and increased diagnosis of preinvasive lesions (see Chap, 32, "Cervical Cytology," for a discussion of preinvasive disease of the uterine cervix).

SYMPTOMS AND DIAGNOSIS

- Abnormal vaginal bleeding is the primary symptom experienced by women with cervical cancer. In particular, many such women experience postcoital bleeding. An ulcerative squamous cell carcinoma is pictured in Fig. 61-1.
- Simple biopsy of a suspicious cervical lesion is usually adequate for diagnosing cervical cancer. Loop electrosurgical excision or cone biopsy is usually not required to establish the diagnosis.

STAGING AND PROGNOSIS

- Staging for carcinoma of the cervix is shown in Table 61-1.
- Survival rates for patients with cervical cancer are shown in Table 61-2.

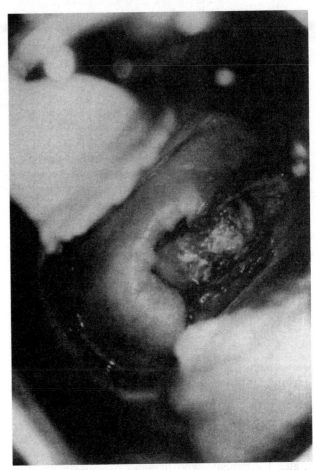

Figure 61-1 Ulcerative squamous cell carcinoma. (From DiSaia PJ, Creasman WT. Clinical Gynecologic Oncology, 4th ed. St. Louis: Mosby-Year Book, 1993: 67. With permission.)

TABLE 61-1   Staging for Carcinoma of the Cervix Uteri

Stage 0	Carcinoma in situ; intraepithelial carcinoma
Stage 1	The carcinoma is strictly confined to the cervix.
Stage IA	Invasive cancer is identified only microscopically. All gross lesions even with superficial invasion are stage IB cancers. Invasion is limited to measured stromal invasion with maximum depth of 5.0 mm and no wider than 7.0 mm.[a]
Stage IA1	Measured invasion of stroma is no greater than 3.0 mm in depth and no wider than 7.0 mm. [Stage IA should be divided into stage IA1 (those lesions with <3 mm of invasion visible only microscopically) and stage IA2 (macroscopically measurable 3- to 5-mm microcarcinomas)], in order to gain further knowledge of the clinical behavior of these lesions. The term *IB occult* should be based on microscopic examination of removed tissue, preferably a cone, which must include the entire lesion. The depth of invasion should not be more than 5 mm taken from the base of the epithelium, either surface or glandular, from which it originates. The second dimension, the horizontal spread, must not exceed 7 mm. Vascular space involvement, either venous or lymphatic, should not alter the staging but should be specifically recorded because it may affect treatment decisions in the future.
Stage IA2	Measured invasion of stroma is greater than 3 mm and no greater than 5 mm in depth and no wider than 7 mm.
Stage IB	Clinical lesions are confined to the cervix or preclinical lesions greater than stage IA. Lesions of greater size should be classified as stage IB. As a rule, it is impossible to estimate clinically whether a cancer of the cervix has extended to the corpus or not. Extension to the corpus should therefore be disregarded.
Stage IB1	Clinical lesions are no greater than 4.0 cm in size.
Stage IB2	Clinical lesions are greater than 4 cm in size.
Stage II	The carcinoma extends beyond the cervix but has not extended to the pelvic wall. The carcinoma involves the vagina but not as far as the lower third. A patient with a growth fixed to the pelvic wall by a short and indurated but not nodular parametrium should be assigned to stage IIB.
Stage IIA	There is no obvious parametrial involvement.
Stage IIB	There is obvious parametrial involvement.
Stage III	The carcinoma has extended to the pelvic wall. On rectal examination, there is no cancer-free space between the tumor and the pelvic wall. It is impossible, at clinical examination, to decide whether a smooth and indurated parametrium is truly cancerous or only inflammatory. Therefore the case should be placed in stage III only if the parametrium is nodular on the pelvic wall or if the growth itself extends to the pelvic wall. The presence of hydronephrosis or nonfunctioning kidney due to stenosis of the ureter by cancer permits a case to be assigned to stage III even if, according to the other findings, the case should be assigned to stage I or stage II. The tumor involves the lower third of the vagina. All cases with a hydronephrosis or nonfunctioning kidney are included unless they are known to be due to other causes.
Stage IIIA	There is no extension to the pelvic wall.
Stage IIIB	There is extension to the pelvic wall and/or hydronephrosis or nonfunctioning kidney.
Stage IV	The carcinoma has extended beyond the true pelvis or has clinically involved the mucosa of the bladder or rectum. The presence of bullous edema, as such, should not permit a case to be assigned to stage IV. Ridges and furrows in the bladder wall should be interpreted as signs of submucous involvement of the bladder if they remain fixed to the growth during palpation (ie, examination from the vagina or the rectum during cystoscopy). A finding of malignant cells in cytologic washings from the urinary bladder requires further examination and a biopsy from the wall of the bladder.
Stage IVA	There is spread of the growth to adjacent organs.
Stage IVB	There is spread to distant organs.

[a]The depth of invasion should not be more than 5 mm taken from the base of the epithelium, either surface or glandular, from which it originates. Vascular space involvement, either venous or lymphatic, should not alter staging.

Source: Modified from International Federation of Gynecology and Obstetrics. *Annual Report on the Results of Treatment in Gynecological Cancer*, 22nd ed. Stockholm: FIGO, 1994.

TABLE 61-2   Approximate 5-Year Survival Rates for Cancer of the Cervix by Stage and Treatment

STAGE	TREATMENT	5-YEAR SURVIVAL (%)
IA1	Surgery	98
IA2	Surgery	98
IB1	Surgery or irradiation	90
IB2	Surgery or irradiation	73
IIA	Irradiation	83
IIA	Surgery	78
IIB	Irradiation	67
IIIA	Irradiation	45
IIIB	Irradiation	36
IVA	Irradiation	14

- Several factors are associated with lower survival rates for patients who undergo radical surgery for invasive cervical cancer. These include lymph node involvement, lesion size >2 cm, lymphatic or vascular space involvement, depth of tumor invasion >1 cm, and small-cell histologic type.

TREATMENT

- Patients with stage IA1 disease have a less than 1 percent risk of lymph node metastases and therefore may be treated with a simple extrafascial hysterectomy. Women who desire future fertility may be treated with a cone biopsy and delay hysterectomy until childbearing is complete.
- Patients with stage IA2 disease have approximately a 5 percent risk of lymph node involvement. Patients with stage IA1 disease with lymphatic or vascular space involvement also are at higher risk for nodal spread. These patients should undergo

radical hysterectomy and pelvic lymphadenectomy (radical hysterectomy involves removal of the uterus, cervix, upper third of the vagina, and the parametrial tissue). Figure 61-2 shows a gross specimen from a patient who underwent a radical hysterectomy.

- Patients with stages IB1, IB2, and IIA disease may be treated with either radical hysterectomy or radiation therapy. Benefits of surgical therapy in patients who are good operative candidates include preservation of ovarian and vaginal function as well as avoidance of long-term complications of radiation therapy (including skin changes, vaginal stenosis, radiation proctitis, and fistula formation).

- Patients with higher-stage disease (IIB, III, and IV) should be treated with radiation therapy. Treatment usually consists of external-beam irradiation to shrink

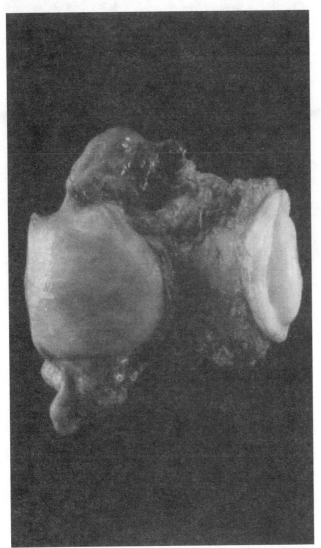

Figure 61-2 Radical hysterectomy specimen. (Courtesy of Robin Foss, Department of Pathology, University of Florida College of Medicine.)

the tumor and treat regional lymph nodes and intra-cavitary brachytherapy directed at the central tumor.

- There is good evidence that patients who receive radiation therapy for cervical cancer, either as primary treatment or as postoperative adjunctive therapy, have lower mortality if they receive platinum-based chemotherapy along with the radiation therapy.

BIBLIOGRAPHY

American College of Obstetricians and Gynecologists. Cervical neoplasia. In: *Precis, Oncology An Update in Obstetrics and Gynecology.* Washington, DC: ACOG, 1998:26–30.

American College of Obstetricians and Gynecologists. *Concurrent Chemoradiation in the Treatment of Cervical Cancer.* ACOG Committee Opinion #242. Washington, DC: ACOG, October 2000.

Hatch K. Cervical cancer. In: Berek JS, Hacker NF, eds. *Practical Gynecologic Oncology.* Baltimore: Williams & Wilkins, 1994:243–284.

Kim RY, Alvarez RD, Omura GA. Advances in the treatment of gynecologic malignancies. *Oncology* 2002;16:1510–1517.

62 ENDOMETRIAL CANCER

John D. Davis

EPIDEMIOLOGY

- Endometrial cancer is the most common female genital tract malignancy. In 2003, approximately 40,000 women were expected to be diagnosed with carcinoma of the endometrium and approximately 6800 of these were expected to die from the disease.

- The incidence of endometrial cancer peaks during the sixth decade of life; however, nearly 25 percent of women diagnosed with endometrial carcinoma are premenopausal.

- Risk factors for endometrial cancer are listed in Table 62-1.

- There are two distinct phenotypes of endometrial cancer. One is related to excess estrogen exposure and

TABLE 62-1   Risk Factors for Endometrial Cancer

Unopposed estrogen use
Late menopause
Obesity
Nulliparity
Tamoxifen therapy for breast cancer

occurs in patients with the above risk factors. Such patients tend to have well-differentiated tumors and high survival rates. The second phenotype tends to occur in thin, multiparous African-American women; these patients have much more aggressive tumors and lower long-term survival rates.

ENDOMETRIAL HYPERPLASIA

- Endometrial hyperplasia is classified as simple or complex, with or without atypia.
- Histopathologically, simple hyperplasia describes an endometrium with dilated glands and abundant stroma (Fig. 62-1). With complex hyperplasia, the glands are crowded with little intervening stroma (Fig. 62-2).
- Histopathologic changes associated with atypia include nuclear pleomorphism and an increase in the nuclear-to-cytoplasmic ratio (Fig. 62-3).
- Patients with complex hyperplasia with atypia have approximately a 25 percent chance of developing

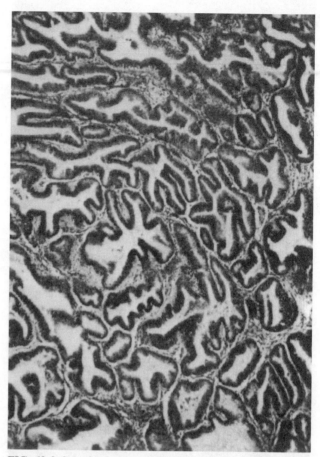

FIG. 62-2 Complex hyperplasia without atypia. (From Kurman RJ. *Blaustein's Pathology of the Female Genital Tract*, 3rd ed. New York: Springer-Verlag, 1987:325. With permission.)

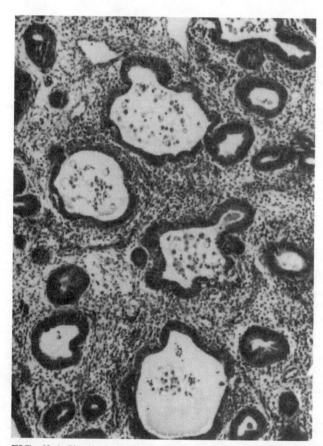

FIG. 62-1 Simple hyperplasia. (From Kurman RJ. *Blaustein's Pathology of the Female Genital Tract*, 3rd ed. New York: Springer-Verlag, 1987:324. With permission.)

invasive cancer. The risk of a patient with endometrial hyperplasia without atypia developing cancer is only 1 to 2 percent.
- Endometrial hyperplasia may be diagnosed by sampling of the endometrium in an outpatient setting. If an endometrial biopsy demonstrates atypical changes, a complete dilation and curettage is indicated to rule out an underlying malignancy.
- Women of any age group who have hyperplasia without atypia may be treated with moderate doses of progestins (for example, medroxyprogesterone acetate 10 mg orally for 10 days of each month, or oral contraceptive pills).
- Reproductive-age women who have hyperplasia with atypia and who desire future childbearing should be treated with more potent progestins (for example, megestrol 40 mg orally once daily).
- Women with hyperplasia who are treated medically should undergo repeat endometrial sampling after 3 to 6 months of therapy to ensure that the hyperplastic changes have regressed.

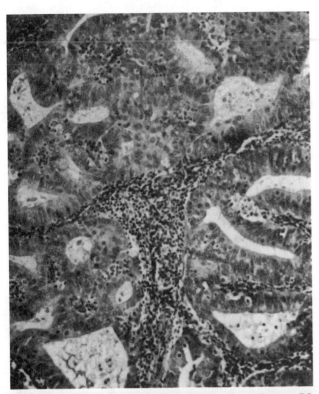

FIG. 62-3 Complex hyperplasia with atypia. (From Kurman RJ. *Blaustein's Pathology of the Female Genital Tract*, 3rd ed. New York: Springer-Verlag, 1987:326. With permission.)

- Medications to induce ovulation may be required for women with successfully treated hyperplasia who wish to conceive.
- Postmenopausal women who have hyperplasia with atypia have approximately a 25 percent chance of having an underlying carcinoma. Such women should undergo hysterectomy and bilateral salpingo-oophorectomy if their medical condition permits.

SYMPTOMS AND DIAGNOSIS

- Postmenopausal bleeding is the classic symptom of endometrial cancer. In pre- and perimenopausal women, abnormal uterine bleeding may signal the presence of malignancy.
- In addition to endometrial cancer, postmenopausal bleeding may be caused by endometrial hyperplasia, other reproductive tract malignancies, endometrial polyps or fibroids, or atrophy of the endometrium or the lower genital tract.
- Transvaginal ultrasound measurements of the endometrial stripe have been used to rule out malignancy (endometrial hyperplasia or cancer is rarely found when the endometrial stripe measures

<5 mm); however, the diagnosis of endometrial cancer is usually made by biopsy of the endomerium.

STAGING AND PROGNOSIS

- Endometrial cancer is staged surgically. The staging system for endometrial cancer developed by the International Federation of Gynecology and Obstetrics (FIGO) is shown in Table 62-2. Figure 62-4 shows a gross specimen of an endometrial carcinoma.
- Table 62-3 shows the 5-year survival rates for endometrial cancer by stage.

TABLE 62-2 Staging for Carcinoma of the Corpus Uteri

Stage 1A G 1, 2, 3	Tumor limited to endometrium
Stage 1B G 1, 2, 3	Invasion to less than one half of the myometrium
Stage 1C G 1, 2, 3	Invasion to more than one half of the myometrium
Stage IIA G 1, 2, 3	Endocervical glandular involvement only
Stage IIB G 1, 2, 3	Cervical stromal invasion
Stage IIIA G 1, 2, 3	Tumor invades serosa and/or adnexa, and/or positive peritoneal cytology
Stage IIIB G 1, 2, 3	Vaginal metastases
Stage IIIC G 1, 2, 3	Metastases to pelvic and/or paraaortic lymph nodes
Stage IVA G 1, 2, 3	Tumor invasion of bladder and/or bowel mucosa
Stage IVB	Distant metastases including intraabdominal and/or inguinal lymph nodes

Histopathology—Degree of Differentiation

Cases of carcinoma of the corpus should be classified (or graded) according to the degree of histologic differentiation as follows:
G1 = 5% or less of a nonsquamous or nonmorular solid growth pattern
G2 = 6–50% of a nonsquamous or nonmorular solid growth pattern
G3 = more than 50% of a nonsquamous or nonmorular solid growth pattern

Notes on Pathologic Grading

1. Notable nuclear atypia, inappropriate for the architectural grade, raises the grade of a grade 1 or grade 2 tumor by 1.
2. In serous adenocarcinomas, clear-cell adenocarcinomas, and squamous cell carcinomas, nuclear grading takes precedence.
3. Adenocarcinomas with benign squamous differentiation are graded according to the nuclear grade of the glandular component.

Rules Related to Staging

1. Because corpus cancer is now staged surgically, procedures previously used for determination of stages are no longer applicable, such as the findings from fractional dilation and curettage to differentiate between stage I and stage II.
2. It is appreciated that there may be a small number of patients with corpus cancer who will be treated primarily with radiation therapy. If that is the case, the clinical staging adopted by FIGO in 1971 would still apply, but designation of that staging system would be noted.
3. Ideally, width of the myometrium should be measured along with the width of tumor invasion.

SOURCE: Modified from International Federation of Gynecology and Obstetrics. *Annual Report on the Results of Treatment in Gynecological Cancer*. 22d ed. Stockholm: FIGO 1994.

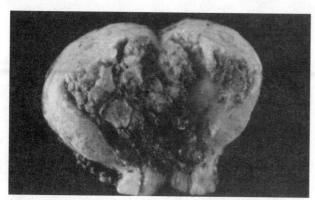

FIG. 62-4 Endometrial cancer (gross specimen). (Courtesy of Robin Foss, Department of Pathology, University of Florida College of Medicine.)

TABLE 62-3   Approximate 5-Year Survival Rates for Endometrial Cancer by Stage

STAGE	5-YEAR SURVIVAL
I	86%
II	66%
III	44%
IV	16%

- The overall survival rate for all patients with endometrial cancer is just over 70 percent.
- Poor prognostic characteristics for patients with endometrial cancer include older age, deep myometrial invasion, poorly differentiated tumor, and advanced surgical stage. Papillary serous- and clear-cell tumor types are associated with a poorer prognosis.

TREATMENT

- The standard surgical staging procedure for patients with endometrial carcinoma includes exploratory laparotomy, abdominal and pelvic washings, complete inspection of the abdomen and removal of any suspicious lesions, total abdominal hysterectomy, bilateral salpingo-oophorectomy, and pelvic and paraaortic lymphadenectomy. In addition, patients with papillary serous- or clear-cell tumor types should undergo omentectomy.
- Surgical staging also may be done laparoscopically, combining laparoscopic assessment of the abdomen and pelvis and laparoscopic lymphadenectomy with vaginal hysterectomy and bilateral salpingo-oophorectomy.
- The indications for lymph node sampling and its extent in patients with presumed early-stage endometrial cancer are controversial. Some authors argue that patients with well-differentiated, superficially invasive tumors should not undergo lymphadenectomy because of the low risk (4 percent) of nodal metastases and the morbidity associated with the lymphadenectomy. Others note the safety of lymphadenectomy when it is performed by an experienced surgeon in a patient who is a good surgical candidate, the potential inaccuracy of preoperative or intraoperative identification of patients at low risk for metastatic disease, and the mounting evidence that survival rates are higher for patients who undergo complete lymphadenectomy.
- Patients with stage I disease at low risk for recurrence (well-differentiated tumor confined to the inner half of the myometrium) require no further therapy.
- Patients with stage I disease at high risk for recurrence (poorly differentiated tumor with deep myometrial invasion) should receive pelvic radiation to reduce the risk of local and distant recurrence.
- Adjuvant treatment for patients determined to have stage II disease has not been studied extensively. The majority of these patients are treated with pelvic irradiation.
- The treatment of patients with stage III or IV endometrial cancer must be individualized. Therapy usually involves surgical resection and radiation. High-dose progestin therapy can be effective for patients with metastatic disease, especially with well-differentiated tumors. Systemic chemotherapy has been used to treat patients with advanced disease, but response rates are low.

BIBLIOGRAPHY

American College of Obstetricians and Gynecologists. Cancer of the uterine corpus. In: *Precis, Oncology: An Update in Obstetrics and Gynecology.* Washington, DC: ACOG, 1998:31–37.

Huh WK, Straughn JM Jr, Kelly FH, Kilgore LC. Endometrial carcinoma. *Curr Treat Options Oncol* 2001; 2:129–135.

Levine DA, Hoskins WJ. Update in the management of endometrial cancer. *Cancer J* 2002; 8:S31–S40.

63   CANCER OF THE FALLOPIAN TUBE

John D. Davis

EPIDEMIOLOGY

- Cancer of the fallopian tube is the least common malignancy of the female genital tract, accounting for less than 1 percent of all gynecologic cancers.
- The mean age of patients with fallopian tube cancer is 55 to 60 years.

- Fallopian tube cancers most frequently arise from the epithelium of the tube and have a serous histology.
- The etiology of fallopian tube cancer is uncertain.

SYMPTOMS

- The most common symptoms and signs of tubal carcinoma are abnormal bleeding, pelvic pain, and a pelvic mass.
- The classic triad of symptoms and signs includes a profuse watery vaginal discharge (hydrops tubae profluens), pelvic pain, and a pelvic mass. Less than 15 percent of women with fallopian tube cancer have this constellation of findings.

DIAGNOSIS

- The diagnosis of fallopian tube carcinoma is rarely made preoperatively. Some tubal cancers have been identified preoperatively by transvaginal ultrasound with Doppler; however, most of these tumors are identified at the time of hysterectomy and bilateral salpingo-oophorectomy.
- It can be difficult to distinguish primary fallopian tube cancer from primary ovarian carcinoma. The pathologic criteria for diagnosing primary fallopian tube cancer include the following:
  ○ The main tumor is located in the tube and arises from the endosalpinx.
  ○ The histologic pattern of the tumor is mucosal tubal epithelium.
  ○ If the tubal wall is involved, the transition from benign to malignant epithelium must be present.
  ○ The endometrium and ovaries are either normal or contain less tumor than the tubes.

STAGING AND PROGNOSIS

- Since the International Federation of Gynecology and Obstetrics (FIGO) has no official staging system for cancer of the fallopian tube, the staging system for tubal carcinoma used here is adapted from the FIGO staging system for ovarian cancer and is shown in Table 63-1.
- The 5-year survival rates for patients with cancer of the fallopian tube are shown in Table 63-2.
- Since most tubal carcinomas are occult and not identified until the surgical specimen is examined histopathologically, many patients with fallopian tube cancer do not undergo complete surgical staging. Thus, patients with apparent stage I disease actually may have occult advanced disease, accounting for the apparently low survival rate for patients categorized in stage I.

TABLE 63-1 Staging of Fallopian Tube Carcinoma

Stage 0	Carcinoma in situ (limited to tubal mucosa).
Stage I	Growth limited to the fallopian tube.
Stage Ia	Growth limited to one tube with extension into the submucosa and/or muscularis but not penetrating the serosal surface; no ascites.
Stage Ib	Growth is limited to both tubes with extension to submucosa and/or muscularis but not penetrating the serosal surface; no ascites.
Stage Ic	Tumor either stage Ia or Ib but with extension through or onto the tubal serosa, or with ascites containing malignant cells or with positive peritoneal washing.
Stage II	Growth involving one or both fallopian tubes with pelvic extension.
Stage IIa	Extension or metastasis to the uterus and/or ovaries.
Stage IIb	Extension to other pelvic tissues.
Stage IIc	Tumor either stage IIa or IIb but with extension through or onto the tubal serosa, or with ascites containing malignant cells or with positive peritoneal washing.
Stage III	Tumor involving one or both fallopian tubes with peritoneal implants outside of the pelvis and/or positive retroperitoneal or inguinal lymph nodes; superficial liver metastasis; tumor limited to the pelvis but with histologically proven malignant extension to the small bowel or omentum.
Stage IIIa	Tumor grossly limited to true pelvis with negative nodes and with histologically confirmed microscopic seeding of the abdominal peritoneal surface.
Stage IIIb	Tumor involving one or both tubes with histologically confirmed implants of abdominal peritoneal surfaces and not exceeding 2 cm in diameter; lymph nodes negative.
Stage IIIc	Abdominal implants more than 2 cm in diameter and/or positive retroperitoneal or inguinal nodes.
Stage IV	Growth involving one or both tubes with distant metastases; if pleural effusion is present, there must be positive cytology to be stage IV; parenchymal liver metastasis equals stage IV.

TABLE 63-2 Approximate 5-Year Survival Rates for Fallopian Tube Cancer by Stage

STAGE	5-YEAR SURVIVAL
I	65%
II	50–60%
III	10–20%
IV	10–20%

- The overall 5-year survival rate for patients with fallopian tube cancer is approximately 40 percent.

TREATMENT

- The treatment of patients with fallopian tube cancer is similar to that of patients with epithelial ovarian cancer: complete surgical staging, including peritoneal washings, total abdominal hysterectomy, bilateral salpingo-oophorectomy, omentectomy, peritoneal sampling, and pelvic and paraaortic lymphadenectomy, followed by combination platinum-based chemotherapy.

BIBLIOGRAPHY

Gadducci A. Current management of fallopian tube carcinoma. *Curr Opin Obstet Gynecol* 2002;14:27–32.

Nikrui N, Duska LR. Fallopian tube carcinoma. *Surg Oncol Clin North Am* 1998;7:363–373.

64 OVARIAN CANCER

John D. Davis

EPIDEMIOLOGY

- Ovarian cancer is the second most common malignancy of the female genital tract, following endometrial cancer. However, ovarian cancer causes more deaths than any other reproductive tract malignancy. In 2003, approximately 25,000 women were expected to be diagnosed with ovarian cancer, and approximately 14,000 of these women were expected to die from the disease.
- The etiology of ovarian cancer is not known. Risk factors include nulliparity, late menopause, delayed childbearing, use of talcum powder on the perineum, family history of ovarian cancer (especially in first-degree relatives), personal history of breast or colon cancer, consumption of a high-fat diet, and residence in North America or western Europe. Oral contraceptive use provides at least some protection against ovarian cancer.
- A woman's lifetime risk of developing ovarian cancer is 1 to 2 percent. Most cases of ovarian cancer are sporadic; fewer than 5 percent are hereditary.
- There are three inherited syndromes that increase a woman's likelihood of developing ovarian cancer:
  - **Site-specific familial ovarian cancer.** The risk of a woman with this syndrome developing ovarian cancer depends on the number of affected first-degree (mother, sister, daughter) and second-degree (grandmother, aunt, first cousin, granddaughter) relatives; it is listed in Table 64-1.
  - **Breast/ovarian familial cancer syndrome.** These women carry the BRCA 1 or BRCA 2 gene and are at increased risk of developing breast and ovarian

cancer. Some 20 to 40 percent of women with the BRCA 1 gene will develop ovarian cancer, while 10 to 20 percent of those with the BRCA 2 gene will develop the disease.
  - **Lynch II syndrome.** Women with this syndrome are at increased risk for developing colon, ovarian, endometrial, and breast cancer.

TABLE 64-1   Risk of Site-Specific Ovarian Cancer

AFFECTED RELATIVE(S)	RISK OF DEVELOPING OVARIAN CANCER
Single first-degree relative	Two-to-fourfold increased risk
Single first-degree relative and single second-degree relative	Three-to-tenfold risk
Two first-degree relatives	50%

SCREENING

- Bimanual examination, pelvic ultrasound, and serum measurements of CA 125 have been used to screen for ovarian cancer. Unfortunately, none of these methods is effective for routine screening of the general population.
- Pelvic ultrasound, especially transvaginal ultrasound, is effective in identifying ovarian abnormalities; however, the majority of abnormalities identified are benign. This lack of specificity results in unnecessary surgical procedures and precludes the use of ultrasound as a screening tool.
- CA 125 is a glycoprotein found on the surface of epithelial cells of tissue derived from coelomic epithelium. Epithelial cells lining the fallopian tube, endometrium, endocervix, peritoneum, pleura, pericardium, and bronchus all normally produce CA 125.
- The use of CA 125 measurements for screening is limited by the poor sensitivity of the test; the test is abnormal in only 50 percent of patients with stage I disease.
- In addition, this test has a high false-positive rate, especially in reproductive-age females. Other causes of elevated CA 125 levels are listed in Tables 64-2 and 64-3.

Table 64-2   Cancers That May Cause Elevated Serum Concentration of CA 125

GYNECOLOGIC CANCERS	NONGYNECOLOGIC CANCERS
Epithelial ovarian cancer	Pancreatic cancer
Some germ-cell tumors	Lung cancer
Some stromal tumors	Breast cancer
Fallopian tube cancer	Colon Cancer
Endometrial cancer	
Endocervical cancer	

TABLE 64-3 Benign Conditions That May Cause Elevated Serum Concentration of CA 125

GYNECOLOGIC CONDITIONS	NONGYNECOLOGIC CONDITIONS
Endometriosis	Pancreatitis
Adenomyosis	Cirrhosis
Leiomyomata uteri	Passive liver congestion
Ectopic pregnancy	Peritonitis
Normal pregnancy	Peritoneal tuberculosis
Pelvic inflammatory disease	Peritoneal sarcoidosis
Menses	Recent laparotomy

HISTOLOGY

- Ovarian tumors may develop from the epithelium lining the ovary (epithelial tumors), the germinal epithelium (germ-cell tumors), or the mesenchyme of the ovary (sex-cord/stromal tumors). In addition, other malignancies may metastasize to the ovary.
- Epithelial, germ-cell, and sex-cord/stromal tumors account for approximately 85, 10, and 5 percent of primary ovarian tumors, respectively. Approximately 50 percent of all epithelial tumors are of the serous type (Fig. 64-1).

- The classification of primary ovarian tumors is given in Table 64-4.

TABLE 64-4 Classification of Ovarian Tumors

Epithelial
  Serous
  Mucinous
  Endometrioid
  Clear-cell
  Transitional-cell (Brenner tumor)
  Mixed epithelial-cell
Germ-cell tumors
  Dysgerminoma
  Yolk sac tumor
  Embryonal carcinoma
  Polyembryoma
  Choriocarcinoma
  Teratomas
Sex-cord/stromal tumors
  Granulosa-stromal cell tumors
  Granulosa cell tumor
  Thecoma-fibroma
  Sertoli–stromal-cell tumors
  Gynandroblastoma
  Steroid- (lipid) cell tumors

- Tumors of low malignant potential, also known as borderline tumors, are a variant of epithelial tumors that grow more slowly and have a better prognosis than frankly invasive cancers.
- Germ-cell tumors occur most commonly in premenarchial and young reproductive-age women. The most common germ-cell tumor is the mature cystic teratoma (Figs. 64-2 and 64-3).
- Granulosa-cell tumors account for more than 90 percent of malignant sex-cord/stromal tumors.
- The tumors that most frequently metastasize to the ovaries arise from the endometrium, breast, and stomach.

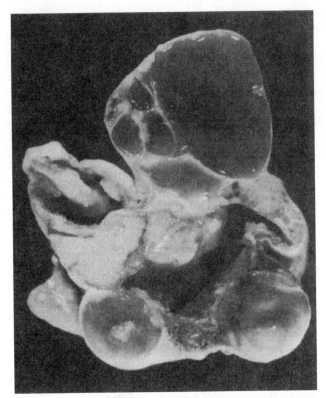

FIG. 64-1 Cut surface of a serous cystadenocarcinoma with cystic, papillary, and solid areas. (From Kurman RJ. *Blaustein's Pathology of the Female Genital Tract,* 3rd ed. New York: Springer-Verlag, 1987:571. With permission.)

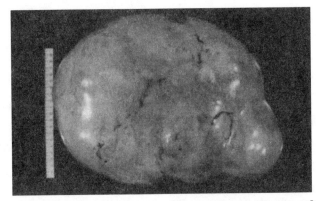

FIG. 64-2 Mature cystic teratoma (gross specimen). (Courtesy of Robin Foss, Department of Pathology, University of Florida College of Medicine.)

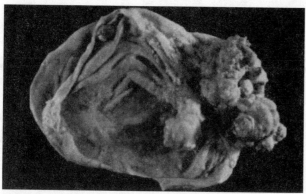

FIG. 64-3 Mature cystic teratoma, sectioned (gross specimen). The nodular growth in the specimen is called Rokitansky's protuberance. (Courtesy of Robin Foss, Department of Pathology, University of Florida College of Medicine.)

PRESENTATION AND DIAGNOSIS

- Most patients with ovarian cancer are not diagnosed until they have advanced disease. Factors that contribute to the delayed diagnosis of ovarian cancer include the intraabdominal location of the ovaries and the nonspecific symptoms experienced by women with the disease.
- Women with advanced-stage ovarian cancer may experience abdominal distention, bloating, early satiety, anorexia, nausea, and constipation.
- While the diagnosis of ovarian cancer is usually made by the histologic evaluation of tissue obtained during surgical exploration, imaging studies and serum tumor markers can be used to identify patients more likely to have a malignant pelvic mass.
- Pelvic ultrasound and CT scan can be used to evaluate patients suspected of having ovarian cancer. Ultrasound findings that may be associated with a malignancy are listed in Table 64-5.
- Serum tumor markers that may be elevated in patients with ovarian malignancies are listed in Table 64-6.

STAGING AND PROGNOSIS

- Ovarian cancer is staged surgically. A staging laparotomy is usually performed through a vertical midline incision and includes collection of ascitic fluid or

TABLE 64-5 Ultrasound Characteristics of Ovarian Malignancy

Large size
Thick septations
Solid components
Papillations or excrescences
Bilateral
Associated ascites
Low impedance to flow (Doppler)

TABLE 64-6 Serum Tumor Markers Associated with Ovarian Malignancies

TUMOR	MARKER
Epithelial	CA 125
Endodermal sinus tumor	AFP
Embryonal carcinoma	AFP, hCG
Choriocarcinoma	hCG
Dysgerminoma	LDH

peritoneal washings for cytologic analysis, hysterectomy, bilateral salpingo-oophorectomy, omentectomy, pelvic and paraaortic lymph node sampling, diaphragmatic biopsies, and random peritoneal biopsies.
- The goal of surgery for ovarian cancer is "optimal reduction," which is defined as leaving no residual tumor >1 cm in size. Patients who have optimal cytoreduction have a more favorable prognosis than those who do not.
- The staging system for ovarian cancer is given in Table 64-7.
- The 5-year survival rates for patients with epithelial ovarian cancer are listed in Table 64-8.

TREATMENT

- The treatment of ovarian cancer depends on the stage and grade of disease and the overall health of the patient. For patients with stage I disease, their desire for future childbearing may influence management.
- The primary treatment for stage I ovarian cancer is a staging laparotomy, as described above.
- Patients with stage IA and B, grade 1 disease do not require postoperative chemotherapy.
- Patients with stage IA, grade 1 disease who desire future fertility may have their uterus and contralateral ovary preserved.
- Patients with stage IA and B, grade 2 or 3 disease and those with stage IC disease should receive 3 to 6 months of chemotherapy postoperatively.
- Patients with stage II, III, and IV disease should undergo complete surgical staging (with optimal cytoreduction if possible) and postoperative chemotherapy. Combination chemotherapy with cisplatin and paclitaxel is recommended for these patients.
- A second-look laparotomy is a procedure performed on a patient who has undergone a staging procedure and completed a course of chemotherapy and has no clinical evidence of residual disease.
- The purpose of a second-look laparotomy is to identify patients without residual disease who require no further therapy and those with persistent disease who may benefit from further chemotherapy.

TABLE 64-7 Staging for Carcinoma of the Ovary

Staging of ovarian carcinoma is based on findings at clinical examination and by surgical exploration. The histologic findings are to be considered in the staging, as are the cytologic findings as far as effusions are concerned. It is desirable that a biopsy be taken from suspicious areas outside of the pelvis.

Stage I	Growth is limited to the ovaries.
Stage IA	Growth is limited to one ovary; no ascites present containing malignant cells. There is no tumor on the external surface; capsule is intact.
Stage IB	Growth is limited to both ovaries; no ascites present containing malignant cells. There is no tumor on the external surfaces; capsules are intact.
Stage IC[a]	Tumor is classified as either stage IA or IB but with tumor on the surface of one or both ovaries; or with ruptured capsule(s); or with ascites containing malignant cells present or with positive peritoneal washings.
Stage II	Growth involves one or both ovaries, with pelvic extension.
Stage IIA	There is extension and/or metastases of the uterus and/or tubes.
Stage IIB	There is extension to other pelvic tissues.
Stage IIC[a]	Tumor is either stage IIA or IIB but with tumor on the surface of one or both ovaries; or with capsule(s) ruptured; or with ascites containing malignant cells present or with positive peritoneal washings.
Stage III	Tumor involves one or both ovaries with peritoneal implants outside the pelvis and/or positive retroperitoneal or inguinal nodes. Superficial liver metastasis equals stage III. Tumor is limited to the true pelvis but with histologically proven malignant extension to small bowel or omentum.
Stage IIIA	Tumor is grossly limited to the true pelvis with negative nodes but with histologically confirmed microscopic seeding of abdominal peritoneal surfaces.
Stage IIIB	Tumor involves one or both ovaries with histologically confirmed implants of abdominal peritoneal surfaces, none exceeding 2 cm in diameter; nodes are negative.
Stage IIIC	There are abdominal implants greater than 2 cm in diameter and/or positive retroperitoneal or inguinal nodes.
Stage IV	Growth involves one or both ovaries, with distant metastases. If pleural effusion is present, there must be positive cytologic findings to assign a case to stage IV. Parenchymal liver metastasis equals stage IV.

[a]To evaluate the impact on prognosis of the different criteria for assigning cases to stage IC or IIC, it would be of value to know whether the rupture of the capsule was spontaneous or caused by the surgeon and if the source of malignant cells detected was peritoneal washings or ascites.

Modified from International Federation of Gynecology and Obstetrics. *Annual Report on the Results of Treatment in Gynecological Cancer*, 22d ed. Stockholm: FIGO, 1994.

TABLE 64-8 Approximate 5-Year Survival Rates for Epithelial Ovarian Cancer by Stage

Stage IA, B: grade 1	95%
Stage IA, B: grades 2, 3, & IC	85%
Stage II	50–60%
Stage III A	30–40%
Stage III B	20%
Stage III C	5%
Stage IV	5%

- Second-look laparotomies do not influence survival of patients with ovarian cancer. Because of this, the procedure is not considered standard of care and is used primarily in clinical trials.

BIBLIOGRAPHY

American College of Obstetricians and Gynecologists. Cancer of the ovary and uterine tube. In: *Precis, Oncology: An Update in Obstetrics and Gynecology.* Washington, DC: ACOG, 1998:37–50.

Berek JS. Epithelial ovarian cancer. In: Berek JS, Hacker NF, eds. *Practical Gynecologic Oncology.* Baltimore: Williams & Wilkins, 1994:327–376.

Ozols RF. Update on the management of ovarian cancer. *Cancer J* 2002; 8:S22–S30.

65 VAGINAL CANCER

John D. Davis

EPIDEMIOLOGY

- Carcinoma of the vagina accounts for approximately 2 percent of all female genital cancers.
- The majority of women who develop vaginal cancer are over 60 years of age.
- Squamous cell carcinoma and adenocarcinoma account for 80 and 15 percent of cases of vaginal cancer respectively. The remaining types of vaginal malignancy include melanoma, clear-cell adenocarcinoma, lymphoma, and sarcoma.
- There is a strong association between squamous-cell cancer of the vagina and infection with human papillomavirus. There also is a strong correlation between vaginal cancer and a previous history of preinvasive or invasive cervical cancer.

PREINVASIVE DISEASE

- The average age of women with **vaginal intraepithelial neoplasia** (VAIN) is 10 to 20 years lower than that of women with invasive vaginal cancer.
- VAIN is frequently associated with past or current cervical or vulvar neoplasia.
- The vast majority of patients with VAIN are asymptomatic; the condition is typically identified by Papanicoulau smear.
- The diagnosis of VAIN is made by colposcopically directed vaginal biopsy of suspicious lesions. Application of a strong iodine solution to the vaginal

walls during the colposcopic examination can assist in the identification of abnormalities.

- Small, focal VAIN lesions may be treated with excisional biopsy. Larger lesions may be treated with wide local excision, upper vaginectomy, or laser ablation. Multifocal lesions may be treated with topical 5-fluorouracil cream applied weekly for 10 weeks.

SYMPTOMS

- The most common symptoms experienced by women with vaginal cancer are abnormal bleeding and an abnormal vaginal discharge.
- Urinary tract symptoms, constipation, and pain may be present in patients with more advanced disease.

DIAGNOSIS, STAGING, AND PROGNOSIS

- The diagnosis of vaginal cancer is made by biopsy of the suspicious lesion.
- The staging classification for vaginal cancer developed by the International Federation of Gynecology and Obstetrics (FIGO) is shown in Table 65-1.
- The 5-year survival rates for vaginal cancer by stage are shown in Table 65-2.

TREATMENT

- Most patients with vaginal cancer are treated with radiation therapy. Patients with stage I disease may be treated with intravaginal brachytherapy, while those with more advanced disease are treated with intravaginal brachytherapy as well as external irradiation.
- Surgical treatment may be chosen for selected patients. For example, patients with small lesions located in the upper third of the vagina may be treated with upper vaginectomy, radical hysterectomy, and

TABLE 65-1   Staging of Vaginal Carcinoma

Stage 0	Carcinoma in situ; intraepithelial carcinoma.
Stage I	Carcinoma limited to vaginal mucosa (wall).
Stage II	Subvaginal infiltration into parametrium, not extending to the pelvic wall.
Stage III	Carcinoma has extended to the pelvic wall.
Stage IV	Carcinoma has extended beyond the true pelvis or involves mucosa of bladder or rectum.
Stage IVA	Carcinoma has spread to adjacent organs and/or direct extension beyond the true pelvis.
Stage IVB	Carcinoma has spread to distant organs.

SOURCE: Modified from International Federation of Gynecology and Obstetrics. *Annual Report on the Results of Treatment in Gynecological Cancer,* 22d ed. Stockholm: FIGO, 1994.

TABLE 65-2   Approximate 5-Year Survival Rates for Vaginal Cancer by Stage

STAGE	5-YEAR SURVIVAL
I	72–90%
II	55%
III	45%
IV A	10–20%
IV B	0%

bilateral pelvic lymph node dissection. Patients with advanced disease or with recurrent disease after radiotherapy may require exenterative surgery.

BIBLIOGRAPHY

American College of Obstetricians and Gynecologists. Cancer of the vagina. In: *Precis, Oncology: An Update in Obstetrics and Gynecology.* Washington, DC: ACOG, 1998:22–25.

Grigsby PW. Vaginal cancer. *Curr Treat Options Oncol* 2002; 3:125–130.

66   VULVAR CANCER

John D. Davis

EPIDEMIOLOGY

- In the United States, vulvar cancer is the fourth most common gynecologic malignancy, following cancer of the endometrium, ovary, and cervix.
- Five percent of all female genital cancers and 1 percent of all malignancies in women are located on the vulva.
- Over the past half century the incidence of vulvar cancer has increased from 5 to 8 percent, possibly due to the increased prevalence of human papillomavirus as well as the increased life span of women.
- Etiologic agents associated with the development of vulvar cancer include **human papillomavirus (HPV)**, **granulomatous diseases**, and **herpes simplex virus** (HSV).
- Squamous-cell carcinoma accounts for 87 percent of cases of vulvar cancer; malignant melanoma accounts for 6 percent. Less common types of vulvar cancer include basal-cell carcinoma, Paget's disease, sarcoma, verrucous carcinoma, and Bartholin's gland adenocarcinoma.

PREINVASIVE DISEASE

- As with squamous cell carcinoma of the vulva, the incidence of **vulvar intraepithelial neoplasia** (VIN) has increased over the past 10 to 15 years. In particular, there has been an increase in the incidence of multifocal disease in young women (Fig. 66-1).
- There is a strong association between VIN and HPV infection.
- VIN may occur as single or multifocal lesions; the condition most frequently involves the lower half of the vulva. VIN lesions may appear white, red, gray, or brown.
- The diagnosis of VIN is made by vulvar biopsy. Other conditions to consider in the differential diagnosis of VIN include condyloma, vulvar cancer, lentigo (a benign condition characterized by darkening of the skin), and vulvar dystrophies and dermatoses (including lichen sclerosus, squamous cell hyperplasia, lichen planus, lichen simplex chronicus, and atrophic dermatitis).
- The standard surgical treatment for VIN is wide local excision. Laser ablation may be used for widespread multifocal disease or for lesions less amenable to surgical resection, such as periclitoral lesions.
- The use of imiquimod cream, an immune modulator, as treatment for VIN is currently under investigation.

SYMPTOMS

- The most common symptom experienced by women with vulvar cancer is pruritus.
- Other manifestations include a vulvar mass, pain, bleeding, vulvovaginal discharge, and dysuria (Fig. 66-2).

DIAGNOSIS

- The differential diagnosis of vulvar cancer includes VIN, vulvar dystrophies and dermatoses, and ulcera-

tive diseases of the vulva (including syphilis, HSV, chancroid, and Crohn's disease).
- Vulvar biopsy should be done on any suspicious vulvar lesion to rule out malignancy.
- In performing a vulvar biopsy to rule out malignancy, the central portion of the lesion should be sampled, since the leading edge of a lesion may demonstrate only premalignant changes.

STAGING AND PROGNOSIS

- Table 66-1 shows the staging system for vulvar cancer developed by the International Federation of Gynecology and Obstetrics (FIGO).

TABLE 66-1 Staging of Vulvar Carcinoma

FIGO Staging	
Stage 0	
Tis	Carcinoma in situ; intraepithelial carcinoma
Stage I	
T1 N0 M0	Tumor confined to the vulva and/or perineum 2 cm or less in greatest dimension, nodes are negative
Stage II	
T2 N0 M0	Tumor confined to the vulva and/or perineum more than 2 cm in greatest dimension, nodes are negative
Stage III	
T3 N0 M0	Tumor of any size with the following:
T3 N1 M0	(1) Adjacent spread to the lower urethra and/or the vagina, or the anus, and/or
T1 N1 M0	(2) Unilateral regional lymph node metastasis
T2 N1 M0	
Stage IVA	
T1 N2 M0	Tumor invades any of the following:
T2 N2 M0	Upper urethra, bladder mucosa, rectal mucosa, pelvic bone, and/or bilateral regional node metastasis
T3 N2 M0	
T4 any N M0	
Stage IVB	
Any T	Any distant metastasis including pelvic lymph nodes
Any N M1	

TNM Classification

T = Primary tumor	
Tis	Preinvasive carcinoma (carcinoma in situ)
T1	Tumor confirmed to the vulva and/or perineum— 2 cm or less in greatest dimension
T2	Tumor confined to the vulva and/or perineum— more than 2 cm in greatest dimension
T3	Tumor of any size with adjacent spread to the urethra, vagina, or anus
T4	Tumor of any size infiltrating the bladder mucosa/rectal mucosa, including the upper part of the urethral mucosa and/or fixed to the bone
N = Regional lymph nodes	
N0	Negative
N1	Unilateral regional lymph node metastasis
N2	Bilateral regional lymph node metastasis
M = Distant metastasis	
M0	None
M1	Distant (including pelvic lymph node metastasis)

SOURCE: Modified from International Federation of Gynecology and Obstetrics. *Annual Report on the Results of Treatment in Gynecological Cancer*, 22d ed. Stockholm: FIGO, 1994.

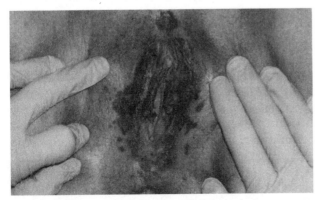

FIG. 66-1 Multifocal vulvar intraepithelial neoplasia.

TABLE 66-2   Approximate 5-Year Survival Rates for Vulvar Cancer by Stage

STAGE	5-YEAR SURVIVAL
I	90%
II	77%
III	51%
IV	18%

- Table 66-2 shows 5-year survival rates for different stages of vulvar cancer.
- The overall 5-year survival rate for patients with vulvar cancer is approximately 70 percent.
- The 5-year survival rate for patients without lymph node involvement is approximately 90 percent; patients with lymph node involvement have an approximate 50 percent 5-year survival rate.

TREATMENT

- Until recently, en bloc radical vulvectomy and bilateral groin node dissection was the standard treatment for most patients with vulvar cancer.
- Disadvantages of this radical surgical procedure include a high incidence of wound breakdown, frequent lower extremity lymphedema, and significant psychosexual sequelae.
- Because of these disadvantages and because of a better understanding of the pattern of lymphatic spread of vulvar cancer, most patients today undergo less radical, less disfiguring surgical procedures. For example:
  ○ Patients with lesions measuring <2 cm in width with <1 mm of invasion do not require lymphadenectomy.
  ○ Patients with well-lateralized lesions (at least 1 cm from the midline) require only unilateral groin node dissection.
  ○ When bilateral groin node dissection is required, the procedure is carried out through separate groin incisions in order to decrease the risk of wound breakdown.
  ○ Radical wide local excision of primary lesions is now preferred over complete radical vulvectomy due to similar cure rates but lower morbidity with the former procedure.
- Sentinel lymph node sampling is currently under investigation in patients with early vulvar cancer. The hypothesis is that, if the first lymph node in the inguinal chain, the sentinel node, is negative for tumor, then all other nodes should be negative and lymphadenectomy can be avoided. Again, this procedure is still investigational.

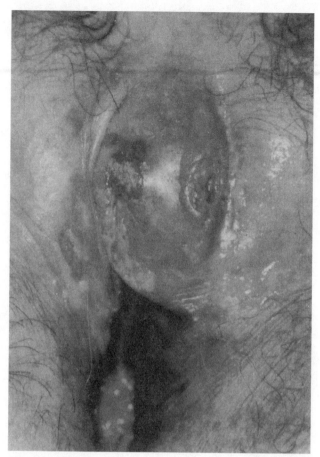

FIG. 66-2 Squamous-cell carcinoma of the vulva. (From Wilkinson EJ, Stone IK. *Atlas of Vulvar Disease*. Baltimore: Williams & Wilkins, 1995:166. With permission.)

OTHER INVASIVE VULVAR LESIONS

- Melanoma is the second most common form of vulvar cancer. Vulvar melanoma is not staged by the FIGO staging system for vulvar cancer but rather by the Breslow or Clark classification. The treatment for melanoma of the vulva is surgical resection (along with lymphadenectomy for higher-stage lesions).
- Basal-cell carcinoma accounts for 2 percent of all vulvar cancers. The tumor is invasive but rarely metastasizes. The treatment for basal-cell carcinoma is wide local excision.
- Invasive Paget's disease is a rare vulvar tumor that occurs in postmenopausal Caucasian women. The lesion has a characteristic red or pink eczematoid appearance. Radical resection with bilateral groin node dissection is the recommended treatment.
- Soft tissue sarcomas account for 2 percent of vulvar malignancies. The recommended treatment for vulvar sarcoma is radical vulvectomy with lymphadenectomy.

Sarcomas have a high recurrence rate, and many patients die rapidly from their disease.

- Verrucous carcinoma is a variant of squamous cell carcinoma that presents as a large cauliflower-like mass. As with basal-cell carcinoma, the disease is invasive, but it rarely metastasizes and may be treated with wide local excision.
- Bartholin's gland adenocarcinoma is a rare form of vulvar cancer. This diagnosis should be considered in any postmenopausal patient who presents with a mass in the area of Bartholin's gland. Treatment is radical vulvectomy with bilateral lymphadenectomy.

BIBLIOGRAPHY

Ghurani GB, Penalver MA. An update on vulvar cancer. *Am J Obstet Gynecol* 2001;185:294–299.

Grendys ED Jr, Fiorica JV. Innovations in the management of vulvar carcinoma. *Curr Opin Obstet Gynecol* 2000;12: 15–20.

67 GESTATIONAL TROPHOBLASTIC DISEASE

Rodney K. Edwards

BACKGROUND

- The term **gestational trophoblastic disease** (GTD) includes multiple tumors, derived from fetal tissue, that range from benign to malignant. Different forms of this disease include hydatidiform mole (complete and partial), invasive mole, choriocarcinoma, and placental site trophoblastic tumor. The term **gestational trophoblastic tumor** has been applied to the last three conditions collectively.
- Although some forms of this disease can be rapidly progressive, cure can usually be achieved with systemic chemotherapy, even if advanced metastatic disease is present.
- The disease presents clinically as a pregnancy. Measurement of serum levels of the beta subunit of human chorionic gonadotropin (β-hCG) allows accurate monitoring of treatment response.
- The overall incidence of GTD is about 1 in 1000 pregnancies. Risk factors include Asian ethnicity, maternal age at the extremes of the reproductive period, and, most importantly, prior GTD. The recurrence rate is approximately 2 percent.

HYDATIDIFORM MOLE

- The vast majority of cases of GTD are hydatidiform molar pregnancies.
- Complete and partial hydatidiform molar pregnancies are differentiated as follows:
  - A **complete hydatidiform mole** involves abnormal overproliferation of the syncytiotrophoblast and replacement of normal trophoblast tissue with hydropic placental villi. No fetus or fetal membranes are present. Genetically, this tissue is entirely paternal in origin, and the karyotype usually is 46 XX. Ninety percent of molar pregnancies are complete moles. The risk of malignant sequelae is 15 to 25 percent.
  - **Partial moles** are characterized by abnormal proliferation of cytotrophoblast tissue. The karyotype usually is triploid, the most common being 69 XXY. An embryo or fetus usually is present but often is markedly growth restricted and/or dead at the time of presentation. The risk of malignant sequelae is 5 to 15 percent.
  - The key features distinguishing complete and partial hydatidiform molar pregnancies are summarized in Table 67-1.
- Features of the clinical presentation are as follows:
  - Women with either type of molar pregnancy most often present with vaginal bleeding and usually have an initial working diagnosis of threatened abortion. With a complete mole, the presentation is most often in the first or early second trimester; women with partial moles usually present later.
  - There is usually a discrepancy between menstrual dates and uterine size; the uterus is commonly larger than expected.
  - The diagnosis of a molar pregnancy is made by ultrasound examination. The ultrasound appearance of a complete mole was previously described as having a "snowstorm" appearance. With more modern equipment, grape-like hydropic villi can be seen filling the uterine cavity (Fig. 67-1).

TABLE 67-1 Comparison of Complete and Partial Hydatidiform Molar Pregnancies

FEATURE	COMPLETE	PARTIAL
Usual time of presentation	First or early second trimester	Second trimester
Embryo or fetus	Absent	Present but abnormal
Serum level of hCG	Markedly elevated	Moderately elevated
Most common karyotype	46 XX	69 XXY
Ovarian theca-lutein cysts	Common	Rare
Malignant potential	15–25%	5–15%

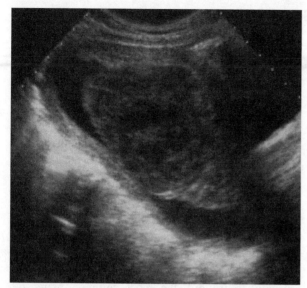

FIG. 67-1 Typical ultrasound appearance of a complete hydatidiform molar pregnancy. (Photograph courtesy of Douglas S. Richards, Department of Obstetrics and Gynecology, University of Florida College of Medicine)

○ Uncommonly, women may have concurrent preeclampsia (otherwise rare in the first 20 weeks of gestation), hyperemesis gravidarum, or hyperthyroidism.

○ Ovarian theca lutein cysts occur in up to 50 percent of cases of complete molar pregnancies, resulting from stimulation by the high levels of β-hCG.

• Treatment comprises the following:

○ After confirmation of the diagnosis of molar pregnancy, a serum β-hCG should be obtained. Particularly with complete moles, levels are much higher than in normal pregnancies. In addition, a baseline chest radiograph should be ordered to evaluate for metastatic disease.

○ Evacuation of the uterus should occur as soon as the diagnosis is made. The procedure of choice for most patients is dilation and curettage. When this procedure is performed for this indication, excessive bleeding and uterine perforation are more likely than usual.

○ Rh-immune globulin should be administered to Rh-negative women who are not sensitized.

○ Respiratory insufficiency, due to embolization of trophoblastic tissue or pulmonary edema, occurs occasionally and is more frequent with increasing uterine size.

○ Hysterectomy is a therapeutic alternative for women who have completed childbearing.

• Postevacuation follow-up:

○ Pregnancy should be avoided for at least 1 year following treatment for a molar pregnancy.

○ During regression, weekly β-hCG levels should be obtained until negative, and pelvic examinations should be performed at least monthly.

○ After remission (three consecutive negative hCG values and uterus not enlarged), hCG levels should be obtained at least every 1 to 3 months until 1 year after uterine evacuation. The average length of time to reach negative hCG values is about 10 weeks.

GESTATIONAL TROPHOBLASTIC TUMORS

• These tumors (invasive mole, choriocarcinoma, and placental site trophoblastic tumor) have cure rates exceeding 90 percent. However, left untreated, they can metastasize and lead to death.

• Presence of a gestational trophoblastic tumor should be suspected when there is continued uterine bleeding after evacuation of a molar pregnancy or if hCG levels plateau or rise during postevacuation follow-up.

• **Invasive mole** is a benign tumor that results from myometrial invasion by a hydatidiform mole. Although benign, these tumors can metastasize, most often to the lungs and vagina. Diagnosis most often is made clinically, based on persistently elevated or rising hCG values after evacuation of a molar pregnancy. Treatment for patients wishing to preserve fertility usually is single-agent chemotherapy with either methotrexate or dactinomycin. Hysterectomy often is used as primary therapy for women who no longer desire fertility.

• **Choriocarcinoma** is a rare malignant disease characterized by invasion of the myometrium and vascular spread to distant sites. The most common sites of metastasis are the lungs, brain, and liver. This malignancy may arise in conjunction with any type of pregnancy, not just hydatidiform moles.

• **Placental site trophoblastic tumors** are very rare. These tumors comprise a cell type that is intermediate between cytotrophoblast and syncytiotrophoblast. Consequently serum hCG levels are only modestly elevated. Unlike other gestational trophoblastic tumors, this lesion is relatively resistant to chemotherapy, and surgery is the mainstay of treatment.

• Patients with "high risk" gestational trophoblastic tumors are those who have very high hCG values (>100,000), sites of metastases other than the pelvis and lungs, and prior failed chemotherapy. These patients should be treated with multiagent chemotherapy and possibly adjuvant radiation therapy or surgery.

- Follow-up of patients treated for gestational trophoblastic tumors is similar to that for patients treated for hydatidiform molar pregnancies, with periodic hCG determinations until negative for 12 months. During a subsequent pregnancy, a first-trimester ultrasound is recommended due to the propensity for recurrent gestational trophoblastic disease. Likewise, histopathologic examination of the products of conception from any future pregnancies and a 6-week-postpartum hCG measurement are recommended.

BIBLIOGRAPHY

Freedman RS, Tortolero-Luna G, Pandey DK, et al. Gestational trophoblastic disease. *Obstet Gynecol Clin North Am* 1996;23:545–571.

Miller BE. Gestational trophoblastic disease. In: Ling FW, Duff P, eds. *Obstetrics & Gynecology: Principles for Practice.* New York: McGraw-Hill, 2001.

Soto-Wright V, Bernstein M, Goldstein DP, Berkowitz RS. The changing clinical presentation of complete molar pregnancy. *Obstet Gynecol* 1995; 86:775–779.

INDEX

Note: Page numbers followed by the letters *f* and *t* indicate figures and tables, respectively.